PRINCIPLES and APPLICATIONS of BIOSTATISTICS

PRINCIPLES and APPLICATIONS of BIOSTATISTICS

RAY M. MERRILL, PhD, MPH, MS, FAAHB, FACE
Professor of Biostatistics and Epidemiology
Director of Gerontology
Brigham Young University

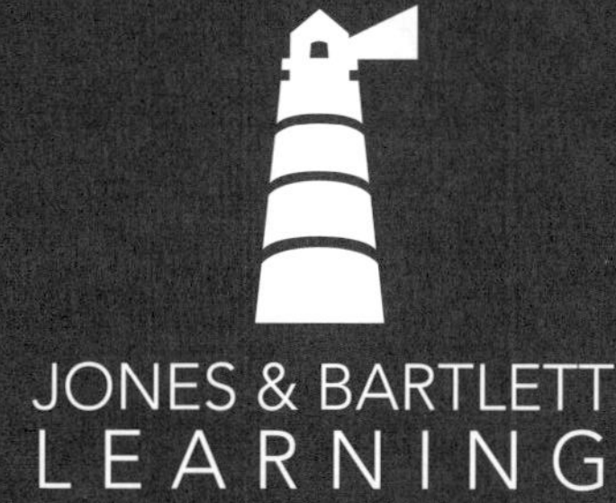

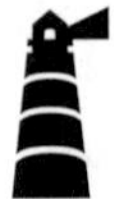

World Headquarters
Jones & Bartlett Learning
25 Mall Road, 6th Floor
Burlington, MA 01803
978-443-5000
info@jblearning.com
www.jblearning.com

Jones & Bartlett Learning books and products are available through most bookstores and online booksellers. To contact Jones & Bartlett Learning directly, call 800-832-0034, fax 978-443-8000, or visit our website, www.jblearning.com.

Substantial discounts on bulk quantities of Jones & Bartlett Learning publications are available to corporations, professional associations, and other qualified organizations. For details and specific discount information, contact the special sales department at Jones & Bartlett Learning via the above contact information or send an email to specialsales@jblearning.com.

24316-1

Production Credits
VP, Product Development: Christine Emerton
Director of Product Management: Matt Kane
Product Manager: Sophie Teague
Content Strategist: Sara Bempkins
Project Manager: Jessica deMartin
Senior Project Specialist: Jennifer Risden
Digital Project Specialist: Rachel DiMaggio
Senior Marketing Manager: Susanne Walker
Content Services Manager: Colleen Lamy
VP, Manufacturing and Inventory Control: Therese Connell
Composition: Straive
Project Management: Straive
Cover Design: Briana Yates
Media Development Editor: Faith Brosnan
Rights Specialist: Maria Leon Maimone
Cover Image (Title Page, Part Opener, Chapter Opener): © MicroStockHub/Getty Images
Printing and Binding: McNaughton & Gunn

Library of Congress Cataloging-in-Publication Data
Names: Merrill, Ray M., author.
Title: Principles and applications of biostatistics / Ray M. Merrill. PhD, MPH, MS, FAAHB, FACE, Professor of Biostatistics and Epidemiology, Director of Gerontology, Brigham Young University.
Description: First edition. | Burlington, Massachusetts : Jones & Bartlett Learning, [2022] | Includes bibliographical references and index.
Identifiers: LCCN 2021009317 | ISBN 9781284225976 (paperback)
Subjects: LCSH: Biometry. | BISAC: EDUCATION / General
Classification: LCC QH323.5 .M467 2022 | DDC 570.1/5195–dc23
LC record available at https://lccn.loc.gov/2021009317

6048

Printed in the United States of America
25 24 23 22 21 10 9 8 7 6 5 4 3 2 1

This book is dedicated with love and appreciation to Marla, Phillip, Dallin, Andrew, Ron, and Cindy.

Contents

Contents

Preface

Statistics is the science of data. It involves collecting, classifying, summarizing, organizing, analyzing, and interpreting data. Data are pieces of information used as a basis for our understanding problems and influencing solutions. In the current era of SARS-Cov-2, we can see that statistics has added to our knowledge of various aspects of the resulting disease, from a description of its frequency and pattern to certain long-term health consequences. A large number of research papers are now being published, rapidly advancing our knowledge of the disease through the help of statistics.

In general, a variety of disciplines rely on statistics: biology, health, medicine, epidemiology, business, psychology, engineering, agriculture, and others. When the focus of statistics is on the biological, health, and medical sciences, it is called biostatistics. Biostatistics involves statistical methods applied to biological data. Biostatistics, along with epidemiology and health services, is the foundation of public health.

All of the primary concepts and methods that are fundamental to our understanding of biostatistics are covered in this text, from data collection and presentation to probability and statistical inference to multiple regression and analysis of variance. Substantive, real-world biological, health, and medical science examples and news files are included, letting the reader see a number of ways biostatistics can help advance knowledge.

This book is written for students and practitioners in the biological, health, and medical sciences. Its primary aim is to present principles and methods of biostatistics in the context of relevant, interesting, and up-to-date applications. The principles and applications are presented with clarity, brevity, and accuracy. Specifically, statistical principles and applications are developed with understandable and focused explanations and practical examples. The aim is to make learning easier for students and pedagogy more effective for instructors.

The book is concise. Key topics in biostatistics are capsulized in order to be manageable in a one-semester course. At the beginning of most chapters is a list of the type of questions that can be addressed using the principles and methods covered in that chapter. Highlighted in the various sections are bolded key words, definitions, and concepts. Concepts and formulas are developed with reasoning suitable for application in biostatistics. Focus is given to the conditions that are necessary to apply the methods correctly.

Excel and SAS computer software will be used to demonstrate data analysis and graphing throughout the book. Other computer software options are readily available.

About the Author

Ray M. Merrill is a professor of biostatistics and epidemiology and program director of gerontology at Brigham Young University. He holds adjunct positions in Family and Preventive Medicine and Health Education at the University of Utah. He is a former Cancer Prevention Fellow at the National Cancer Institute and visiting scientist at the International Agency for Research on Cancer, Lyon, France. He is currently a fellow of the American Academy of Health Behavior and the American College of Epidemiology. He teaches introductory and advanced level courses in biostatistics and epidemiology. He is the author of more than 300 peer-reviewed research articles and text books (*Environmental Epidemiology*, *Reproductive Epidemiology*, *Behavioral Epidemiology*, *Principles of Epidemiology Workbook*, *Fundamentals of Epidemiology and Biostatistics*, *Statistical Methods in Epidemiologic Research*, *Fundamental Mathematics for Epidemiology Study*, and *Introduction to Epidemiology*). In his spare time he hikes mountains and runs marathons.

Reviewers

Chakra Budhathoki, PhD
Associate Professor
Johns Hopkins University
School of Nursing
Baltimore, Maryland

Macey Buker, PhD, CPA
Assistant Professor, Program Director
Dixie State University

Susan Draine, EdD, MSN, CNS, MBA, RN

Lenis Chen-Edinboro, PhD
Assistant Professor in Public Health
University of North Carolina Wilmington

Sarbani Ghoshal, MPH, PhD
Assistant Professor
Queensborough Community College, CUNY

Jayanta Gupta, MD, PhD
Florida Gulf Coast University

Shayesteh Jahanfar, PhD
Professor
Central Michigan University

Maureen K. Johnson, PhD
Associate Professor
Department of Applied Health Sciences
Indiana State University

Seung-Hwan Kim, PhD
Merrimack College

Bernadette McCrory, PhD, MPE, PE, CHFP
Mechanical and Industrial Engineering
Montana State University

Mary Moore, PhD
Colorado State University Global

Ramzi W. Nahhas, PhD
Professor
Department of Population and Public Health Sciences
Department of Psychiatry
Boonshoft School of Medicine,
Wright State University

Oluwatomi Oluwasanmi, MPH
Hunter College Urban School of Public Health

Erin Reynolds, PhD, MPH
Associate Professor
University of Southern Indiana

Ramona Stone, PhD, MPH
West Chester University of Pennsylvania

Jing Xu, PhD, MHA
University of North Florida

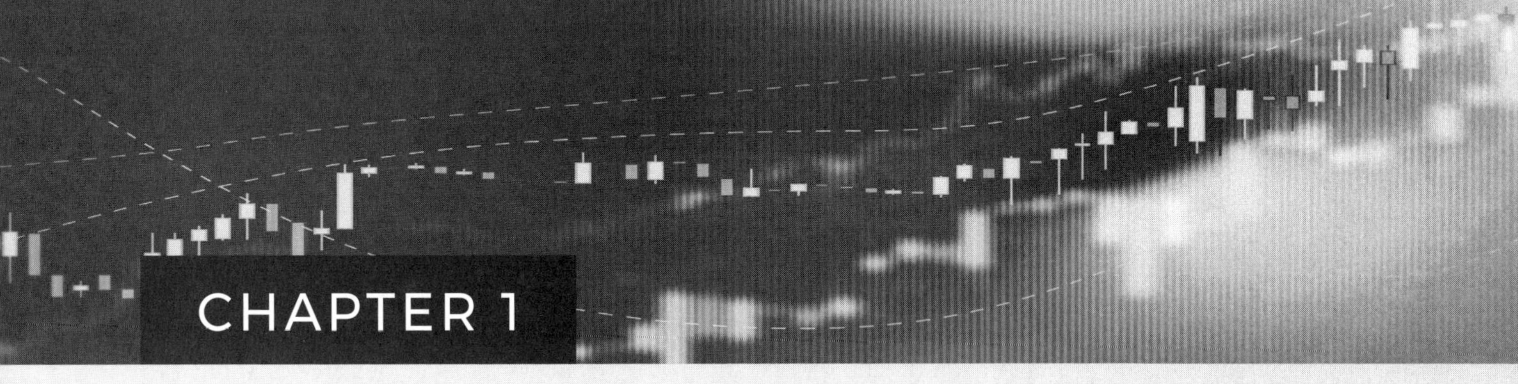

Introduction to Biostatistics

KEY CONCEPTS

- Biostatistics is the branch of statistics concerned with the development and application of methods for collecting, analyzing, and interpreting biological data to assist decision-making.
- Problems in the biological sciences lead to research questions (representing uncertainty to be resolved), which may be addressed using biostatistics.
- Data are information taken from variables.
- A variable is a characteristic that varies from one subject to the next and can take on a specified set of values.
- Quantitative data are information about quantities or numbers.
- Qualitative data are information about the quality, nature, or essence of something.
- Nominal scale refers to data that fall into categories with no logical order or structure.
- Ordinal scale refers to data that fall into categories with an inherent order.
- Interval scale refers to measurements where the difference between the intervals is meaningful, but there is no true definition of zero.
- Ratio scale has the same properties as interval scale, but there is a true zero.
- The four broad areas of biostatistics are descriptive statistics, probability, inference, and statistical techniques.
- Descriptive biostatistics are measures of frequency (e.g., count, percent), central tendency (e.g., mean, median), dispersion (variation) (e.g., standard deviation, range, interquartile range), and position (e.g., percentile, rank) that represent either a sample or a population.
- Probability provides a basis for evaluating the reliability of the conclusions we reach and the inferences we make under uncertainty.
- Inferential statistics draw conclusions about a population based on sample information taken from that population.
- Statistical techniques are analytic approaches that utilize statistical methods to investigate a range of questions.
- Application of statistical software is essential as we address research questions in biostatistics.

This chapter provides an introduction to biostatistics. First, the meaning of the term biostatistics is discussed. Second, the research question and its importance for motivating the application of biostatistics is developed. Third, basic concepts related to data collection, analysis, presentation, and interpretation are covered. Fourth, the four broad areas of biostatistics, upon which this book is organized, are presented: descriptive statistics, probability, inference, and statistical techniques. Fifth, a brief introduction to statistical software and coding is given.

1.1 What Is Biostatistics?

The word statistics is from the German word *statistik*, which derives from the Latin word *statisticum* ("of the state") and the Italian word *statista* ("statesman," "politician"). In 1749, it was used to refer to the science dealing with data about the condition of a community or state.[1] Today we refer to statistics as the area of mathematics that involves the collection, analysis, presentation, and interpretation of data. Biostatistics is the science or practice of statistics applied to data that relate to living organisms, which primarily involves human biology, health, and medicine. In other words, it is a contraction of biology and statistics. Biostatistics contributes to a number of fields, including health, medicine, nutrition, genetics, biology, epidemiology, and many more. It is important in the health sciences for a number of reasons, including helping us identify the natural course of a disease; individuals at greatest risk for disease, injury, or death; risk factors for disease, injury, or death; and the value of new drugs, medical procedures, and healthcare interventions.

Biostatistics is the branch of statistics concerned with the development and application of methods for collecting, analyzing, and interpreting biological data to assist decision-making.

Biostatistics finds application in many areas, including clinical trials to evaluate the safety and efficacy of medications or medical devices. In clinical trials, biostatistics plays an important role at all levels: designing the study; determining the sample size; and collecting, analyzing, and interpreting the data. In public health programs, biostatistics is often used to evaluate a program's efficacy, effectiveness, and potential for replication in other areas. In literature reviews and meta-analyses, biostatistics provides the tools for quantifying patterns and trends, thus showing evidence for medical delivery and treatment practices. There are yet several other examples of application areas for biostatistics, many of which will be discussed in this book.

1.2 Questions for Biostatistics

When a problem is identified in the biological sciences, it leads to a research question or questions. A research question reflects the uncertainty that the investigator wishes to resolve by conducting a study. The application of methods in biostatistics allows us to effectively address questions arising in the biological sciences.

Consider the question, "Does physical activity increase your life expectancy?" A study showed that more leisure-time physical activity leads to longer life expectancy.[2] Physical activity equivalent to brisk walking for approximately 75 minutes per week resulted in 1.8 more years in life expectancy compared with no physical activity. Brisk walking for 450+ minutes per week resulted in 4.5 additional years in life expectancy compared with being inactive. Improvements in life expectancy with greater physical activity were found across weight classifications (normal, overweight, and obese). Individuals of normal weight with physical activity equivalent to 150+ minutes per week of brisk walking had 7.2 more years in life expectancy compared to those who were physically inactive and obese. Other questions about physical activity and

Table 1.1 Selected Questions Related to COVID-19

What is the frequency and pattern of this disease?
What are the clinical characteristics of this disease?
How do the symptoms vary by age group?
How does population density affect this disease?
How does comorbid health problems affect this disease?
How does nutrition and obesity affect this disease?
How does climate influence the virus?
Who is at the greatest risk?
What is the length of time after exposure before clinical symptoms appear (i.e., incubation period)?
When are infected people most contagious?
How is the disease spread?
How long is an asymptomatic carrier contagious?
What is the probability of reinfection of the disease following recovery?
What is the probability of false negatives and false positives for the test?
How effective is wearing a mask at preventing the spread of the disease?
What is the death-to-case ratio, and how does it vary by selected groups?
What are the long-term health consequences of the disease?
Is there an effective treatment for the disease?
Is there an effective vaccine for the disease?

health have also been addressed in recent years with the application of biostatistics.[3–7]

With the current COVID-19 pandemic, several research questions are being investigated, some of which are listed in **Table 1.1**. As answers are discovered, the disease can be better managed. For example, identifying the duration of time from exposure to first symptoms (incubation period) for COVID-19 tells us about the possible source of the virus, the appropriate length of time for quarantine, and the time a person can spread the virus prior to knowing they have it. Consider the question about the incubation period for COVID-19. One study found that the median incubation period is 5 days (range 1–14 days).[8] Incubation periods for several other infectious diseases are listed elsewhere.[9]

The Centers for Disease Control and Prevention has presented a general list of questions and answers related to COVID-19.[10] In the coming months, data will become increasingly more available to address such questions.

1.3 Data

The heart of biostatistics is data. Data are information and may be thought of as observations or measurements of something of interest.

> **Data** are information obtained through observation, experiment, or measurement of a phenomenon of interest.

Data are either quantitative or qualitative.

> **Quantitative data** are information about quantities or numbers, measured on a numerical scale.

Identifying additional years of life associated with increased exercise is an example of quantitative data.

Qualitative data are information about the quality, nature, or essence of something, with information gathered and ordered into larger themes as the researcher works from the specific to the general.

Describing how regular exercise makes people feel is an example of qualitative data.

Qualitative data are also called categorical data when the levels of the variable fit into categories. The levels of categorical data have no logical order. For example, males versus females or disagree, neutral, agree.

Data consist of measurements taken from variables. A variable is a characteristic that varies from one entity to another and can be measured or categorized. A variable can take on a specified set of values. A random variable is any outcome of a variable that occurs by chance, such as for every 1000 COVID-19 patients, how many are hospitalized.

Data measurements are made on different scales: nominal, ordinal, interval, and ratio, listed in **Table 1.2**. The statistical techniques presented and applied in this book depend on the type of data involved.

Interval and ratio data can be divided into one of two types: discrete or continuous. Discrete data have a finite number of measurements based on counts. Continuous data have a theoretically infinite number of measurements; there are no limits in the area between measurements. While discrete data represent things that are counted, continuous data represent things that are measured. Continuous data are more precise and provide more information than discrete data.

1.3.1 Data Collection

Data collection is the systematic approach in which information is gathered and measured in order to obtain an accurate picture of a phenomenon of interest. Data collection involves various methods, depending on whether quantitative or qualitative data are desired. Quantitative data collection methods consist of scales, tests, questionnaires, and surveys, whereas qualitative data collection

Table 1.2 **Measurement Scales**

Scale	Description	Example
Nominal	Refers to placing data into categories, where there is no logical order or structure	Exposed ("Yes" or "No") Diseased ("Yes" or "No") Sex, race, marital status, educational status
Ordinal	Refers to placing data into categories where the gross order of the categories is informative but the relative positional distances are not quantitatively meaningful	Preference rating (e.g., agree, neutral, disagree) Rank-order scale
Interval	Refers to a measurement where the difference between the intervals is meaningful, but there is no true definition of zero	Temperature, since zero on Fahrenheit or Celsius scales does not mean no temperature Calendar year
Ratio	Has the same properties as interval scale data, but has a clear definition of zero (e.g., height, weight, and blood pressure)	Height, weight, blood pressure Length, duration

methods consist of interviews, observations, and documents. In the physical activity and life expectancy study, leisure-time physical activity was associated with life expectancy according to six large cohort studies comprising 654,827 individuals, ages 21–90 years. Physical activity was measured as metabolic equivalent hours per week (Met-h/week). An approximate 10-year follow-up period occurred in the study with the main outcome, variable life expectancy, measured in years.

1.3.2 Data Analysis

Data analysis is the process of evaluating data to discover useful information. While quantitative data can be statistically analyzed, qualitative data are generally used to build concepts, hypotheses, or theories. In the physical activity and life expectancy study, the data were quantitatively assessed using a statistical technique called proportional hazards regression.

1.3.3 Data Presentation

Data presentation is the method in which we summarize, organize, and communicate information. These methods may be textual, tabular, or graphical. Textual methods include ranking data and the stem-and-leaf plot; tabular methods include the frequency distribution table and contingency table; and graphical methods include the bar chart, histogram, frequency polygon, and **pie chart**. In general, graphs and tables are effective ways to communicate data so that they can be easily understood.

1.3.4 Data Interpretation

Once data are collected, they are analyzed and presented in various forms, such as statistics, tables, graphs, diagrams, maps, and so on. At this point, the findings need to be interpreted. Data interpretation is the process of assessing and determining the meaning and importance of the results. Data interpretation involves consideration of questions about the data as they relate to your study questions. The answer to these questions should be organized as results and conclusions. Implications and recommendations may follow.

Data may be interpreted with perspective by comparing the results among groups or with what is typically known. In clinical trials, a control group is critical for assessing new drugs and medical procedures. The control group is also an effective way to control for confounding factors. Controlling for confounding allows us to have confidence that intervention effects are not explained by extrinsic factors. In the physical activity and life expectancy study, meaning and importance of leisure-time physical activity in terms of greater life expectancy was made by comparing life expectancy among people classified into groups according to physical activity and body weight.

1.4 Methods in Biostatistics

Biostatistics has four general method areas: descriptive, probability, inferential, and statistical techniques. They do not stand alone; for example, descriptive biostatistics often requires the use of probability and statistical techniques; inferential biostatistics relies on probability; and statistical techniques often involve inference.

1.4.1 Descriptive Biostatistics

Descriptive biostatistics involves methods of organizing, summarizing, and describing biological data. Suppose we want to describe our data so that we can answer who is at greatest risk for disease and where is the disease risk greatest. In recent months, several reports have answered questions about the frequency and pattern of COVID-19. As of July 27, 2020, the observed death-to-case ratio for COVID-19 was 15.2% in the United Kingdom, 14.3% in Italy, 13.9% in France, 10.4% in Spain, 7.2% in Sweden, 6.8% in Ireland, 5.7% in Switzerland, 3.9% in Poland, 3.5% in the United States, and 2.3% in India.[11]

Descriptive biostatistics are measures of frequency (e.g., count, percent, rate), central tendency (e.g., mean, median, mode), dispersion (variation) (e.g., standard deviation, range, interquartile range), and position (e.g., percentile, rank) representing either a sample or a population.

In a study involving 5700 hospitalized COVID-19 patients in New York, the median age was 63 years. The patients were more likely male (60.3% versus 39.7%) and had at least one comorbid condition (88% versus 6.3% with one and 6.1% with none). An estimated 56.6% had hypertension, 41.7% were obese, and 33.8% had diabetes.[12]

However, another study that controlled for underlying conditions and patient characteristics found that hypertension was no longer associated with hospitalization, indicating that underlying factors associated with hypertension (e.g., obesity and diabetes) were explaining the positive association.[13]

1.4.2 Probability

Probability provides a basis for evaluating the reliability of the conclusions we reach and the inferences we make under uncertainty. Biostatistics applies probability in several areas, such as in risk assessment, sampling and evaluating the reliability of an estimator, validity of a diagnostic test, and the chance of survival over a given time period.

Probability is a numerical description of the likelihood of an events occurrence.

A common question in biological health research is whether the probability of an event is related to the levels of a given variable, like exposure status, age, race and Hispanic origin, marital status, treatment, and so on. For example, in the United States, the probability of COVID-19 cases dying from the disease varies considerably by age (**Figure 1.1**).[14]

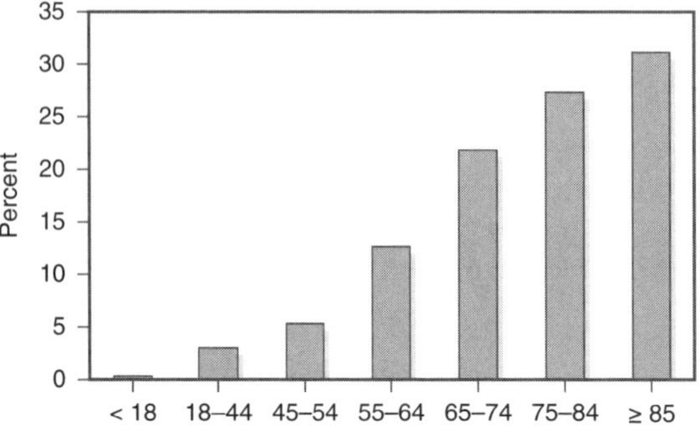

Figure 1.1 Mortality from COVID-19 in the United States by Age, February 12 through May 18, 2020

Among hospitalized cases in New York City, the probability of dying is greater among males than females in each age group (**Figure 1.2**).[12] The higher probability of death in males than females is more pronounced in the younger age groups. For example, the risk of death is 3.9 times greater in males compared with females in the age group 20–29 years and 1.4 times greater in the age group ≥ 90 years.

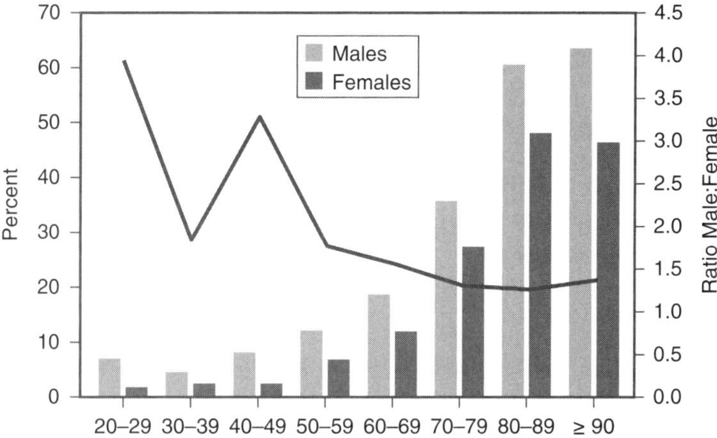

Figure 1.2 Deaths in COVID-19 Patients Hospitalized in the New York City Area by Sex and Age

1.4.3 Inferential Statistics

Inferential statistics involves a process of drawing conclusions about some aspect of a population, typically based on random sampling. For example, according to an observed subset of all customers who shop at a given store, females are more likely than males to wear a mask to prevent the spread of COVID-19.

Inferential statistics is the theory, methods, and practice of drawing conclusions about the parameters of a population based on sample information taken from the population.

The population is all customers.

A **population** is a set or collection of items of interest in a study.

The sample should be a sufficiently large, representative group from the population.

A **sample** is a subset of items that have been selected from the population.

Two methods are commonly used in inferential statistics: estimation and hypothesis testing. We may wish to infer something about a population, based on an estimated value from a sample. The estimated statistic is hopefully close to the true population parameter. Because our estimate contains some uncertainty, an accompanying statement of confidence (confidence interval) should be included.

A **statistic** is a measure from a sample that is used in statistics.

A **parameter** is a measure from a population that is often unknown. We are usually not able to calculate its value.

A **confidence interval** is a range of values wherein there is a **level of confidence** that the true parameter value lies within it.

Sampling is the process of selecting participants for the study when the number of people in the population of interest is larger than the required sample size. A number of sampling methods will be considered in this book. We will also address ways to minimize sampling bias where systematic error causes the sample of people in the study to not represent the target population.

An example of estimation, in which an estimate is derived from a sample and a statement of confidence is associated with the estimate, involves the death-to-case ratio for COVID-19. What is the death-to-case ratio for COVID-19? On March 5, 2020, researchers estimated the death-to-case ratio for China, including Hong Kong, Macau, and Taiwan, to be 3.48% (95% confidence interval [CI] 3.35–3.61%).[15]

In some cases, we may wish to infer that an estimated value is significantly different from another value. To assess this difference, we employ the process of hypothesis testing. For example, suppose you want to know whether the death-to-case ratio of COVID-19 is different between the United States and the United Kingdom. Your research hypothesis is that the ratios are different. On July 27, 2020, the number of confirmed cases and deaths in the United States was 4,288,012 and 148,009, respectively.[16] Corresponding values in the United Kingdom were 301,706 and 45,844.[16] The death-to-case ratio was 15.19% in the United Kingdom and 3.45% in the United States. The ratio of these two death-to-case estimates is 4.40 (95% CI = 4.36–4.45). In other words, the death-to-case ratio was 4.40 times greater in the United Kingdom than in the United States. Because the 95% confidence interval does not overlap 1, we conclude that this result is statistically significant at the 0.05 level.

1.4.4 Statistical Techniques

A variety of statistical techniques will be presented in this book. These statistical techniques are often applied to questions in the biological sciences. For example, rate ratios were used to address questions as to whether pregnancy associates with hospitalization and increased risk for intensive care unit admission, receipt of mechanical ventilation, and death among reproductive age women with COVID-19 infection.[17] Rate ratios are commonly used to compare the risk of an outcome in one group with another group. After adjusting for age, race and Hispanic origin, and underlying health conditions, pregnant women were 5.4 (95% CI = 5.1–5.6) times more likely to be hospitalized, 1.5 (95% CI = 1.2–1.8) times more likely to be admitted to the ICU, and 1.7 (95% CI = 1.2–2.4) times more likely to receive mechanical ventilation. Each of these estimates are statistically significant because the confidence intervals do not overlap 1. On the other hand, pregnant women were 0.9 (95% CI = 0.5–1.5) times as likely to die, which is not statistically significant.

Statistical techniques are analytic approaches that utilize statistical methods to investigate a range of questions.

News File

During March 27–28, 2020, three University of Texas students showed symptoms and tested positive for severe acute respiratory syndrome coronavirus 2 (SARS-CoV-2). Each of these students had gone to Cabo San Lucas, Mexico for spring break (March 14–19). Symptoms for the students did not manifest until March 22–25. Other student travelers were identified by contact tracing interviews and flight manifests. Of 183 students who traveled to Cabo San Lucas and who were evaluated for SARS-CoV-2, 60 (33%) tested positive. In addition, there was 1 of 13 (8%) household contacts of the travelers and 3 of 35 community contacts of the travelers who tested positive. Of those with positive tests, 20% were asymptomatic, and no one needed hospitalization or died. Testing of all those who were at risk allowed public health officials to identify those who could spread the virus, even asymptomatic people, in an effort to control further COVID-19 outbreaks.[18]

1.5 Statistical Software

Throughout this text, we will give examples of programs and output from computer packages designed to assess statistical data. Common statistical software used to analyze data include Statistical Analysis System (SAS), Statistical Package for the Social Sciences (SPSS), Stata, R, and Microsoft Excel. Although we will concentrate on SAS and Excel, the supplementary content for this class will be programs and output for SPSS, STATA, and R. In this section, we will provide introductions to both SAS and Excel.

SAS has three interactive windows: the Editor, Log, and Output. Each will be briefly described here. SAS programs involve SAS statements. Each SAS statement ends with a semicolon. The semicolon completes the SAS statement. SAS statements are used to create SAS data sets and to run predefined statistical or other routines. A group of SAS statements used to define and create your SAS data set is called a Data Step. A Data Step tells SAS programs about the data. For example,

```
DATA Example;
  INPUT Age Sex $;
DATALINES;
  17 Male
  18 Female
  20 Male
  24 Male
  24 Female
  30 Male
  32 Male
  ;
```

The name of the data set is arbitrary but must begin with a letter. For categorical variables, follow the variable name on the INPUT line with "$".

"DATALINES" comes prior to entering the data. Following the data set is a semicolon. It does not matter whether you choose to type words in uppercase or lowercase.

PROC (meaning procedure) begins several predefined routines. Each PROC is followed by a specific option, like PRINT, UNIVARIATE, MEAN, FREQ, REG, and so on. We end the procedure statements with "RUN". For example, to obtain the mean age for males and females separately, we first sort the data according to sex:

```
PROC SORT DATA=Example;
   Title 'Sorted Data by Sex';
   BY Sex;
RUN;
```

Then run PROC MEANS, with the variable that the means are to be computed for preceded by VAR and, because the means are to be computed for males and females, "BY Sex" is added. The MAXDEC option allows you to specify the number of decimal values.

```
PROC MEANS DATA=Example MAXDEC=2;
   TITLE 'Mean Age by Sex';
   VAR Age;
   BY Sex;
RUN;
```

SAS programs are entered into the SAS Editor and then run by clicking "Submit" on the toolbar. When the procedure is executed, it produces a LOG and OUTPUT. The LOG is an annotated copy of the original program, with the data excluded. Any procedure coding errors and information about the data set (e.g., number of observations and variables) will be identified there. The OUTPUT provides the results requested by the PROC statement, which for our example appear as follows:

The MEANS Procedure

Sex=Female

Analysis Variable : Age				
N	Mean	Std Dev	Minimum	Maximum
2	21.00	4.24	18.00	24.00

Sex=Male

Analysis Variable : Age				
N	Mean	Std Dev	Minimum	Maximum
5	24.60	6.39	17.00	32.00

Microsoft Excel features the ability to store, organize, and manipulate data (i.e., make calculations, graphs, and more). It is used to create spreadsheets, which are special documents that allow us to store and organize data in rows (horizontal sets of boxes labeled as 1, 2, 3, etc.) and columns (vertical sets of boxes labeled as A, B, C, etc.). The data can then be read and manipulated. The interaction of each row and column is a cell wherein we enter numbers, text, or formulas.

An Excel document is a workbook. A workbook consists of one or more worksheets. Worksheets are the grid where we store and calculate data. Simple and complex formulas can be calculated in Excel. Excel also offers a variety of charts (e.g., line graph, bar chart, scatter plot) to assess data. To introduce you to Excel, consider the partial table shown here. The data are the same as used in the SAS example. To obtain the statistics in Column B, we entered in cell B8 =COUNT(B2:B6), in cell B9 =AVERAGE(B2:B6), in cell B10 =STDEV.S(B2:B6), in cell B11 =MIN(B2:B6), and in cell B12 =MAX(B2:B6). Statistics for the data in column C are computed similarly.

	A	B	C
1		Male	Female
2		17	18
3		20	24
4		24	
5		30	
6		32	
7			
8	Number	5	2
9	Mean	24.6	21
10	Standard Deviation	6.4	4.2
11	Minimum	17	18
12	Maximum	32	24

Excel also has an add-in feature for performing data analysis. To add this feature, go to the File tab and select Options. Then select Add-ins and choose Analysis ToolPak. In the Manage box, select Excel Add-ins and click Go. Check the Analysis ToolPak and then select OK. Now, in the Excel spreadsheet under the Data tab on the far right of the toolbar, the Data Analysis option will appear.

To use the Data Analysis option, choose the Descriptive Statistics option, identify the input range, check the summary statistics option, and select OK. This will return the summary statistics shown in the previous table, and more.

1.6 Summary

This chapter provides an introduction to the meaning of biostatistics and the role it plays in addressing research questions. In biostatistics, data are the numerical values from variables. A variable is an attribute which describes something and can vary from one entity to another. Variables are quantitative if the values are quantities or numbers, and qualitative if the information is about quality. Data are measured on different scales: nominal, ordinal, interval, and ratio. The scale of measurement determines how the values should be collected, analyzed, and presented.

Four broad areas of biostatistics are descriptive, probability, inference, and statistical techniques. Descriptive statistics are important because they present data in a more manageable, meaningful way that leads to simpler interpretation. Probability is important because it serves as a basis for evaluating the reliability of the conclusions we reach and the inferences we make under uncertainty. Inferential statistics is important because it allows us to draw conclusions about a population based on sample information. Statistical techniques are important because they allow us to explore and answer a range of research questions. Statistical software is an efficient tool for conducting thorough analysis of each of these areas of biostatistics.

Exercises

1. List and briefly describe the four broad areas of biostatistics.
2. Classify the following as (A) nominal data, (B) ordinal data, (C) discrete data, or (D) continuous data.

   ___ Integers of counts that differ by fixed amounts, with no intermediate values possible

   ___ Measurable quantities not restricted to taking on integer values

   ___ Ordered categories or classes

   ___ Unordered categories or classes
3. Classify the following as either (A) quantitative or (B) qualitative data.

   ___ Age

   ___ Hometown

   ___ Cholesterol level

   ___ Eye color

   ___ Number of siblings
4. Discuss whether discrete or continuous data provide more precision and information.
5. Descriptive biostatistics involves four types of statistics. List and define these.
6. Define probability and list some of its applications.
7. In what way does inferential statistics involve probability?
8. Classify the following as either (A) a statistic, (B) a parameter, or (C) a confidence interval.

   ___ Gives a range of values for an unknown parameter

   ___ Measure from a sample

   ___ Measure from a population

   ___ A numerical characteristic of a population

   ___ A number that represents a property of a sample
9. The length of stay for a sample of eight patients admitted to the hospital were recorded: 3, 16, 12, 3, 2, 5, 4, 1. Use a statistical software package to compute the number of patients, mean, standard deviation, minimum, and maximum. For the mean and standard deviation, express your answers to the nearest hundredth. For the others, do not round.
10. In this chapter we spoke briefly about confidence intervals. Much more will be said about confidence intervals later in this book. For now, try calculating a confidence interval for the population mean based on data in the previous exercise. Express your answer to the nearest hundredth. (Hint: In SAS use the procedure MEANS and the option CLM. In Excel, go into Data Analysis, choose Descriptive Statistics, identify the input range of your data and select summary statistics and confidence level for the mean. Use the estimated mean and confidence level in the output to derive the confidence interval.)

References

1. Van der Zande J. Statistik and history in the German enlightenment. *J Hist Ideas.* 2010;*71*(3):411–432.
2. Moore SC, Patel AV, Matthews CE, et al. Leisure time physical activity of moderate to vigorous intensity and mortality: A large pooled cohort analysis. *PloS Med* 2012;*9*(11):e1001335.
3. US Department of Health and Human Services. *Physical activity and health: A report of the Surgeon General*. Atlanta, GA: CDC; 1996.
4. American Heart Association. Physical activity improves quality of life; 2018. http://www.heart.org/HEARTORG/HealthyLiving/PhysicalActivity/FitnessBasics/Physical-activity-improves-quality-of-life_UCM_307977_Article.jsp#.W2CQd9VKiUk. Accessed July 24, 2020.
5. Holme I, Anderssen SA. [Physical activity, smoking and mortality among men who participated in the Oslo studies of 1972 and 2000]. *Tidsskr Nor Laegeforen.* 2014;*134*(18): 1743–1748.
6. US Department of Health and Human Services. *2008 Physical Activity Guidelines for Americans.* Washington, DC: US Department of Health and Human Services; 2008. https://health.gov/paguidelines/pdf/paguide.pdf. Accessed May 3, 2021.
7. US Department of Health and Human Services. *Physical Activity Guidelines Advisory Committee Report*, 2008. Washington, DC: US Department of Health and Human Services; 2008. https://health.gov/sites/default/files/2019-10/CommitteeReport_7.pdf instead? Accessed May 3, 2021.
8. Lauer SA, Grantz KH, Bi Q, et al. The incubation period of coronavirus disease 2019 (COVID-19) from publicly reported confirmed cases: Estimation and application. *Ann Intern Med.* 2020;*172*(9):577–582.
9. Merrill, RM. *Introduction to Epidemiology,* Eighth Edition. Chapter 3. Burlington, MA: Jones & Bartlett Learning; 2021.
10. Centers for Disease Control and Prevention. Clinical questions about COVID-19: Questions and answers. https://www.cdc.gov/coronavirus/2019-ncov/hcp/faq.html. Accessed July 24, 2020.
11. Mortality analysis. Johns Hopkins University & Medicine. https://coronavirus.jhu.edu/data/mortality. Accessed July 27, 2020.
12. Richardson S, Hirsch JS, Narasimhan M, et al. Presenting characteristics, comorbidities, and outcomes among 5700 patients hospitalized with COVID-19 in the New York City area. *JAMA.* 2020;*323*(20):2052–2059.
13. Killerby ME, Link-Gelles R, Haight SC, et al. Characteristics associated with hospitalization among patients with COVID-19—metropolitan Atlanta, Georgia, March–April 2020. *MMWR.* 2020;*69*:790–794.
14. Wortham JM, Lee JT, Athomsons S, et al. Characteristics of persons who died with COVID-19—United States. February 12–May 19, 2020. *MMWR* 2020;*69*(28):923–929.
15. Wilson N, Kvalsvig A, Barnard LT, Baker MG. Case-fatality risk estimates for COVID-19 calculated using a late time for fatality. *Emerg Infect Dis.* 2020;*26*(6):1339–1441.
16. COVID-19 Dashboard by the Center for Systems Science and Engineering (CSSE) at Johns Hopkins University (JHU). Johns Hopkins University & Medicine. https://coronavirus.jhu.edu/map.html. Accessed July 27, 2020.
17. Ellington S, Strid P, Tong VT, et al. Characteristics of women of reproductive age with laboratory-confirmed SARS-CoV-2 infection by pregnancy status—United States, January 22–June 7, 2020. *MMWR.* 2020;*69*:769–775.
18. Lewis M, Sanchez R, Auerbach S, et al. COVID-19 outbreak among college students after a spring break trip to Mexico—Austin, Texas, March 26–April 5, 2020. *MMWR.* 2020;*69*(26):830–835.

CHAPTER 2

Descriptive Summaries of Data

KEY CONCEPTS

- A research design is a formal approach of scientific investigation.
- Three general types of research designs are descriptive, exploratory, and analytic.
- A descriptive design is used to provide information about patterns and frequencies in data; it is used to describe what is occurring.
- An exploratory design is the least structured of the three research designs, with a high level of uncertainty and poor understanding about the biological problem.
- An analytic design is used to measure associations and test whether those associations are statistically significant.
- A frequency distribution is a display, either tabular or graphical, of the number of observations a variable takes at each level.
- A proportion is a number compared to the whole.
- A rate is a proportion with the added dimension of time.
- A ratio is the relationship between two quantities, normally expressed as the quotient of one divided by the other.
- Greek letters are used to represent population characteristics (parameters), and Roman letters are used to represent sample characteristics (statistics).
- Measurements on a nominal or ordinal scale are evaluated using frequency, relative frequency, proportions, and rates.
- Measurements on an interval or ratio scale are evaluated using measures of central tendency and variation.
- Measures of central tendency describe what is typical for a distribution of data, such as the geometric mean, arithmetic mean, median, and mode.
- Measures of variation capture the extent of spread over the values of a data set, such as variance, standard deviation, coefficient of variation, range, and interquartile range.
- Tables and graphs are used to present information, typically involving a large number of observations, in a concise and comprehendible way.

In the previous chapter, we emphasized that studies in biostatistics begin with a research question, which represents an unknown issue to be resolved by carrying out the study. A research design reflects the purpose of the study, whether descriptive, exploratory, or analytic. It is an overall plan that describes the approach that will be taken to answer the research question—it is a formal approach of scientific investigation. We will cover descriptive research designs in this chapter and emphasize the first major topic area in biostatistics—descriptive biostatistics.

In this chapter, you will become familiar with questions for descriptive biostatistics, and selected tabular and graphical approaches will be shown for summarizing and presenting numerical data. Numerical descriptions of data obtained through arithmetic operations will be presented. These are called descriptive statistics. They measure frequency (e.g., count, percent, rate), central tendency (e.g., mean, median), dispersion or variation (e.g., standard deviation, range, interquartile range), and position (e.g., percentile, rank). Rate calculations and adjustment methods of rates will be presented.

2.1 Questions for Descriptive Biostatistics

A descriptive study design in biostatistics should provide an accurate and valid representation of the variables that are relevant to the research question. This type of research is less structured than the analytic study design, but more structured than the exploratory study design. The analytic study design investigates why and how a phenomenon occurred. The exploratory study design proceeds with a high level of uncertainty and poor understanding about a biological problem.

Descriptive measures describe and summarize numerical data. A descriptive study design aims to provide information about patterns and frequencies in the data. Descriptive statistics allow us to present the data so that simple interpretation might occur. For example, if we had the race results of all the athletes from the Boston marathon, we may be interested in how many started the race, how many finished the race, the fastest time, the average time, how spread out the times were, how the results varied according to age, sex, and race and Hispanic origin, and so on. These descriptive statistics, therefore, help us summarize the race information in a meaningful way so that patterns might emerge from the data. Descriptive statistics, however, do not allow us to draw conclusions beyond the data we have assessed or test specific hypotheses. We are simply describing what occurred in our data.

The descriptive research design, with accompanying possible questions and examples, is presented in **Table 2.1**. To help emphasize the distinct role descriptive research plays, the descriptive study design is contrasted with the exploratory and analytic study designs. Later chapters will cover the analytic study design, but briefly it involves techniques for measuring associations between variables and testing hypotheses of association.

Table 2.1 Questions and Examples Associated with Descriptive, Exploratory, and Analytic Biostatistics Study Designs

Type of Design	Question	Examples
Descriptive	What is the number of cases? What is the proportion of cases? What is the rate of cases? Are selected variables related?	How many COVID-19 cases were identified today? What proportion of COVID-19 cases resulted in death? What is the rate of COVID-19 per 100,000 in July 2020? Is the death rate for COVID-19 cases related to age?

Table 2.1 Questions and Examples Associated with Descriptive, Exploratory, and Analytic Biostatistics Study Designs ***(Continued)***

Type of Design	Question	Examples
Exploratory	What is a case? What are the key factors involved?	What clinical characteristics tend to manifest among patients exposed to COVID-19? What reasons are there for the high percentage of students being absent from school today?
Analytic	Why? What are the causes of the health problem?	Do differences in comorbid diseases among racial/ethnic groups explain the high racial/ethnic disparity in case-fatality rates? Will a new treatment lower the risk of death among COVID-19 patients?

News File

In order to rapidly monitor changes in mental health, the Census Bureau partnered with the National Center for Health Statistics to conduct the Household Pulse Survey.[1] The survey was intended to provide relevant information about how COVID-19 affects the U.S. population. It covered April 23 through July 21, 2020.

Questions were included to assess the frequency of anxiety and depressive symptoms. The questions collected information from participants regarding the previous 7 days. It identified the percentage of adults who experienced symptoms of anxiety or depression more than half of the time.

Results from the survey are presented in **Table 2.2**. The overall increase in anxiety or depression was 14%. The greatest increase was among individuals 30–39 years, males, non-Hispanic Asians, and in those with at least a high school diploma. An increase in anxiety or depression occurred in each age group except for those 80 years and older, where it decreased by 17%. Although other reports have shown that the death-to-case ratio of COVID-19 increases with age, other factors (e.g., social isolation, unemployment) seem to be affecting younger people disproportionately hard. Although we might expect an increase in percentages of depression or anxiety in the older age groups because they are more vulnerable to dying from the disease, the reason for the decrease in percentages among ages 80 and older is unclear.

For age, sex, race and Hispanic origin, and education, the greatest increase tends to be in those groups that started with the lowest levels of anxiety or depression, and vice versa. Social isolation, employment, and economic concerns are certainly contributors to the increase, but where anxiety or depression was initially higher, some or all of these concerns may have already been greater. For example, Hispanics, non-Hispanic blacks, and non-Hispanic other or multiple race began with higher levels of anxiety or depression, but the increase during the COVID-19 pandemic was smaller than the increase among non-Hispanic whites and non-Hispanic Asians. In addition, among the education groups those with less than a high school education began with the highest level of anxiety or depression, but only increased 4% during the COVID-19 pandemic.

Table 2.2 Anxiety or Depression in the United States During April 23 through July 16

	Week Beginning April 23	Week Beginning July 16	Ratio
United States	35.9%	40.9	1.14
Age Group			
18–29 years	46.8%	53.4%	1.14
30–39 years	39.6%	47.1%	1.19
40–49 years	38.9%	44.5%	1.14
50–59 years	35.8%	40.0%	1.12
60–69 years	28.9%	32.1%	1.11
70–79 years	21.5%	24.3%	1.13
80 years and above	21.1%	17.5%	0.83
Sex			
Male	31.0%	37.0%	1.19
Female	40.7%	44.6%	1.10
Race and Hispanic Origin			
Hispanic or Latino	42.7%	46.3%	1.08
Non-Hispanic white, single race	33.6%	38.8%	1.15
Non-Hispanic black, single race	38.9%	42.6%	1.10
Non-Hispanic Asian, single race	31.9%	40.3%	1.26
Non-Hispanic, other or multiple race	43.9%	48.8%	1.11
Education			
Less than a high school diploma	45.4%	47.3%	1.04
High school diploma or GED	36.7%	42.2%	1.15
Some college/ associate's degree	38.5%	43.3%	1.12
Bachelor's degree or higher	30.7%	35.7%	1.16

2.2 Empirical Frequency Distributions

Tabular and graphical presentations of the data are generally known as empirical frequency distributions. It is often of interest to know the pattern or grouping into which data fall. In this section, we will present the frequency distribution and corresponding statistical measures.

2.2.1 Frequency Distribution

A **frequency distribution** is a display, either tabular or graphical, of the number of occurrences at each possible level of a variable. For example, the number of deaths from COVID-19 in the United States during the week ending July 25, 2020,[2] is distributed across selected age groups as follows:

	< 45	45–54	55–64	65–74	75–84	≥ 85
Frequency of deaths	933	834	1968	3311	4434	5925

2.2.2 Relative Frequency

Relative frequency is the number for the specific level of a variable compared with the total number across the levels of the variable. For example, the frequency distribution table is expanded to include the relative frequencies. If you sum the relative frequencies, they total to 1. The relative frequencies here tell us the proportion of cases in each age group.

	< 45	45–54	55–64	65–74	75–84	≥ 85
Frequency of deaths	933	834	1968	3311	4434	5925
Relative frequency	0.054	0.048	0.113	0.190	0.255	0.340

2.2.3 Proportion

Each of the relative frequencies just shown is a proportion. They range from 0 to 1. Proportions are often presented as a percentage (per 100) of the whole. Thus we can make statements like 0.340 (or 34.0%) of the cases of COVID-19 in the United States are in the age group 85 years and older, as of July 25, 2020.

A **proportion** is a part or number in comparative relation to a whole.

2.2.4 Rate

A related measure is a rate. A rate is the number of cases compared with the population at risk of becoming a case from which the cases derived. A rate specifies some period of time in which cases were generated. In biostatistics a rate may reflect a disease (e.g., hemophilia, meningococcal meningitis, COVID-19), an event (e.g., domestic violence, premature birth, pulmonary embolism), or a behavior or condition (e.g., social distancing during an infectious disease outbreak, nutrition, vaccination, use of health services). In other words, rather than representing the magnitude of something, it represents the risk of something.

A **rate** is a proportion with the added dimension of time.

For example, a measure of the magnitude of COVID-19 is the number of cases. A measure of the risk of COVID-19 is the rate of the illness. Extending the distribution table to include age-specific rates per 100,000 people in the United States population is as follows:

	< 45	45–54	55–64	65–74	75–84	≥ 85
Frequency of death	933	834	1968	3311	4434	5925
Relative frequency	0.054	0.048	0.113	0.190	0.255	0.340
Rate per 100,000	0.48	2.05	4.60	10.10	26.77	88.42

In one report identifying COVID-19 hospitalization rates by race and Hispanic origin for March 1–July 18, 2020, the authors were able to make meaningful comparisons because the rates accounted for differential population sizes. The rates were further adjusted for age differences among the racial/ethnic groups, also making the comparisons more meaningful. The rate estimates (per 100,000 population) were 281 for non-Hispanic American Indians or Alaska Natives, 247 for non-Hispanic black or African American, 242 for Hispanic or Latino, 67 for non-Hispanic Asian or Pacific Islander, and 53 for non-Hispanic white.[3] It would have been less informative had just the counts been reported since race/ethnicity population sizes from which cases derived vary considerably. According to population estimates for race and Hispanic origin in the United States on July 1, 2019, 76.3% were white only, 13.4% were black only, 5.9% were Asian only, 1.3% were American Indians/Alaska Natives only, 0.2% were native Hawaiians and other Pacific Islanders only, 2.8% were two or more races, and 18.5% were Hispanic or Latino.[4]

2.2.5 Adjusting Rates

If crude rates are compared between populations who have different age distributions, and if age is related to the rate variable, then the comparison of rates will be confounded. Essentially, any variable that varies across the population distributions being compared, if related to the rate variable, will make the comparison in rates potentially misleading. To account for the potential confounder and make the comparison of rates valid, the rates should be adjusted. Two methods will be presented in this section: direct and indirect. These will be illustrated for the situation where age is a potential confounder.

Sometimes age-adjusted rates are also applied to a single group where rates are being compared over time, but the age distribution is changing. For example, cancer rates tend to increase with age. In the United States, life expectancy increased from about 50 years in 1900 to about 79 years today. So some of the higher cancer rates now are because people are living to older ages where cancer is more common. To account for this, when the National Cancer Institute reports cancer rates over time, they are age-adjusted to some standard population, such as the U.S. age distribution in 2000.

Applying the direct method of age adjustment to rates over time assumes that the age-specific rates have a similar trend. If age-specific trends are not somewhat parallel, then an age-adjusted rate can mask important information. In the situation of nonparallel trends in age-specific rates, reporting trends in age-specific rates is more appropriate.

In practice, the direct method of standardizing rates is more common than the indirect method. With computer software such as Excel, it is fairly easy to compute age-adjusted rates using either the direct method or the indirect method. One rule of thumb is to use the direct method when subgroup-specific rates are available for all the groups being compared. If not, or if the subgroup rates are based on small numbers and therefore are unstable, the indirect method should be used.

2.2.5.1 Direct Method of Adjusting Rates

A comparison of the crude mortality rate of COVID-19 in the United States between males and females is appropriate if the rate is not dependent on age and the age distribution is similar between males and females. Mortality rates increase with age, and the age distribution differs between males and females (**Table 2.3**).[2,3]

The crude mortality rate (per 100,000) of COVID-19 during the week ending in July 25, 2020, was 5.40 for males and 5.07 for females. To obtain the age-adjusted rate, for each population, we need to know the age-group specific rates. These are calculated in the table. The crude rate in each population is just a weighted average of the age-group specific rates. For example, the crude mortality rate for males is

$$\frac{\sum(\text{Rate} \times n)}{\text{Total } n} = \frac{(1.69 \times 138{,}890{,}329) + (12.49 \times 15{,}328{,}874) + (30.89 \times 7{,}267{,}187) + (96.73 \times 2{,}418{,}086)}{138{,}890{,}329 + 15{,}328{,}874 + 7{,}267{,}187 + 2{,}418{,}086}$$
$$= 5.40 \text{ per } 100{,}000.$$

Because we are interested in obtaining rates that reflect similar age-distributions, the numbers in each category from one of the populations can be selected as the reference population and used as the weights to form weighted averages for both populations. It does not matter which of the two populations

Table 2.3 Death Rate from COVID-19 in the United States for Males and Females, During the Week Ending July 25, 2020

	Male				Female			
Age Group	Population	%	Cases	Rate per 100,000	Population	%	Cases	Rate per 100,000
< 65 years	138,890,329	84.74	2345	1.69	137,697,207	81.61	1390	1.01
65–74 years	15,328,874	9.35	1915	12.49	17,460,563	10.35	1396	8.00
75–84 years	7,267,187	4.43	2245	30.89	9,294,062	5.51	2189	23.55
⩾ 85 years	2,418,086	1.48	2339	96.73	4,282,794	2.54	3586	83.73
Total	163,904,476	100.00	8844	5.40	168,734,626	100.00	8561	5.07

is selected as the reference, but it is important to note the reference population in the interpretation of the rate. Sometimes a set of age-specific frequencies from a totally separate reference population is used. What is important is that the same set of numbers (standard) is applied to both populations.

For this example, we will select the male population as our standard and apply it to the age-group specific rates in the female population, as follows:

$$\begin{aligned}\text{Age-Adjusted Rate} &= \frac{\sum(\text{Rate} \times n \text{ in standard})}{\text{Total } n \text{ in standard}} \\ &= \frac{(1.01 \times 138{,}890{,}329) + (8.00 \times 15{,}328{,}874) + (23.55 \times 7{,}267{,}187) + (83.73 \times 2{,}418{,}086)}{138{,}890{,}329 + 15{,}328{,}874 + 7{,}267{,}187 + 2{,}418{,}086} \\ &= 3.88 \text{ per } 100{,}000\end{aligned}$$

So, if females had the same age-distribution as males, their mortality rate (per 100,000) of COVID-19 during the week ending July 25, 2020, would be 3.88 instead of 5.07.

Therefore, the direct method of age-adjustment involves a weighted average of the age-specific rates, where the weights are the proportions of persons in the corresponding age groups of the standard population.

2.2.5.2 *Indirect Method of Adjusting Rates*

In situations where age-group specific rates are unstable because of small numbers or unavailable altogether in the populations being compared, the indirect method may be useful for adjusting rates.

As was the case with the direct method, a standard population is selected. Age-group specific rates are calculated according to age-group specific values from a standard population. These rates are then multiplied by the age-group specific population value in the comparison population to obtain the expected number of cases in each age group. The total number of cases observed in the comparison population is then divided by the total number of expected cases. This ratio is referred to as the standard morbidity/mortality ratio (SMR).

$$\text{SMR} = \frac{\text{Observed}}{\text{Expected}}$$

To illustrate, refer again to Table 2.3. Suppose that some or all of the female age-group specific deaths are unavailable but that the total is available. Further, suppose that the age-group specific rates for males have been calculated. Multiply the age-group specific rates in the male population by the age-group specific female population values to obtain the age-group specific number of COVID-19 deaths for females, assuming they have the same rates as males. Sum the expected counts to obtain the total number of expected deaths in the comparison population. Then divide the observed count for females by the expected count for females.

$$\begin{aligned}\text{Expected} = &(0.0000169 \times 137{,}607{,}207) + (0.0001249 \times 17{,}460{,}563) \\ &+ (0.0003089 \times 9{,}294{,}062) + (0.0009673 \times 4{,}282{,}794) = 11{,}520\end{aligned}$$

Then

$$\text{SMR} = \frac{8561}{11{,}520} = 0.74$$

The SMR indicates that females have a 36% lower mortality rate from COVID-19 than males in the week ending in July 25, 2020.

2.2.6 Ratio

Finally, ratios can be used for descriptive and analytic purposes. As a descriptive measure, a ratio can describe comparisons among groups. For example, the rate of hospitalization for COVID-19 for each racial/ethnic group (presented in Section 2.2.4) can be compared using ratios.[3] Hospitalization rates for each of the racial/ethnic groups compared with non-Hispanic whites are 5.30, 4.66, 4.57, and 1.26, respectively.

A **ratio** is the relationship between two quantities, normally expressed as the quotient of one divided by the other.

We can now apply the following equations to ratios to calculate percent greater or less than the reference group.

If Ratio > 1 then (Ratio – 1) × 100%
If Ratio ≤ 1 then (1 – Ratio) × 100%

Therefore, the rate of hospitalization is 430% greater for non-Hispanic American Indians or Alaska Natives, 366% greater for non-Hispanic blacks, 357% greater for Hispanic or Latino, and 26% greater for non-Hispanic Asian or Pacific Islander compared with non-Hispanic white.

Using the ratio as an analytic tool in which hypotheses are considered is also common in biostatistics. A hypothesis could be that the rate of hospitalization is greater for Hispanics than non-Hispanic whites. This hypothesis would be tested against there being no difference in rates. We would then apply a statistical test to the data in order to evaluate whether the difference in rates is statistically significant.

2.3 Notation

Recall that data are information obtained through observation, experiment, or measurement of a phenomenon of interests, such as the weekly case-fatality rate of COVID-19 for all U.S. states, the average age of COVID-19 patients for each census tract within a given state, or the proportion of COVID-19 hospital patients requiring invasive mechanical ventilation at selected hospitals. A capital letter or symbol like X is used to represent the characteristic of interest. If two characteristics are measured, we represent them by X and Y, and so on. By convention a subscript is added to the variable so that each subscript number identifies a specific item in the data set. For example, x_i represents a specific characteristic of interest for the ith person or item in the population. The number in the population is denoted by N, and the number in the sample is denoted by n. Other common statistical notation includes f_i = frequency of x_i, f = total number of observations in an interval, and Σ = sum.

Greek letters are used to represent population characteristics (parameters), and Roman letters are used to represent sample characteristics (statistics). Some examples appear as follows:

Parameter		Statistic	
Symbol	**Name**	**Symbol**	**Name**
μ	Population mean	$\overline{x}$	Sample mean
σ^2	Population variance	s^2	Sample variance
σ	Population standard deviation	s	Sample standard deviation

2.4 Measures of Central Tendency

For numerical data and their frequency distributions, the observed values usually tend to group toward a center. In other words, some central measure best characterizes the data. This phenomenon is called central tendency.

A **measure of central tendency** is a typical value for a distribution of data. Measures of central tendency include the geometric mean, arithmetic mean, median, and mode.

2.4.1 Geometric Mean

The geometric mean applies to positive numbers. It is used for variables measured on an exponential or logarithmic scale, such as dilution assays (1/2, 1/4, 1/8, 1/16, etc.). It is often used for environmental samples, where the levels of the variable can range over several orders of magnitude (e.g., coliforms in sample taken from a lake can range from less than 100 to greater than 100,000).

The **geometric mean** is an average that indicates the typical value of a set of numbers by taking the *n*th root of the product of their values.

$$\text{Geometric mean} = \sqrt[N]{(x_1)(x_2)\ldots(x_N)} \quad \text{Population}$$

$$\text{Geometric mean} = \sqrt[n]{(x_1)(x_2)\ldots(x_n)} \quad \text{Sample}$$

For example, suppose you are monitoring the level of *Enterococci* bacteria per 100 mL of sample over time and obtain the following data: 5, 25, 50, 100 per 100 mL. The geometric mean is $\sqrt[4]{5 \times 25 \times 50 \times 100} = 28.1$.

Now suppose two types of face masks are compared. The first has a protection score against SARS-CoV-2 of 65 and gets a 7 in reviews. The second has a protection score of 80 and gets a 5 in reviews. Comparing using the arithmetic mean gives (65 + 7)/2 = 36 versus (80 + 5)/2 = 42.5. On the other hand, the geometric means of the two face masks are: $\sqrt{65 \times 7} = 21.3$ and $\sqrt{80 \times 5} = 20$. Therefore, even though the protection is 15 points better for the second mask, the lower user rating of 5 is still important.

For data measured on an exponential or logarithmic scale, the median may be a better summary measure than the geometric mean if the data contains a negative number or a zero observation. Otherwise, when the data have a multiplicative or propagative nature, the geometric mean has some nice mathematical properties and should be used.

2.4.2 Arithmetic Mean

The **arithmetic mean** or average indicates the typical value of a set of numbers by taking their sum divided by either the population or sample size.

$$\mu = \frac{1}{N}\sum_{i=1}^{N} x_i \quad \text{Population}$$

$$\bar{x} = \frac{1}{n}\sum_{i=1}^{n} x_i \quad \text{Sample}$$

For example, you observe a sample of 10 ages: 24, 24, 25, 25, 25, 25, 26, 26, 26, 27. The mean age is

$$\bar{x} = \frac{1}{10}(24 + 24 + 25 + 25 + 25 + 25 + 26 + 26 + 26 + 27) = \frac{253}{10} = 25.3.$$

2.4.3 Weighted Mean

In some situations where the numbers are not equally important, the numbers may be weighted.

$$\mu = \frac{\sum_{i=1}^{N} w_i x_i}{\sum_{i=1}^{N} w_i} \quad \text{Population}$$

$$\bar{x} = \frac{\sum_{i=1}^{n} w_i x_i}{\sum_{i=1}^{n} w_i} \quad \text{Sample}$$

For example, the weighted mean for the data in the previous example is

$$\bar{x} = \frac{2 \times 24 + 4 \times 25 + 3 \times 26 + 1 \times 27}{2 + 4 + 3 + 1} = \frac{253}{10} = 25.3$$

2.4.4 Median

The **median** is a number in which half the data are greater than that number and half the values are less than that number. If the number of observations is an odd number, then the median is the middle value. If the number of observations is an even number, then the median is the average of the two middle values.

For example, the number of people performing COVID-19 tests at each of the nine locations is

2 3 3 5 **5** 9 9 10 10.

The median is 5 people. Consider if there were 10 locations in our data, such as

2 3 3 5 **5** **9** 9 9 10 10.

The observations 5 and 9 occupy two center positions, so the median is (5 + 9)/2, or 7.

2.4.5 Mode

The **mode** of a set of data is the number that most frequently occurs. The mode is a desirable measure when we desire to know which number occurs most frequently. In the previous example, the mode is 9.

2.4.6 Choosing a Measure of Central Tendency

In general, the shape of the frequency distribution influences the relationship among the measures of central tendency. If the distribution consists of a symmetrical bell-shaped curve, then the mean, median, and mode will coincide. If the frequency distribution is not symmetric (skewed) then the measures of central tendency will not coincide. The mean is most sensitive to extreme values. For example, if the average age of a group of individuals was estimated in a group of 10 or so people, and one of the people was 100, then the average age might not be characteristic of most of the people's ages. Hence, the median or mode may be preferred.

Conceptually, if we took a large number of sets of data from the same population and the mean, median, and mode were computed each time, less variation will result in the means than in the medians or the modes. Therefore, the mean is more stable. This fact, along with the mean being more amenable to mathematical treatment, makes the mean most widely chosen for statistical purposes, with the exception of some exploratory and descriptive assessment. The order of their statistical desirability is usually first the mean, second the median, and third the mode.[5]

2.5 Measures of Variation

A **measure of variation** (also called dispersion, scatter, or spread) is the extent to which a distribution is spread over the data range. Common measures of variation include the variance, standard deviation, range, interquartile range, and coefficient of variation.

2.5.1 Variance and Standard Deviation

To begin, consider the deviations from the mean as equal to $(x_1 - \mu)$, $(x_2 - \mu)$,... $(x_N - \mu)$. The average of the deviations from the mean is then

$$\frac{1}{N}\sum_{i=1}^{N}(x_i - \mu) = 0.$$

The average of the deviations from the mean will always be 0 because

$$\sum_{i=1}^{N}(x_i - \mu) = 0.$$

This is also true when sample data are involved:

$$\sum_{i=1}^{n}(x_i - \bar{x}) = 0.$$

Because the average of the deviations from the mean do not capture variation in the data, the average squared deviations from the mean is used as a dispersion measure. This is called the variance.

$$\sigma^2 = \frac{1}{N}\sum_{i=1}^{N}(x_i - \mu)^2 \quad \text{Population}$$

$$s^2 = \frac{1}{n-1}\sum_{i=1}^{n}(x_i - \bar{x})^2 \quad \text{Sample}$$

The standard deviation is the square root of the variance.

$$\sigma = \sqrt{\sigma^2} = \sqrt{\frac{1}{N}\sum_{i=1}^{N}(x_i - \mu)^2} \quad \text{Population}$$

$$s = \sqrt{s^2} = \sqrt{\frac{1}{n-1}\sum_{i=1}^{n}(x_i - \bar{x})^2} \quad \text{Sample}$$

For example, recall the random sample of 10 ages. The standard deviation is

$$s = \sqrt{s^2} = \sqrt{\frac{1}{10-1}\left[(24-25.3)^2 + (24-25.3)^2 + \cdots + (27-25.3)^2\right]}$$
$$= \sqrt{0.9} = 0.949.$$

You likely noticed the differences between the population and sample formulas for the variance. The population variance uses μ, and the sample variance uses $\overline{x}$. This is only a difference in notation. The population variance divides by N, and the sample variance divides by $n - 1$. The variance is a measure of dispersion or scatter of observations around the mean. Given that a sample is a subset of the population, the range of sample data is going to be smaller than the range of population data. Hence, the mean of the deviations about the mean will be smaller for sample data than it will be for population data. To adjust the variance up to where it better estimates the population variance, we divide by $n - 1$ instead of N. In addition to presenting the standard deviation for the arithmetic mean, the standard deviation for the geometric mean is shown in the following definition box.

The geometric standard deviation for a set of numbers $(x_1, x_2, \ldots, x_n)$ is denoted as

$$\sigma_g = \exp\left(\sqrt{\frac{\sum_{i=1}^{N}\left(\ln\frac{x_i}{\mu_g}\right)^2}{N}}\right) \quad \text{Population}$$

$$s_g = \exp\left(\sqrt{\frac{\sum_{i=1}^{n}\left(\ln\frac{x_i}{\overline{x}_g}\right)^2}{n-1}}\right) \quad \text{Sample}$$

For the example in 2.4.1, $s_g = \exp\left(\sqrt{\frac{\left(\ln\frac{5}{28.1}\right)^2 + \left(\ln\frac{25}{28.1}\right)^2 + \left(\ln\frac{50}{28.1}\right)^2 + \left(\ln\frac{100}{28.1}\right)^2}{4-1}}\right)$

$= 3.61.$

2.5.2 Degrees of Freedom

Degrees of freedom of an estimate is the number of independent pieces of information used to obtain the estimate. For the variance, several sums of squared quantities make up the estimate. In the above example, we had 10 squares of deviations from the mean. However, these 10 values are not independent because each of the sampled observations were used to obtain an estimate of the mean. Therefore, the sum of squares of deviations of the n values from their mean has $n - 1$ degrees of freedom, or in our example, nine degrees of freedom. In general, the degrees of freedom for an estimate equals the number of observed values minus the number of parameters estimated in order to obtain the estimate in question.

2.5.3 More on the Standard Deviation

Because the units of the variance are squared, it is no longer in the same unit of measurement as the original data. Taking the square root of the variance, which yields the standard deviation, is a way to provide a measure of variation that is restored to the original unit of measurement. It is also important to note that when the frequency distribution is symmetrical and bell-shaped, which is called a normal distribution, the Empirical Rule in statistics applies.

The **Empirical Rule** states that for a normal distribution, almost all the data lie within three standard deviations of the mean. Under this rule, about 68% of the observations lie within the interval $\mu \pm \sigma$; about 95% of the observations lie within the interval $\mu \pm 2\sigma$; and about 99.7% of observations lie within the interval $\mu \pm 3\sigma$.

The empirical rule is one way to define an outlier when the data have an approximately symmetric distribution. Approximately 0.3% of data account for outliers. Another approach to identify outliers, useful when the data are not symmetric, will be described in section 2.7.

2.5.4 Coefficient of Variation

The **coefficient of variation** is the ratio of the standard deviation to the mean. It is a measure of relative variability that should only be derived for data measured on a ratio scale. It allows us to compare the variability between groups when the unit of measurement differs between groups.

$$CV = \frac{\sigma}{\mu} \times 100\% \quad \text{Population}$$

$$CV = \frac{s}{\overline{x}} \times 100\% \quad \text{Sample}$$

Consider two measures used to screen for depression, *A* and *B*. If we take a random sample of individuals who were assessed for depression based on these two measures we might find the following standard deviations:

$$s_A = 3 \quad s_B = 12$$

This might cause us to want to avoid the second depression measure because of its relatively high variability in scores. Before we do so, note that the range of *A* is 1–10 and the range of *B* is 1–100. Let $\overline{x}_A = 7.5$ and $\overline{x}_B = 75$.

To convert the standard deviation so that we can compare between two sets of numbers with different units of measurement, we apply the coefficient of variation. The coefficient of variation expresses the standard deviation as a percentage of the mean. It is a unitless quantity.

$$CV_A = \frac{3}{7.5} \times 100\% = 40\%$$

$$CV_B = \frac{12}{75} \times 100\% = 16\%$$

From these results, we now see that the second depression measure is preferred in terms of having smaller spread of scores scattered around its mean.

2.5.5 Range and Interquartile Range

The **range** is the difference between the largest and smallest values in the data. In a previous example (2.4.4), the range is 8 (10 – 2). In reporting the range, it is often informative to include the maximum and minimum values upon which it is based.

However, reasons have been given as to why this may be a less preferred measure of variation. First, it only uses a small part of the available information about variation in the data. It fails to capture the extent to which most of the observations are dispersed. Second, with larger data sets, the range tends to increase. Hence, a comparison of ranges between data sets is inappropriate unless the data sets are equal in size. Third, the range is a less stable measure than the other measures of variation considered in this section. In other words, from sample to sample, the range will vary the most.[5] Nevertheless, when the median is used rather than the mean to represent the center of a data distribution, we tend to report with it the range, or the interquartile range.

The **interquartile range** represents the middle 50% of the data, extending from the first quartile to the third quartile. Two common approaches for calculating interquartile range are the exclusive and inclusive methods. The exclusive method does not include the median when identifying the first and third quartiles, whereas the inclusive method does include the median when identifying the quartiles. For example, for the data set referred to above that has an odd number of values (i.e., 2, 3, 3, 5, 5, 9, 9, 10, 10), to obtain the interquartile range using the exclusive method, place parentheses around the numbers above and below the median: (2, 3, 3, 5), 5, (9, 9, 10, 10). Think of the first quartile as the median of the first group of numbers and the third quartile as the median of the second group of numbers, or Q1 = (3 + 3)/2 = 3 and Q3 = (9 + 10)/2 = 9.5. Subtract Q1 from Q3 to obtain the interquartile range as 9.5 – 3 = 6.5. Using the inclusive method, Q1 = 3 and Q3 = 9, hence the interquartile range is 9 – 3 = 6.

2.6 Describing Data with Statistics and Graphs

As with frequency distribution tables and summary statistics, **graphs** can present a large amount of data in a concise and understandable way. Graphs often do a nice job clarifying biological health problems. They identify patterns, trends, aberrations, similarities, and differences in the data. They are important for communicating information according to selected factors like age, sex, and race and Hispanic origin, geographic location, and across time. They should be accompanied with descriptive titles, labels, and legends.

A summary of the statistical methods that we have considered in this chapter for describing data is presented in **Table 2.4**. The approach depends on the measurement scale of our data. A number of graphical approaches useful for describing data are described in **Table 2.5**.

Table 2.4 Scales of Measurement and Corresponding Statistics and Graphs

Scale	Statistics	Graphs
Nominal	Frequency Relative frequency Proportion Rate	Line graphs Bar chart/pie chart Spot map Area map
Ordinal	Frequency Relative frequency Proportion	Bar chart/pie chart
Interval or Ratio	Geometric mean Arithmetic mean Median Mode Range Variance Standard deviation Coefficient of variation	Bar chart/pie chart Histogram or frequency polygon Box plot Scatter plot Stem-and-leaf plot

Reference 6.

Table 2.5 Graphs for Describing Data

Type of Graph	Description
Arithmetic-scale line graph	Line graphs are used mostly for data plotted against time. An arithmetic graph has equal quantities along the y-axis. An arithmetic graph shows actual changes in magnitude of the number or rate of something across time.
Logarithmic-scale line graph	The y-axis is changed to a logarithmic scale. In other words, the axis is divided into cycles, with each being 10 times greater than the previous cycle. Focus is on the rate of change. A straight line reflects a constant rate of change.
Simple bar chart	A visual display of the magnitude of the different categories of a single variable is shown, with each category or value of the variable represented by a bar.
Grouped bar chart	Multiple sets of data are displayed as side-by-side bars.
Stacked bar chart	Although similar to a grouped bar chart, each of the segments in which the bar or column is divided belongs to a different data series. It shows how a total entity is subdivided into parts.
Deviation bar chart	Differences, both positive and negative, from the baseline are illustrated.
100% component bar chart	The bar is divided into proportions that are the same as the proportions of each category of the variable; it compares how components contribute to the whole in different groups.
Pie chart	Components of a whole are shown.
Population pyramid	This graphical illustration shows the distribution of age groups in a population for males and females.

Table 2.5 Graphs for Describing Data *(Continued)*

Type of Graph	Description
Histogram	A graphic representation of the frequency distribution of a variable, rectangles are drawn in such a way that their bases lie on a linear scale representing different intervals and their heights are proportional to the frequencies of the values within each of the intervals.
Frequency polygon	A graphical display of a frequency table, the intervals are shown on the *x*-axis, and the frequency in each interval is represented by the height of a point located above the middle of the interval. The points are connected so that together with the *x*-axis they form a polygon.
Cumulative frequency	A running total of frequencies is shown. A cumulative frequency polygon is used to graphically represent it.
Spot map	A map that indicates the location of each case of a rare health-related state or event that is potentially relevant to the health event being investigated, such as where each case lived or worked.
Area map	A map that indicates the number or rate of something, using different colors or shadings to represent the various levels of it in each place.
Stem-and-leaf plot	A method of organizing numerical data in order of place value. The stem of the number includes all but the last digit. The leaf of the number will always be one digit.
Box plot	Also called a box-and-whisker plot, it is a graphical depiction of numerical data through five-number summaries: the smallest observation, the first quartile, the median, the third quartile, and the largest observation. Sometimes the mean is added to the plot. The box portion of the graph represents the middle 50% of the data. The plot is useful for describing the distribution of the data, whether it is skewed, and if outliers are present.
Scatter plot	This graph is a useful summary of the association between two numerical variables. It is usually drawn before calculating a Pearson correlation coefficient or fitting a regression line because these statistics assume a linear relationship in the data.

Reference 6.

Excel is an excellent tool for constructing high-quality graphs. For example, suppose we identify 15 individuals with staphylococcal food poisoning who ate at a particular location. We want to construct a histogram identifying the incubation times for these individuals. The incubation times were 2 hours for four individuals, 3 hours for five individuals, 4 hours for three individuals, 5 hours for two individuals, and 6 hours for one individual. Now, in an Excel worksheet, enter this data into cells A1:A15 and highlight it. On the Insert tab, in the Charts, click the Histogram symbol.

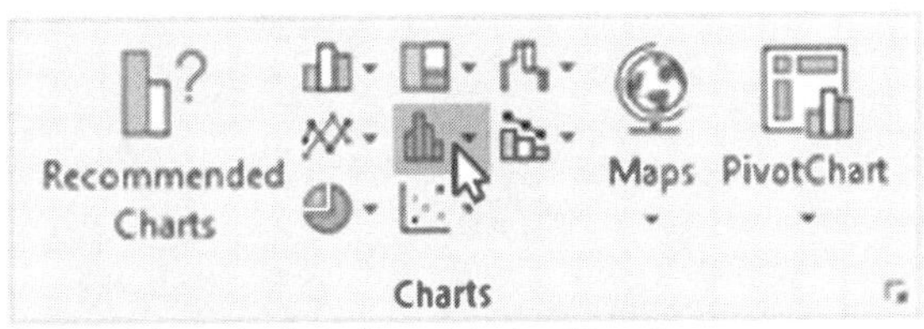

Click Histogram.

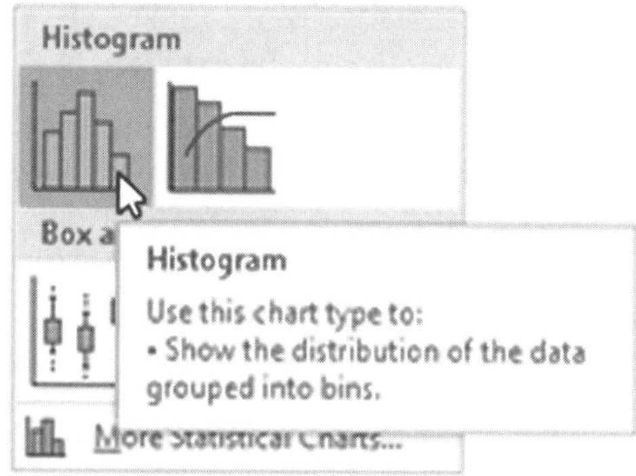

A histogram with three bins appears in the spreadsheet next to the data.

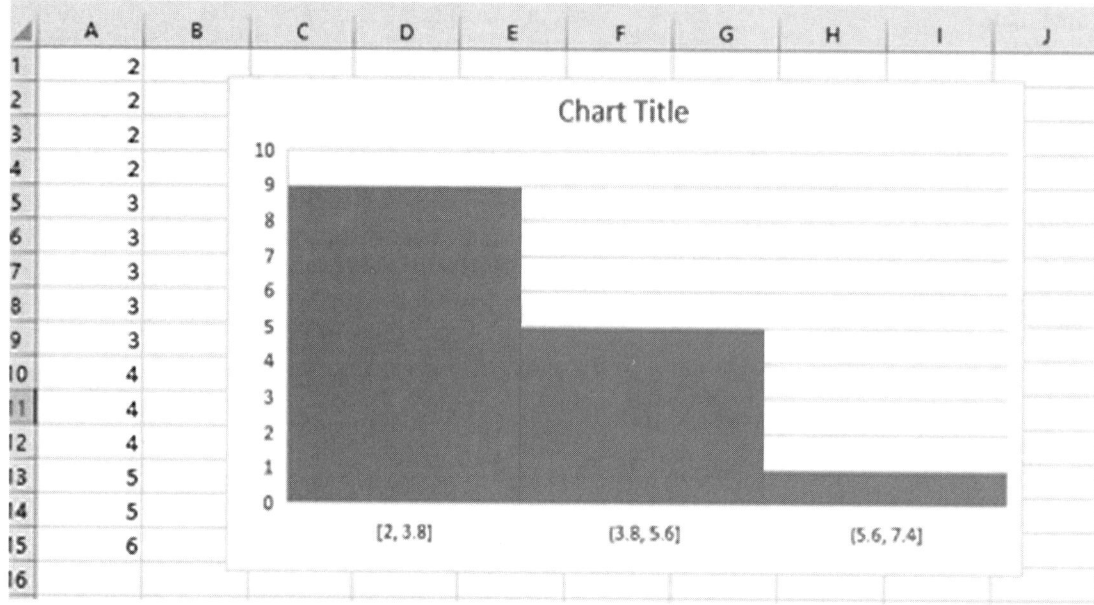

Double click the horizontal axis on the graph, and the Format Axis will appear on the right side of the screen. Select Number of bins and enter 5.

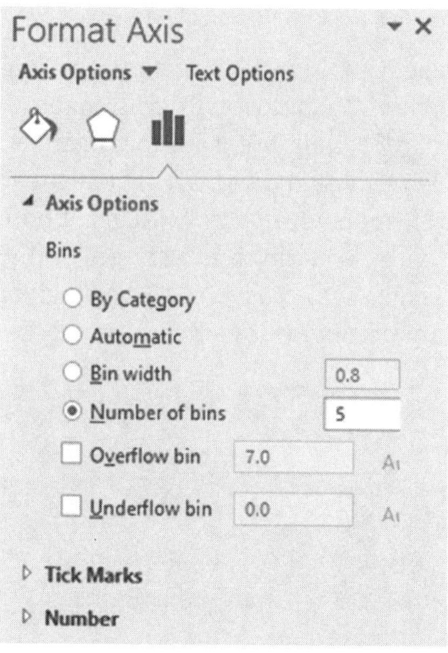

You can adjust the gap width so that the histogram appears as follows:

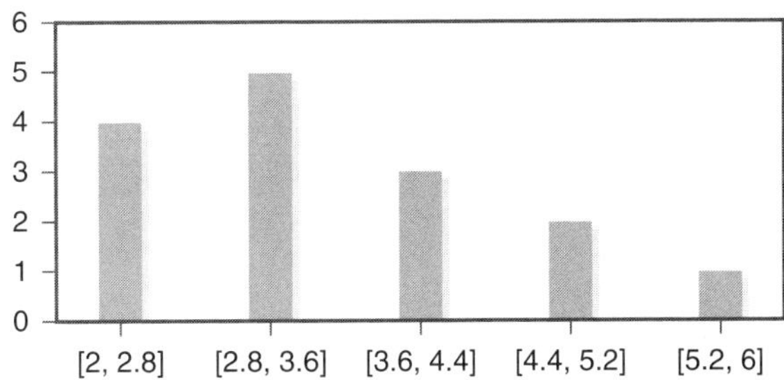

Other examples of graphs will be shown throughout this book.

2.7 Misleading Graphs

Graphs are sometimes misleading when the baseline is omitted, the horizontal axis is manipulated, certain data are cherry picked, or when the wrong graph is used. Examples of these situations are as follows:

1. Omitting the baseline

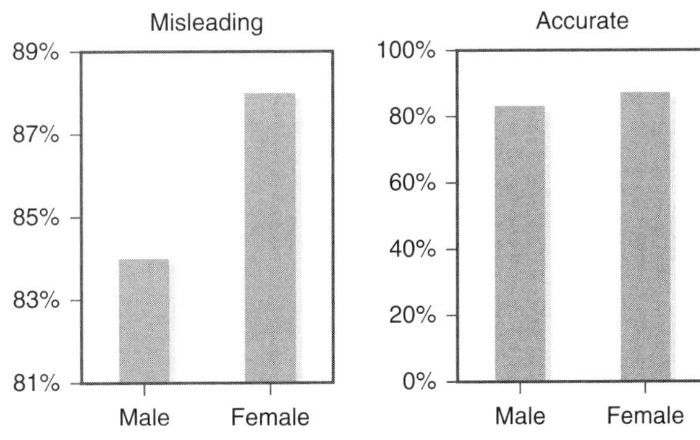

2. Manipulating the vertical axis

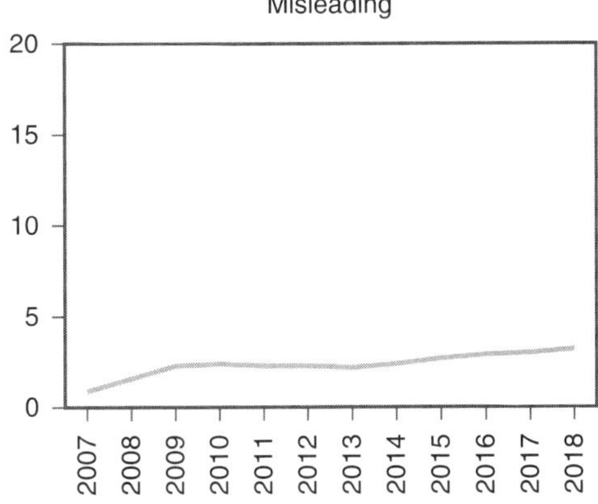

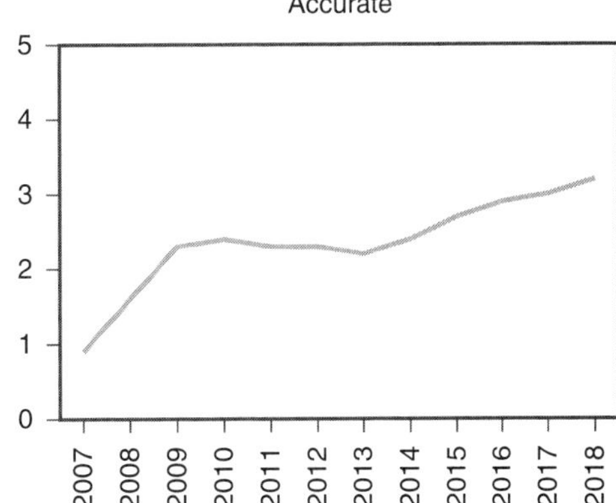

3. Cherry picking data

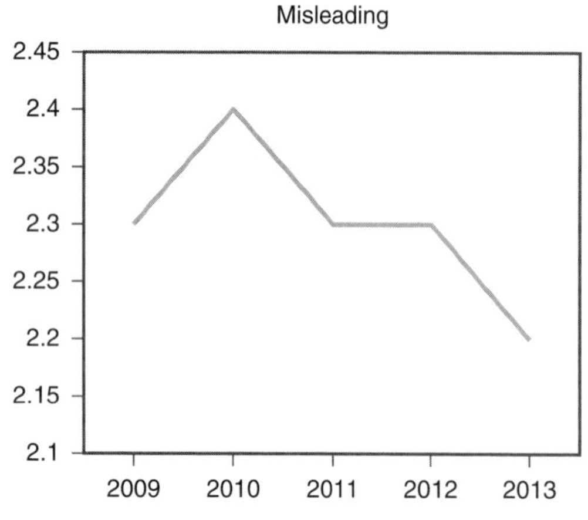

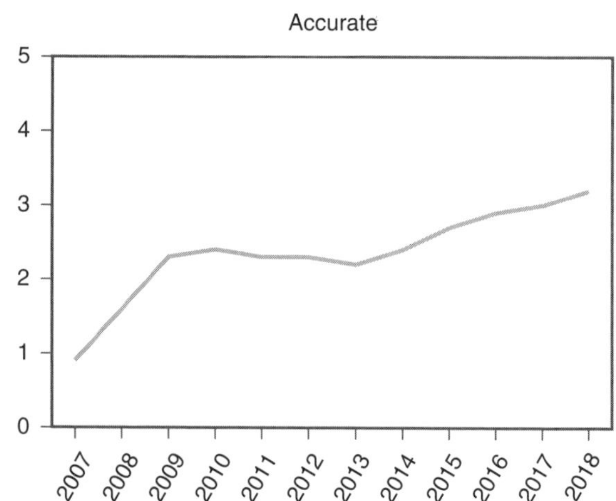

4. Using the wrong graph

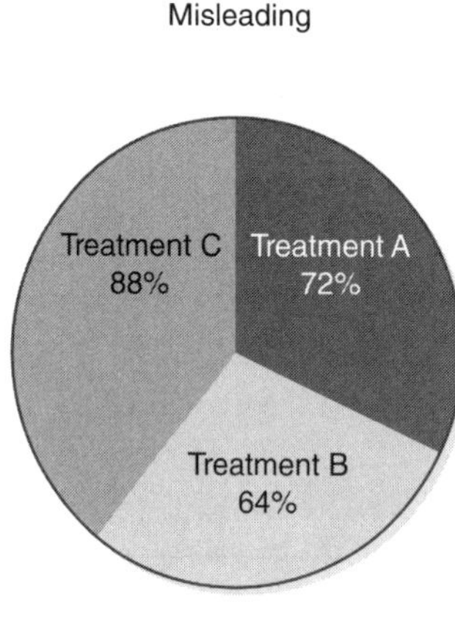

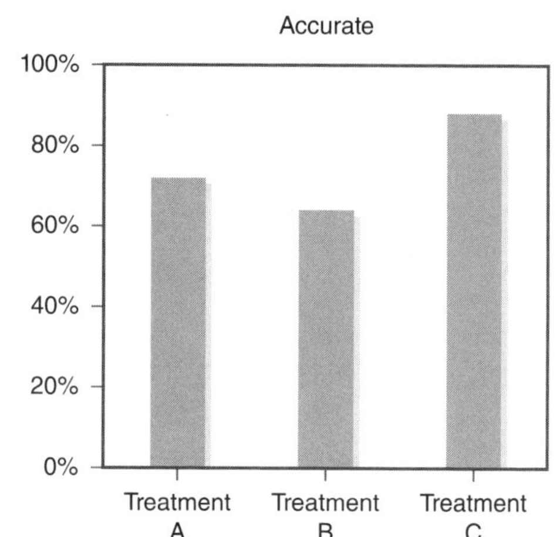

Note that pie charts are used to compare parts of a whole, not the difference between groups.

2.8 Five-Number Summary

The five-number summary provides a rough idea about what the data set looks like. The **five-number summary** includes the minimum, the first quartile (25th percentile), the median (50th percentile), the third quartile (75th percentile), and the maximum. A box plot can represent the five-number summary:

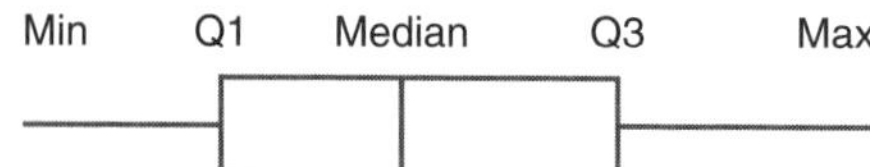

In addition to saying something about the distribution of the data, these numbers are used for calculating the range (max – min) and the interquartile range (IQR) (Q3 – Q1).

When the data distribution is not symmetric, outliers may be identified as < Q1 – (1.5 × IQR) or > Q3 + (1.5 × IQR). For example, in the data set 1, 3, 6, 7, 9, 15, and 100, the first quartile is 3, and the third quartile is 15. The interquartile range is 15 – 3 = 12. To check for outliers, 3 – 1.5 × 12 = –15 and 15 + 1.5 × 12 = 33. So, 100 is an outlier.

2.9 Statistical Software

In Table 2.3, age-specific mortality and population data for males and females were presented for COVID-19 in the United States. The "male" portion of that table is shown here, as it appears in Excel. The formulas for obtaining the age-distribution and rates are shown.

	A	B	C	D	E
1	Age Group	Population	%	Cases	Rate per 100,000
2	< 65 years	138,890,329	=B2/$B$6*100	2,345	=D2/B2*100000
3	65-74 years	15,328,874	=B3/$B$6*100	1,915	=D3/B3*100000
4	75-84 years	7,267,187	=B4/$B$6*100	2,245	=D4/B4*100000
5	≥ 85 years	2,418,086	=B5/$B$6*100	2,339	=D5/B5*100000
6	Total	163,904,476	=B6/$B$6*100	8,844	=D6/B6*100000

To calculate the geometric mean in Excel for the data in 2.4.1, enter 5 in cell A1, 25 in cell A2, 50 in cell A3, and 100 in cell A4. Then enter the formula in another cell as =GEOMEAN(A1:A4). An alternative is the formula =(A1*A2*A3*A4)^(1/4). Note that A1:A4 is called an array (a structure that holds a collection of values) in Excel.

For the example involving the arithmetic mean in 2.4.2, enter 24 in cell A1, 24 in cell A2, etc. Then enter the formula in another cell =AVERAGE(A1:A10). If the data are in the form shown in the following table, then the mean is calculated as:

	A	B	C
1	Age	Frequency	Weighted Age
2	24	2	=A2*B2
3	25	4	=A3*B3
4	26	3	=A4*B4
5	27	1	=A5*B5
6	Total	=sum(B2:B5)	=sum(C2:C5)
7	Mean		=C6/B6

To obtain the median for the numbers in 2.4.4, enter 2 in cell A1, 3 in cell A2, etc., then in another cell enter =MEDIAN(A1:A9) for the first example and =MEDIAN(A1:A10) for the second example. To obtain the mode for the numbers in the second example, use the formula =MODE(A1:A10).

To obtain the sample standard deviation for the 10 ages in 2.4.2, if the data are in cells A1 through A10, then use the formula =STDEV.S(A1:A10). If this was not sample data, but represented an entire population, we would have used the formula =STDEV.P(A1:A10). If we were interested in obtaining the coefficient of variation for these data, then use the formula =STDEV.S(A1:A10)/AVERAGE(A1:A10). To obtain the range, use the formula =MAX(A1:A10)-MIN(A1:A10).

To use the Data Analysis option, choose the Descriptive Statistics option, identify the input range, check the summary statistics option, and select OK.

To use SAS to evaluate these data, apply the following code. Note that the symbols @@ tells SAS to read the data across the row versus the default, which is by column. Some PROC MEANS options available in SAS are n (sample size), Mean (average), STD (standard deviation), CV (coefficient of variation), Median (middle or 50th percentile), Min (smallest value), Max (largest value), Range (max – min), Q1 (lower quartile or 25th percentile), Q3 (upper quartile or 75th percentile), QRange (q3 – q1), p10 (10th percentile), and p90 (90th percentile).

```
DATA E2_4_2;
   INPUT AGE @@;
   DATALINES;
24 24 25 25 25 25 26 26 26 27
;

PROC MEANS DATA=E2_4_2 MAXDEC=2 N MEAN STD CV MEDIAN
MIN MAX RANGE Q1 Q3 QRANGE P10 P90;
   VAR Age;
RUN;
```

Analysis Variable : Age												
N	Mean	Std Dev	Coeff of Variation	Median	Minimum	Maximum	Range	Lower Quartile	Upper Quartile	Quartile Range	10th Pctl	90th Pctl
10	25.30	0.95	3.75	25.00	24.00	27.00	3.00	25.00	26.00	1.00	24.00	26.50

If we are interested in the five-number summary to describe the data, we see in this output the minimum, Q1, median, Q3, and maximum are 24, 25, 25, 26, and 27, respectively. The range is 27 – 24 = 3. The IQR is Q3 – Q1 = 26 – 25 = 1. Outliers would be below Q1 – (1.5 × IQR) (i.e., 25 – 1.5 × 1 = 23.5) and above Q3 + (1.5 × IQR) (i.e., 26 – 1.5 × 1 = 27.5). There are no outliers in this dataset.

These statistics can also be computed in Excel. Following are some useful commands in Excel to obtain the five number summary:

MIN(*array*)
QUARTILE.INC(*array*, 1); PERCENTILE.INC(*array*, .25)
MEDIAN(*array*); QUARTILE.INC(*array*, 2); PERCENTILE.INC(*array*, .50)
QUARTILE.INC(*array*, 3); PERCENTILE.INC(*array*, .75)
MAX(*array*)

From these statistics we can easily calculate the range and IQR. If the exclusive method is desired, then use .EXC instead of .INC.

2.10 Summary

This chapter presented the descriptive study design as a means to provide information about patterns and frequencies in data. This design is used to describe what is happening. The different scales of measurement influence the statistics and graphs for summarizing and displaying information.

Nominal or ordinal scaled measurements are evaluated using frequency, relative frequency, proportions, and rates. Interval or ratio scaled measurements are evaluated using central tendency and variation. Measures of central tendency capture what is typical for a distribution of data. These measures include the geometric mean, arithmetic mean, median, and mode. The geometric mean is appropriate for a set of positive numbers in which the values are meant to be multiplied or have an exponential distribution (e.g., a set of growth figures). For data that are normally distributed, the arithmetic mean, median, and mode fall at the same location, otherwise they will not coincide. Of these measures, the mean is the most sensitive to outliers. When the distribution is not a symmetric bell shaped curve, a measure such as the median will better reflect where the data are most common.

A measure of variation captures the extent to which a distribution is spread over the data range. The standard deviation is a particularly important measure of variation, and we will see later that it is used in constructing confidence intervals and hypothesis tests. The coefficient of variation allows us to compare the variability between groups when their unit of measurement differs.

Tables and graph are ways to present information in a concise and comprehensible way. They should be simple, easy to understand, and stand on their own.

A summary of the formulas for descriptive measures is shown in **Table 2.6**.

Table 2.6 Selected Formulas for Descriptive Measures

	Population	Sample
Geometric mean	$GM = \sqrt[N]{(x_1)(x_2)\ldots(x_N)}$	$GM = \sqrt[n]{(x_1)(x_2)\ldots(x_n)}$
Arithmetic mean	$\mu = \frac{1}{N}\sum_{i=1}^{N} x_i$	$\overline{x} = \frac{1}{n}\sum_{i=1}^{n} x_i$
Weighted mean	$\mu = \frac{\sum_{i=1}^{N} w_i x_i}{\sum_{i=1}^{N} w_i}$	$\overline{x} = \frac{\sum_{i=1}^{n} w_i x_i}{\sum_{i=1}^{n} w_i}$
Variance	$\sigma^2 = \frac{1}{N}\sum_{i=1}^{N}(x_i - \mu)^2$	$s^2 = \frac{1}{n-1}\sum_{i=1}^{n}(x_i - \overline{x})^2$
Standard deviation	$\sigma = \sqrt{\sigma^2} = \sqrt{\frac{1}{N}\sum_{i=1}^{N}(x_i - \mu)^2}$	$s = \sqrt{s^2} = \sqrt{\frac{1}{n-1}\sum_{i=1}^{n}(x_i - \overline{x})^2}$
Coefficient of variation	$CV = \frac{\sigma}{\mu} \times 100\%$	$CV = \frac{s}{\overline{x}} \times 100\%$

Exercises

1. The fraction $\frac{\text{Number of deaths from COVID-19 in 2020}}{\text{Number of deaths from cancer in 2020}}$ is a
   a. ratio
   b. proportion
   c. rate
2. The fraction $\frac{\text{Number of deaths from COVID-19 in 2020}}{\text{Number of all deaths in 2020}}$ is a
   a. ratio
   b. proportion
   c. rate
3. The fraction $\frac{\text{Number of deaths from COVID-19 in 2020}}{\text{Total population, midyear in 2020}}$ is a
   a. ratio
   b. proportion
   c. rate

4. In a recent survey, investigators found that the prevalence (new and existing cases) of disease A was higher than that of disease B. The incidence (new cases) and seasonal pattern of both diseases is similar. Which factors may explain the higher prevalence of disease A?

5. In a community of 460 residents, 63 individuals attended a church social event that included a meal prepared by some of its members. Within 3 days, 34 of those attending the social became ill with a condition diagnosed as *salmonellosis*. What is the rate of illness? Express your answer to the nearest tenth.

6. Which of the following is not true of a rate?
   a. The cases in the numerator are included in the denominator.
   b. The cases in the denominator must be at risk of being in the numerator.
   c. Subjects in the numerator and denominator must cover the same time period.
   d. The numerator must consist of disease cases.

7. Classify the following as (A) descriptive design, (B) exploratory design, or (C) analytic design.
   a. ___ What is the case-fatality rate?
   b. ___ What constitutes a case?
   c. ___ How many new cases occurred today?
   d. ___ What are some reasons for not agreeing with the requirements?
   e. ___ Does diabetes increase the risk of death for patients with COVID-19?

For exercises 8–12 refer to the following table of age-group specific deaths and population sizes in Florida and Utah in 2016.[7]

	Florida		Utah	
Ages (years)	**All Deaths**	**Population**	**All Deaths**	**Population**
0–19	2617	4,612,753	523	1,012,075
20–39	5359	3,957,007	780	701,826
40–59	16,982	5,220,599	1795	724,993
60–79	61,285	5,004,747	5115	482,361
80+	111,056	1,817,333	9700	129,962
Total	197,299	20,612,439	17,913	3,051,217

8. Calculate the crude mortality rates (per 100,000) in Florida and Utah. Then divide the rate in Florida by the rate in Utah. What is your conclusion about the risk of death in the two populations?

9. Calculate the relative frequency of the population in each age group for Florida and Utah. Comment on any differences you see in the age distributions between the two states.

10. Compare the age-specific rates between Florida and Utah and interpret your results.

11. Using the direct method, calculate the age-adjusted rate for Utah using Florida as the standard.

12. Now compare the age-adjusted rate in Utah to the crude Florida rate and interpret your results.

For exercises 13–14 refer to the age-group specific deaths from malnutrition, along with corresponding population values in Texas, 2014–2016, for whites and blacks.[7]

	Whites		Blacks	
Ages (years)	**Deaths from Malnutrition**	**Population**	**Deaths from Malnutrition**	**Population**
45–54	43	8,452,525	0	1,353,830
55–64	85	7,532,374	31	1,099,882
65–74	166	4,922,068	28	559,349
75–84	315	2,441,907	42	236,797
85+	588	1,006,805	62	88,869
Total	1197	24,355,679	163	3,338,727

ICD 10 codes E40-E46.

13. What is the age-specific expected number of cases in blacks, assuming they had the same rates as whites?
14. Apply the indirect method of standardization to this data, assuming blacks had the same age-group specific death rates as whites. Interpret your results.
15. Is there ever a time that you would not want to age-adjust rates when comparing rates between or among groups?
16. What is an important assumption behind age-adjusted rates that are calculated for the same population over time?
17. Age-adjusted rates have been referred to as hypothetical constructs, with critics considering the actual age-adjusted rates meaningless. How would you respond to these critics?
18. Is the choice of the standard population for age-adjustment really arbitrary?
19. The number of cases of COVID-19 from July 25 through August 3, 2020, in Utah were 381, 438, 421, 354, 490, 503, 483, 477, 339, and 361, respectively. Corresponding numbers in Arizona were 3740, 1973, 1813, 2107, 2339, 2525, 3212, 2992, 1465, and 1030.[8] For each state, calculate the mean, median, variance, standard deviation, range, interquartile range, and coefficient of variation. Which state has the greatest relative variability in cases?
20. During the first week of December in Utah, the rates of COVID-19 were 2516, 3960, 4035, 3003, 3586, 2563, and 2231. Calculate the five-number summary statistics, along with the range and interquartile range.
21. Continuing with the previous exercise, are there any outliers?
22. What is a typical graph that is used to represent rates over time?
23. What is an appropriate graph for describing the percentage of a population according to race and Hispanic origin?

   a. Pie chart
   b. Histogram
   c. Box plot
   d. Scatter plot

24. When might it be better to assess data using the geometric mean instead of the arithmetic mean?
25. A new drug had a sensitivity of 0.75 and a tolerability rating of 8 (on a scale from 1 to 10). The currently used drug had a sensitivity of 0.8 and a tolerability rating of 5. Compare these drugs taking into account both sensitivity and tolerability using the geometric mean. Should the new drug be adopted?
26. In the equation for the population variance we divide by N, but for the sample variance we divide by $n - 1$. Why?
27. What is the meaning of degrees of freedom?
28. The Empirical Rule in statistics applies under what conditions?
29. For a normal distribution, what percentage of data lies within 1, 2, or 3 standard deviation of the mean?
30. Based on the Empirical Rule, what percentage of data account for outliers in a normal distribution of data?

References

1. Mental Health: Household Pulse Survey. Centers for Diseases Control and Prevention. https://www.cdc.gov/nchs/covid19/pulse/mental-health.htm. Updated March 10, 2021. Accessed May 23, 2020.
2. Provisional Covid-19 death counts by sex, age, and week. Centers for Disease Control and Prevention. https://data.cdc.gov/NCHS/Provisional-COVID-19-Death-Counts-by-Sex-Age-and-W/vsak-wrfu. Updated March 17, 2021. Accessed March 17, 2021.
3. United States Census Bureau. Age-adjusted COVID-19 associated hospitalization rates by race and ethnicity, COVID-NET, March 1–July 18, 2020. https://www.cdc.gov/coronavirus/2019-ncov/covid-data/covidview/index.html. Accessed July 24, 2020.
4. United States Census Bureau. Population estimates, July 1, 2019. https://www.census.gov/quickfacts/fact/table/US/PST045219. Accessed May 23, 2020.
5. Watson CJ, Billingsley P, Croft DJ, Huntsberger DV. *Brief Business Statistics*. Needham Heights, MA: Allyn and Bacon, Inc.; 1988.
6. Merrill RM. *Fundamentals of Epidemiology and Biostatistics: Combining the Basics*. Burlington, MA: Jones & Bartlett Learning; 2013.
7. Centers for Disease Control and Prevention, National Center for Health Statistics. Compressed Mortality File 1999–2016 on CDC WONDER Online Database, released June 2017. Data are from the Compressed Mortality File 1999–2016 Series 20 No. 2U, 2016, as compiled from data provided by the 57 vital statistics jurisdictions through the Vital Statistics Cooperative Program. http://wonder.cdc.gov/cmf-icd10.html. Accessed August 5, 2020.
8. Coronavirus disease. Daily change. https://www.google.com/search?q=covid+19+cases+arizona&oq=co&aqs=chrome.0.69i59j014.3868j0j9&sourceid=chrome&es_sm=91&ie=UTF-8. Accessed August 5, 2020.

CHAPTER 3

Probability

KEY CONCEPTS

- Probability is useful for evaluating the reliability of conclusions made under conditions of uncertainty.
- Probability sampling allows us to obtain a more representative sample from the population.
- A random experiment is a process that is repeatable under stable conditions, with a set of possible outcomes that cannot be predicted with certainty.
- A trial is any process that can be infinitely repeated with a specific set of possible outcomes.
- A sample space *S* is an exhaustive list of all possible outcomes of an experiment.
- An event is one or more outcomes of an experiment.
- Frequentist probability of an event is a proportion of times the event occurs as the limit of its relative frequency in a large number of independent trials.
- Classical probability measures the likelihood of something happening, with each outcome being equally likely to occur and the outcomes mutually exclusive.
- Subjective probability is a type of probability based on a person's judgment about the likely occurrence of an event.
- Rules are presented that apply to computing probabilities for certain types of events.
- Bayes' theorem reflects the concept of conditional probability—the probability of an event depending on an earlier event.
- Sampling is a process in which a subset of a larger population is selected for statistical analysis.
- A sampling frame is a complete list of people or items in a population from which a sample will be drawn.

Probability is the second general topic in the area of biostatistics. Probability provides a basis for evaluating the reliability of the conclusions we make under conditions of uncertainty. It is the foundation upon which we evaluate estimates and make inferences when applying statistical methods to the collection, analysis, and interpretation of data. In this chapter, we will present probability concepts, classifications, and properties. Probability concepts include random experiments, outcomes, sample space, and events. Probability classifications include frequentist probability, classical probability, and subjective probability. Probability properties include the addition rule, multiplication rule, and modifications to these rules when events are not mutually exclusive or independent. Bayes' theorem will be presented for assessing conditional events. Finally, conventional sampling methods will be discussed.

3.1 Probability Questions in Biostatistics

Research questions addressed using probability may involve the frequentist concept of probability in which the probability of an event is investigated in the context of relative frequency in the sequence of trials in the long run. For example, to answer the question, "What is the probability of death among COVID-19 patients who require mechanical ventilation?" several days of accrued data may be required. Yet not all research questions require repeated experiments over time to establish the probability of an event. With classical probability, every experiment will result in outcomes that are equally likely, and the research question may ask something like, "What is the probability of being randomly selected into a study?" or "What is the probability of being assigned a given level of an intervention?" An answer to a research question that is not based on repeated trials, relative frequencies stabilized over time, or equally likely events is subjective. For example, a person may believe that wearing a cloth mask while in public will reduce the probability of exposure to severe acute respiratory syndrome coronavirus 2 (SARS-CoV-2) to no more than 10%.

A research question may involve the probability of a single event, the event's complement, two or more mutually exclusive events, two or more independent events, or conditional events. Examples of how to address these types of questions using probability will be covered in this chapter. Finally, sampling plays an important role in biostatistics. To obtain a representative sample of a larger population requires probability sampling. Answers to research questions based on probability sampling are more representative of the larger population.

3.2 Probability Concepts

Consider a process that may result in a definite set of possible outcomes. The process is governed by chance, such that we cannot predict the outcome with complete certainty. Further, suppose the process is repeatable under stable conditions, such as, an adverse drug reaction for a group of coronavirus disease 2019 (COVID-19) patients. A repeatable outcome like this is referred to as a random experiment.

A random experiment is any planned process of data collection. A random experiment consists of a number of independent trials under the same conditions, such as treating 10 COVID-19 patients with a new drug and evaluating whether each patient has a favorable response. To qualify as a random experiment, the process must produce observations or measurements. All possible outcomes of an experiment make up the outcome space or, as it has become more commonly called, the sample space.

> A **random experiment** is a process that is repeatable under stable conditions, with a set of possible outcomes that cannot be predicted with certainty.

> A **trial** is any process that can be infinitely repeated with a specific set of possible outcomes.

> A **sample space** S is an exhaustive list of all possible outcomes of an experiment.

For a COVID-19 patient, the sample space consists of the possible outcomes—recovery, disability, or death. Suppose we identified 100 COVID-19 patients in which 80 fully recover, 15 have long-term health consequences, and 5 die from the disease. The sample space here is made up of three possible events.

An **event** is one or more outcomes of an experiment.

There are three different conceptual approaches to study probability: frequentist, classical, and subjective.

3.2.1 Frequentist Probability

The frequentist definition of probability is that if an experiment is repeated n times under the same conditions, and if the event A occurs m times, then as n grows large, the ratio of $\frac{m}{n}$ approaches a fixed limit that is the probability of A. Mathematically we can write this as

$$P(A) = \frac{m}{n}.$$

Frequentist probability of an event is a proportion of times the event occurs as the limit of its relative frequency in a large number of independent trials.

Suppose that for each COVID-19 patient admitted to a given hospital, we keep track of the event of invasive mechanical ventilation use. For each person, we assess the relative frequency with which the event occurs, in the sequence of patients admitted to the hospital over the long run. The relative frequency in the sequence of trials will eventually stabilize, which is the probability of the event. It is likely that the probability of receiving invasive mechanical ventilation is initially higher or lower than what it levels off to be.

Therefore, under the frequentist concept of probability, the probability of an event is defined in the context of relative frequency in the sequence of trials in the long run. In our hospital example, it may have taken several days to have sufficient data points to get a stable estimate of the probability of receiving invasive mechanical ventilation among COVID-19 patients.

3.2.2 Classical Probability

Classical probability is a concept in statistics that measures the likelihood of something happening. It also means that every experiment will result in outcomes that are equally likely to occur. It is not always necessary to repeat an experiment several times and observe the outcomes in order to establish the probability of an event. For example, the probability of being randomly selected from a group of 10 is 0.10; the probability of tossing a fair coin and getting heads is 0.50; or the probability of being randomly assigned to a treatment versus a control group is 0.50.

In addition to each outcome being equally likely to occur, the outcomes are mutually exclusive.

Mutually exclusive events are outcomes that cannot occur at the same time.

Classical probability measures the likelihood of something happening, with each outcome being equally likely to occur and the outcomes being mutually exclusive.

Mathematically, the probability of an event under the classical concept of probability is written the same as under the relative frequency concept of probability, but the meaning of the numerator and denominator in the computation is different. Under classical probability, m is the number of outcomes of an experiment that are favorable to the event, and n is the total number of outcomes of the experiment. A limitation of classical probability is that for some experiments not all events are equally likely and mutually exclusive.

3.2.3 Subjective Probability

A personal conception of probability is subjective. Subjective probability is probability of events based on our own personal judgment or experience. It is not based on mathematical data and contains no formal calculations. Subjective probability is variable among people and is limited by personal bias. Yet subjective probability plays a primary role in how we make choices. For example, currently more scientific research is needed to show the full effectiveness of wearing a cloth face covering in preventing transmission of SARS-CoV-2 when social distancing is not possible. Although wearing a mask is a means of source control and helps prevent respiratory droplets from traveling into the air and onto other people, how effective is it really? How effective we perceive wearing masks to be in controlling the spread of SARS-CoV-2 is likely to influence if we wear a mask.

Subjective probability is a type of probability based on a person's judgment about the likely occurrence of an event.

Therefore, subjective probability is not based on fact but is created according to an individual's judgment or experience of whether an event is likely to occur.

3.3 Properties of Probabilities

Events are denoted by upper case letters A, B, etc., with their probabilities expressed as $P(A)$, $P(B)$, and so on. There are four basic properties of probability. First, the probability of an event is 0 to 1, inclusive. The probability of any event, say $P(A)$, is a marginal probability.

Property 1

For event A,

$$0 \le P(A) \le 1.$$

Second, the sample space S contains all possible outcomes of the experiment; the probabilities of the sample space sum to 1. Therefore, each outcome of an experiment will be in the sample space. For example, the sum of the three racial groups in the United States is 1.

$$P(\text{White}) + P(\text{Black}) + P(\text{Other}) = 0.782 + 0.14 + 0.078 = 1$$

Property 2

$$P(S) = 1$$

Third, the probability of the complement is equal to 1 minus the probability of the event. The complement of event A is what happens if A does not occur. The complement of event A is denoted as $\bar{A}$. For example, as of August 10, 2020, in the United States, 5,220,545 individuals out of 331,214,010 had been diagnosed with COVID-19.[1]

$$P(\text{Case in USA}) = \frac{5{,}220{,}545}{331{,}214{,}010} = 0.0158$$

So 1.6% of the population had been diagnosed with COVID-19. The complement of this event indicates that 98.4% of the population had not been diagnosed with the disease.

$$P(\overline{\text{Case in USA}}) = 1 - 0.0158 = 0.9842$$

Property 3

The probability of the complement of A is

$$P(\bar{A}) = 1 - P(A).$$

Fourth, events are mutually exclusive if they cannot exist concurrently; two events are mutually exclusive if the probability of them both occurring is zero. For example, the probability of a person having blood type B and blood type AB is zero. Therefore, the probability of having one or the other blood type (BT) is the sum of their probabilities;

$$P(\text{BT} = B \text{ or BT} = AB) = P(\text{BT} = B) + P(\text{BT} = AB) = 0.10 + 0.04 = 0.14.$$

Property 4

If event A is mutually exclusive of event B, then

$$P(A \text{ or } B) = P(A) + P(B).$$

Note that the probability that events A and B both occur at the same time is written as $P(A \text{ and } B)$. This is the union of event A with event B and is referred to as a joint probability.

3.4 Calculating Probabilities

In this section, we will present rules that apply to calculating probabilities for certain types of events.

The addition rule for computing probabilities differs according to whether the events are mutually exclusive.

Rule for Addition of Probabilities

$P(A \text{ or } B) = P(A) + P(B)$	Events *A* and *B* are mutually exclusive.
$P(A \text{ or } B) = P(A) + P(B) - P(A \text{ and } B)$	Events *A* and *B* are NOT mutually exclusive.

As of August 10, 2020, for example, 20,147,024 individuals had been diagnosed worldwide with COVID-19 (**Table 3.1**). A diagnosis of COVID-19 in each country is mutually exclusive because if a person is a case in one country they will not be a case in another country. The table shows that among all COVID-19 cases, 25.9% are in the United States, 15.1% are in Brazil, and so on. The table also shows that among all COVID-19 deaths, 22.5% are in the United States, 13.8% are in Brazil, and so on. Of all COVID-19 cases, more than half (i.e., 52.5%) are in the United States, Brazil, and India. Of all COVID-19 deaths, less than half (42.5%) are in the United States, Brazil, and India.

Table 3.1 **Sample Space for 16 Countries Leading the World in COVID-19 Cases and Deaths, as of August 10, 2020**

	Total Cases	Relative Frequency	Cum Relative Frequency	Total Deaths	Relative Frequency	Cum Relative Frequency	Death-to-Case Ratio
World	20,147,024			736,098			
United States	5,220,545	0.259	0.259	165,855	0.225	0.225	0.032
Brazil	3,039,349	0.151	0.410	101,269	0.138	0.363	0.033
India	2,266,954	0.113	0.523	45,352	0.062	0.425	0.020
Russia	892,654	0.044	0.567	15,001	0.020	0.445	0.017
South Africa	559,859	0.028	0.595	10,408	0.014	0.459	0.019
Mexico	480,278	0.024	0.618	52,298	0.071	0.530	0.109
Peru	478,024	0.024	0.642	21,072	0.029	0.559	0.044
Colombia	387,481	0.019	0.661	12,842	0.017	0.576	0.033
Chile	375,044	0.019	0.680	10,139	0.014	0.590	0.027
Spain	361,442	0.018	0.698	28,503	0.039	0.629	0.079
Iran	328,844	0.016	0.714	18,616	0.025	0.654	0.057
United Kingdom	311,641	0.015	0.730	46,526	0.063	0.717	0.149
Saudi Arabia	289,947	0.014	0.744	3199	0.004	0.721	0.011
Pakistan	284,660	0.014	0.758	6097	0.008	0.730	0.021
Bangladesh	260,507	0.013	0.771	3438	0.005	0.734	0.013
Italy	250,825	0.012	0.784	35,209	0.048	0.782	0.140
Other Countries	4,358,970	0.216	1.000	160,274	0.218	1.000	0.037

Reference 1.

The **death-to-case** ratio is the number of deaths attributed to the disease divided by the number of new cases of the disease during the same time period. It ranges from 1.1% in Saudi Arabia to 14.9% in the United Kingdom.

Now refer to the marginal and joint probabilities for race and Hispanic origin in the United States in 2016, shown in **Table 3.2**.[2] The marginal probabilities are represented in the row and column totals. The joint probabilities are the values in the body of the table. For example, 78.2% of the population is white, 82.2% are non-Hispanic, and 62.3% are white, non-Hispanic.

Table 3.2 Sample Space for Race and Hispanic Origin in the United States, 2016

	Hispanic	Not Hispanic	Total
White	0.159	0.623	0.782
Black	0.010	0.130	0.140
Asian or Pacific Islander	0.003	0.061	0.064
American Indian or Alaska Native	0.006	0.008	0.014
Total	0.178	0.822	1.000

Data from Compressed Mortality File 1999–2016. Centers for Disease Control and Prevention. http://wonder.cdc.gov/cmf-icd10.html. Accessed August 10, 2020.

We are often interested in determining the probability of one event conditional on another event. In other words, the probability of an event is based on a reduced sample space. In our notation, the vertical bar | represents conditional.

The **conditional probability** of event B given event A has occurred, denoted as $P(B|A)$, is

$$P(B|A) = \frac{P(A \text{ and } B)}{P(A)} \text{ where } P(A) > 0.$$

For example, suppose we want to know the probability of being classified a certain race among those with Hispanic origin. Applying the conditional formula gives probability of white, black, Asian or Pacific Islander, and American Indian or Alaska Native conditioned on being Hispanic as 0.89, 0.06, 0.02, and 0.03, respectively.

In order to compute joint probabilities, we can rearrange the equation, using the general rule for multiplication of probabilities. If we know two terms, we can solve for the other.

Rule for Multiplication of Probabilities

$$P(A \text{ and } B) = P(A) \times P(B \mid A)$$

It is also true that because $P(A \text{ and } B) = P(B \text{ and } A)$ that $P(A \text{ and } B) = P(B) \times P(A \mid B)$.

Now consider the concept of independent events. If events A and B are independent, then

$$P(A \mid B) = P(A).$$

In other words, B gives no information about the probability of A. For example, the probability of a COVID-19 patient entering the hospital requiring mechanical ventilation should be independent of another COVID-19 patient requiring mechanical ventilation. On the other hand, the probability of a given race is dependent on Hispanic origin. According to the rule for multiplication of independent events shown in the next box, if race and Hispanic origin were independent, then the joint probability would equal the product of the marginal probabilities. This does not hold for any of the race and Hispanic origin combinations (see Table 3.2). For example, the probability of being black and Hispanic origin is 0.010, but the product of the marginal probabilities is $0.140 \times 0.178 = 0.025$.

Rule for Multiplication of Independent Events

If A and B are independent events, then

$$P(A \text{ and } B) = P(A) \times P(B).$$

The distribution of blood types is presented according to Rh disease status in **Table 3.3**.[3] Blood type and Rh status are independent events because the product of each combination of marginal probabilities equals the corresponding joint probability; for example,

$$\begin{aligned} P(\text{Blood Type AB and Rh positive}) &= P(\text{Blood Type AB}) \times P(\text{Rh positive}) \\ &= 0.85 \times 0.04 = 0.034 \end{aligned}$$

Therefore, while some racial groups are more likely to reflect Hispanic origin than others, Rh status is not influenced by blood type.

3.5 Bayes' Theorem

Thomas Bayes (1702–1761) was an English theologian and mathematician. He studied probability and statistical inference and developed the law of inverse probability, called Bayes' theorem. The theorem relates the probability of an

Table 3.3 **Blood Type by Rh Disease Status**

Blood Type	Rh Positive	Rh Negative	Total
O	0.374	0.066	0.44
A	0.357	0.063	0.42
B	0.085	0.015	0.10
AB	0.034	0.006	0.04
Total	0.85	0.15	1.00

Data from Stanford Blood Center. Blood Types: What's Your Type? https://stanfordbloodcenter.org/donate-blood/blood-donation-facts/blood-types/. Accessed July 11, 2020.

event (yes versus no) to the probability of an associated event (yes versus no). In other words, the theorem says that we can find a probability if we know other specific probabilities. Given the properties of probabilities, which we discussed earlier, $P(B \mid A)$ tells us the probability of B given A, when we know $P(A \mid B)$, $P(A)$, and $P(B)$.

Bayes' Theorem 1

$$P(B \mid A) = \frac{P(A \mid B) \times P(B)}{P(A)}$$

$P(B \mid A)$ is called the posterior probability because it is derived from or depends on the specific value of A; $P(A \mid B)$ is the conditional probability of A given B; $P(B)$ is the prior probability (or prevalence) of B. It is called the "prior" because it does not consider any information about A.

Imagine 100 people are shopping at the grocery store and you tally how many are wearing a cloth face mask and how many are male. You get the following hypothetical numbers.

	Mask	No Mask	Total
Male	18	24	42
Female	38	20	58
Total	56	44	100

The probability of being male is $P(\text{Male}) = 42/100 = 0.42$; the probability of wearing a mask is $P(\text{Mask}) = 56/100 = 0.56$; and the probability of wearing a mask if male is $P(\text{Mask} \mid \text{Male}) = 18/42 = 0.429$. Then, applying Bayes' theorem, the probability that a person wearing a mask is male is

$$P(\text{Male} \mid \text{Mask}) = \frac{P(\text{Mask} \mid \text{Male}) \times P(\text{Male})}{P(\text{Mask})} = \frac{0.429 \times 0.42}{0.56} = 0.32.$$

Now, note that $P(A)$ occurs if events B and A both occur or if events $\overline{B}$ and A both occur. Then, according to the properties of probability, $P(A) = P(B \text{ and } A) + P(\overline{B} \text{ and } A) = P(B) \times P(A \mid B) + P(\overline{B}) \times P(A \mid \overline{B})$. Bayes' theorem can also be expressed as follows:

Bayes' Theorem 2

$$P(B \mid A) = \frac{P(A \mid B) \times P(B)}{P(A \mid B) \times P(B) + P(A \mid \overline{B}) \times P(\overline{B})}$$

Now let us apply the mask wearing data to this expanded equation. Two additional probabilities need to be computed: $P(\text{Mask} \mid \overline{\text{Male}}) = 38/58 = 0.655$ and $P(\overline{\text{Male}}) = 58/100 = 0.58$.

$$P(\text{Male} \mid \text{Mask}) = \frac{P(\text{Mask} \mid \text{Male}) \times P(\text{Male})}{P(\text{Mask} \mid \text{Male}) \times P(\text{Male}) + P(\text{Mask} \mid \overline{\text{Male}}) \times P(\overline{\text{Male}})}$$
$$= \frac{0.429 \times 0.42}{0.429 \times 0.42 + 0.655 \times 0.58} = 0.32$$

So why would we use the more complicated formula if both approaches give us the same answer? The answer is in the prior probability. Sometimes it is nice to use our knowledge about the past in our calculation. For example, perhaps long-term data say that for that store, $P(\text{Male}) = 0.35$. Choosing this prior probability for our calculation rather than what we get in our particular sample requires that we use the latter equation. Using this prior probability in the calculation allows us to take advantage of our better knowledge of the prevalence of male shoppers:

$$P(\text{Male} \mid \text{Mask}) = \frac{P(\text{Mask} \mid \text{Male}) \times P(\text{Male})}{P(\text{Mask} \mid \text{Male}) \times P(\text{Male}) + P(\text{Mask} \mid \overline{\text{Male}}) \times P(\overline{\text{Male}})}$$
$$= \frac{0.429 \times 0.35}{0.429 \times 0.35 + 0.655 \times 0.65} = 0.26$$

News File

A letter to the editor published on July 1, 2020, in *American Family Physician* talked about the sensitivity and specificity of SARS-CoV-2 antibody testing as depending on the prevalence of the virus in the population. SARS-CoV-2 antibody testing is important in identifying the extent of the infection. This information is important for determining the pace of relaxing physical distancing measures, and clinicians can use antibody testing to counsel patients about whether they are infectious and their immune status.[4]

Antibody tests provide either a positive or negative test result. The sensitivity of a test is the probability of a positive test given a person has the virus. If a large number of people who have the virus test positive (true positive), the test has high sensitivity. If a large number of people who have the virus test negative (false negative), the test has low sensitivity. The specificity of a test is the probability of a negative test given a person does not have the virus. If a large number of people who do not have the virus test negative (true negative), the test has high specificity. If a large number of people who do not have the virus test positive (false positive), then the test has low specificity. Low sensitivity (high false negative) is problematic because people are falsely reassured and appropriate contact tracing and isolation is hindered. Low specificity (high false positive) is problematic because people who do not have the virus but think they do may make decisions that can hurt their economic situation.

The first antibody test (called Cellex) approved by the U.S. Food and Drug Administration for the virus reports a sensitivity of 94% and a specificity of 96%.[5] The probability that an individual with a positive test has SARS-CoV-2 is 85%, 95%, and 97% if the prevalence of the virus in the population is 1%, 3%, or 5%, respectively.

3.6 Evaluating Screening and Diagnostic Tests

An important application area of Bayes' theorem is in evaluating the validity of screening and diagnostic tests. Bayes' theorem may be used to evaluate the validity of a screening test. The validity of a test is shown by how well the test actually measures what it is supposed to measure. Validity is determined by the sensitivity and specificity of the test. If a person has the disease and tests positive, she is classified as a true positive (*TP*); if a person does not have the disease and tests negative, she is classified as a true negative (*TN*); if a person has the disease and tests negative, she is classified as a false negative (*FN*); and if a person does not have the disease and tests positive, she is classified as a false positive (*FP*). Sensitivity is the proportion of people with the disease who have a positive test. Specificity is the proportion of people without the disease who have a negative test. Disease status by test results is presented in the following table:

	True Disease Status	
Test Result	**Present**	**Not Present**
Positive	TP	FP
Negative	FN	TN

$$\text{Sensitivity} = P(T^+ \mid D) = \frac{\text{TP}}{\text{TP} + \text{FN}}$$

$$\text{Specificity} = P(T^- \mid \bar{D}) \frac{\text{TN}}{\text{FP} + \text{TN}}$$

Now suppose we are interested in knowing the probability that an individual with a positive test (T^+) actually has the disease (D). The equation for the predictive value of a positive test, based on Bayes' theorem, is

$$PV^+ = P(D \mid T^+) = \frac{P(T^+ \mid D) \times P(D)}{P(T^+ \mid D) \times P(D) + P(T^+ \mid \bar{D}) \times P(\bar{D})}$$
$$= \frac{\text{Sensitivity} \times \text{Prior Probability}}{\text{Sensitivity} \times \text{Prior Probability} + (1 - \text{Specificity}) \times (1 - \text{Prior Probability})}.$$

We may also be interested in knowing the probability that an individual with a negative test (T^-) does not have the disease ($\bar{D}$). The equation for the predictive value of a negative test is

$$PV^- = P(\bar{D} \mid T^-) = \frac{P(T^- \mid \bar{D}) \times P(\bar{D})}{P(T^- \mid \bar{D}) \times P(\bar{D}) + P(T^- \mid D) \times P(D)}$$
$$= \frac{\text{Specificity} \times (1 - \text{Prior Probability})}{\text{Specificity} \times (1 - \text{Prior Probability}) + (1 - \text{Sensitivity}) \times \text{Prior Probability}}$$

Suppose we are interested in evaluating the validity of the COVID-19 test for identifying SARS-CoV-2 infection. Consider the following hypothetical data. If we calculate the prior (prevalence) from the data in the table, the simpler equation may be used.

	True Disease Status		
Test Result	**Present**	**Not Present**	**Total**
Positive	80	20	100
Negative	20	1000	1020
Total	100	1020	1120

$$\text{Sensitivity} = \frac{80}{100} = 0.80$$

$$\text{Specificity} = \frac{1000}{1020} = 0.98$$

$$\text{Prior Probability} = \frac{1000}{1020} = 0.089$$

$$P(D \mid T^{+}) = \frac{TP}{(TP + FP)} = \frac{80}{(80 + 20)} = \frac{80}{100} = 0.80$$

$$P(\bar{D} \mid T^{-}) = \frac{TN}{(FN + TN)} = \frac{1000}{(20 + 1000)} = \frac{1000}{1020} = 0.980$$

Therefore, the proportion of tests positive for COVID-19 is 0.80. The proportion of tests negative for COVID-19 is 0.98. You can try the more complicated equation to see if you get the same results. Now suppose a study in a larger sample from the same population gave a prevalence of COVID-19 of 0.05. Applying this to the equations gives

$$P(D \mid T^{+}) = \frac{0.80 \times 0.05}{0.80 \times 0.05 + (1 - 0.98) \times (1 - 0.05)} = 0.68$$

$$P(\bar{D} \mid T^{-}) = \frac{0.98 \times (1 - 0.05)}{0.98 \times (1 - 0.05) + (1 - 0.80) \times 0.05} = 0.99.$$

In a general sense, a valid screening test minimizes the threat of a false positive test, which may cause unnecessary stress, anxiety, and treatment. It also minimizes the threat of a false negative test, which may cause an individual to not take appropriate action. Screening and diagnostic tests are intended to improve the prognosis of an illness.

A **prognosis** is a prediction of the likely course and outcome of a disease. It is generally based on selected prognostic indicators (signs, symptoms, and circumstances). Clinical exams and laboratory testing provide important prognostic information.

3.7 Sampling

Sampling is a process in which a subset of a larger population is selected for statistical analysis. We then infer or generalize from the assessment of our sample to a larger population. Samples are preferred to trying to assess the entire population for a number of reasons (**Table 3.4**).

Table 3.4 **Why We Sample**

1. A sample is often evaluated more quickly than large populations.
2. Samples are less expensive than studying entire populations.
3. Studying the entire population may be impossible.
4. Sample results may be more accurate than results based on populations (given more time and resources can be spent on training the people who observe and collect the data and on procedures that improve accuracy).
5. Samples of the population that reflect specific characteristics rather than the entire population may be more appropriate for studying a certain health outcome.[6]

There are two broad types of sampling: nonprobability and probability. Convenience sampling is an example of nonprobability sampling and consists of subjects that meet the selection criteria and are easily accessible. It is often less expensive and not as logistically challenging. For example, asking individuals at a student union building to answer questions is convenience sampling. Convenience sampling may be a good choice for pilot testing. However, to be valid, it must be representative of the target population, which involves a subjective judgment. Convenience sampling is susceptible to selection bias.

Another type of nonprobability sampling is voluntary sampling. Here interested individuals volunteer to participate in a survey. This type of sampling is also prone to selection bias.

To ensure that the sample represents the population of interest, in that measures characterizing sample data can be generalized to the total population, we use probability sampling. The best way to obtain a sample in which the results produce valid inferences is probability sampling. Probability sampling uses random sampling techniques to obtain a representative sample. There are four types of probability sampling: simple random sampling, systematic sampling, stratified random sampling, and cluster sampling.

Simple random sampling is a random process of selecting elements. The sample is obtained by assigning a number to each subject in the population and then selecting a subset using a random number generator. The sampling frame is the actual set of units from which a sample will be drawn. It is a list that contains every member of the population from which a sample is selected. Each subject has an equal chance of being selected. The process may be considered a random experiment. For example, suppose a local hospital has 200 COVID-19 patients. To take a random sample of COVID-19 patients, say 20, assign each COVID-19 patient a number from 1 to 200 and use a random number generator to select 20 numbers. Excel provides a way to randomly select a subset of numbers from a larger population. To illustrate, if the patients were assigned unique numbers from 1 through 200, then in Excel we can type into a cell =RANDBETWEEN(1,200). This formula returns a random integer in the specified range. Then, copy and paste this function into the next several cells.

It is a good idea to obtain a few more than the desired number, in case there are duplicates.

A **sampling frame** is a complete list of people or items in a population from which a sample will be drawn.

Systematic sampling involves selecting elements from an ordered sampling frame. It is similar to simple random sampling in that there is a random starting point, but every kth member is selected thereafter at regular intervals. To determine k, the number of items in the sampling frame is divided by the desired sample size. For example, in the previous example 200/20 = 10, so every 10th patient is selected. The starting point depends on a randomly selected number from 1 to 10.

Stratified random sampling involves dividing the population into a few heterogeneous subgroups, called strata, and then taking a simple random sample in each stratum. There is homogeneity within subgroups. This type of sampling is also called proportional or quota random sampling. Stratified random sampling guarantees that we represent particular strata in the sample; even small subgroups in the population can be represented. It is also useful if we desire to observe relationships between two or more strata. Greater statistical precision occurs for stratified random sampling compared with simple random sampling because the variability with the strata is lower. The required sample size is also lower. For example, in studying the association between COVID-19 death and diabetes, we could stratify the population according to race and age groups and then sample equal numbers from each stratum.

Cluster sampling divides the entire population into many externally homogeneous strata, with each cluster as a smaller representation of the entire population. Once the clusters are identified, certain clusters are chosen through simple random sampling. Two methods can be used for sampling the elements of a cluster: one stage and two stage. With one-stage sampling, all the elements in the selected clusters are sampled. With two-stage sampling, simple random sampling is used to obtain a subset of the elements in each cluster. It is important to not confuse stratified sampling and cluster sampling. In stratified sampling, the population is divided into a few heterogeneous mutually exclusive groups. In cluster sampling, the clusters are similar, but their internal composition varies. For example, we want to conduct a survey about COVID-19 among hospitals in the United States. The United States has 5627 registered hospitals. The employees at each hospital represent a cluster. Using simple random sampling, we can select 100 hospitals from the 5627. We have saved time and money by using cluster sampling. In addition, a smaller number of hospitals to visit may improve the quality of data collection (e.g., more time and resources are available for providing incentives for people to participate and for training people who observe and collect the data).

In cluster sampling, the cluster is the primary sampling unit, and the units within the cluster are the secondary sampling units. It is important to make this distinction when calculating standard errors. Treating the cluster sample as a simple random sample would cause the estimated standard errors to be biased downward. This is because the units in a cluster are typically more similar than the units in a random sample of the entire population. For a cluster sample to provide the same level of precision as a random sample, the sample size needs to be increased.[7]

3.8 Summary

This chapter focused on probability as an essential tool in statistics. Important probability concepts, classifications, and properties were presented. Probability concepts included random experiments, outcomes, sample space, and events. A random experiment is a process that is repeatable under stable conditions. The set of possible outcomes or the experimental process cannot be predicted with certainty. An exhaustive list of all possible outcomes of the experiment is referred to as the sample space. The specific performance of a random experiment is called a trial. One or more outcomes of an experiment is called an event.

Probability was classified as frequentist, classical, and subjective. Frequentist probability is an interpretation of probability that defines the probability of an event as the proportion of times it occurs as the limit of its relative frequency in a large number of independent trials. Classical probability is a statistical concept that measures the likelihood of something happening. Each outcome is equally likely to happen, and the outcomes are mutually exclusive. Mutually exclusive is a statistical term that describes two or more events that cannot occur simultaneously. Subjective probability involves using one's own experience, judgment, or opinion to find probabilities.

We presented certain properties of probability. These included the addition rule, multiplication rule, and modifications of these rules for nonmutually exclusive events and nonindependent events. The addition rule is used to sum the probabilities of two or more events that are mutually exclusive. For nonmutually exclusive events, we subtract the probability of their joint occurrence from their sum. The multiplication rule involves multiplying the probabilities of two or more independent events. For nonindependent events, they are considered to be conditional. To obtain the probability of conditional events, we can use Bayes' theorem. A useful application of Bayes' theorem is for evaluating screening and diagnostic tests.

Researchers do not generally study populations, but rather they study samples, subsets of the population. Selected reasons were given for why sampling might be preferred, such as quicker evaluation, less expense, greater accuracy, and better focus. Two general types of sampling were presented: nonprobability and probability. Nonprobability sampling may involve convenience sampling and voluntary sampling, both of which are susceptible to selection bias. Probability sampling allows us to obtain a sample that is representative of the population, where the results produce valid inferences. Probability sampling employs random sampling techniques: simple random sampling, systematic sampling, stratified random sampling, and cluster sampling.

A simple random sample is a sample in which each subject in the population has an equal chance of being selected. A systematic sample is a sample in which subjects from the population are selected according to a random starting point and then every fixed, period interval. The interval is determined by dividing the size of the population by the desired size of the sample. A stratified sample is a sample in which a simple random sample is taken from a number of distinct strata of the population. Cluster sampling is used when natural groups exist in the population. The population is divided into clusters, and a simple random selection is taken of each cluster.

Equations for computing probabilities with their definitions, properties, and rules are summarized in **Table 3.5**.

Table 3.5 Summary of Equations for Computing Probabilities

1. Events are written in uppercase Roman letters *A*, *B*, and *C*. *P*(*A*) refers to the probability that event *A* will occur. It is referred to as a marginal probability.
2. Probability that events *A* or *B* occur is written *P*(*A* or *B*) or $P(A \cup B)$.
3. In conditional probability the vertical bar | means given.
4. Probability that events *A* and *B* both occur is written *P*(*A* and *B*) or $P(A \cap B)$, and is referred to as a joint probability.
5. Property 1 says that the probability of event *A* ranges from 0 to 1, inclusive; $0 \le P(A) \le 1$.
6. Property 2 says the sample space *S* contains all possible outcomes of the experiment; $P(S) = 1$.
7. Property 3 say the probability of the complement of *A* is $P(\bar{A}) = 1 - P(A)$.
8. Property 4 says that if events *A* and *B* are mutually exclusive (meaning they cannot both occur at the same time), then $P(A \text{ or } B) = P(A) + P(B)$.
9. If *A* and *B* are mutually exclusive events, then $P(A \text{ and } B) = 0$.
10. The rule for complementary events says that if *A* and $\bar{A}$ are complementary events, then the $P(\bar{A}) = 1 - P(A)$.
11. The rule for the addition of probabilities says that if *A* and *B* are not mutually exclusive, then $P(A \text{ or } B) = P(A) + P(B) - P(A \text{ and } B)$.
12. The conditional probability of *B*, given *A*, is defined as $P(B \mid A) = \dfrac{P(A \text{ and } B)}{P(A)}$, where $P(A) > 0$.
13. The rule for multiplication of probabilities is $P(A \text{ and } B) = P(A) \times P(B \mid A)$. The expression on the left is the joint probability of events *A* and *B*.
14. The rule for multiplication of independent events says if *A* and *B* are independent events (one event does not influence the other), then $P(A \text{ and } B) = P(A) \times P(B)$.
15. Independence of events means $P(B \mid A) = P(B)$, and also $P(A \mid B) = P(A)$.
16. Bayes' theorem is used to compute posterior probabilities from prior and observed probabilities; $P(B \mid A) = \dfrac{P(A \mid B) \times P(B)}{P(A \mid B) \times P(B) + P(A \mid \bar{B}) \times P(\bar{B})}$.

Exercises

1. What is the frequentist definition of probability?
2. What is the classical definition of probability?
3. What is the subjective definition of probability?
4. Classify the following as (A) frequentist probability, (B) classical probability, or (C) subjective probability.

   ___ Each outcome is equally likely to occur, and the outcomes are mutually exclusive.

   ___ It is not necessary to repeat an experiment several times.

   ___ Relative frequency occurs in the sequence of trials in the long run.

   ___ The probability of events is based on personal judgment or experience.

5. Describe the difference between mutually exclusive and independent events.
6. When does the $P(A \text{ or } B) = P(A) + P(B)$?
7. If two events are not mutually exclusive, how would you express $P(A \cup B)$?
8. Suppose that the probability of hypertension if you are obese is 0.15 and the probability of hypertension if you are overweight is 0.10. What is the probability of one or the other of these events occurring?
9. When does the $P(A \text{ and } B) = P(A)P(B)$?
10. Among seniors competing at the World Senior Games, 461 completed a survey investigating the relationship between selected quality of life indicators and a history of voice disorders. Individuals were asked whether they had ever had a voice problem in which their voice did not work, perform, or sound as they felt it normally should, such that it interfered with their ability to communicate. Comment on the dependence or independence of the event being a man and not having a previous voice disorder for these data.

    Here are the data reflecting the history of a voice disorder in a group of elderly adults.[8]

	Previous Voice Disorder		
Classification	**Yes**	**No**	**Total**
Man	30	189	219
Woman	47	195	242
Total	77	384	461

For exercises 11–18 refer to the following table of women in the United States giving birth in 2018 according to age and plurality.[9]

Age	Total	Singleton	Twin	Triplet and Higher
< 15	1736	1715	21	0
15–19	179,871	176,756	3084	31
20–24	726,175	709,046	16,835	294
25–29	1,099,491	1,065,264	33,394	833
30–34	1,090,697	1,050,006	39,441	1250
35–39	566,786	541,686	24,268	832
40–44	117,381	111,902	5269	210
45–54	9575	8276	1224	75
Total	3,791,712	3,664,651	123,536	3525

11. What is the probability that a woman who gave birth in 2018 had one child, twins, triplets, or higher?

12. How does the probability of having twins change with increasing age?
13. Is having triplets or higher independent of age?
14. What percentage of women giving birth at age 30 or older will have a single child? Round your answer to the nearest hundredth.
15. What percentage of women giving birth at age 30 or older will have twins? Round your answer to the nearest hundredth.
16. What percentage of women giving birth at age 30 or older will have triplets or higher? Round your answer to the nearest hundredth.
17. What is the joint probability of being 25–29 and having twins?
18. What is the marginal probability of having twins?
19. Describe Bayes' theorem.

For exercises 20–21 refer to the following table, which reflects physical abuse from parents and a physical exam conducted under the direction of school officials.

Test Result	Abused	Not Abused	Total
Positive for abuse	285	970	1255
Negative for abuse	15	8730	8745
Total	300	9700	10,000

20. Calculate the sensitivity and specificity of the physical exam to detect abuse and interpret your results.
21. Assuming the prior probability of abuse is 3%, what is the predictive value positive and predictive value negative for these data? Interpret your results.
22. List some possible advantages of collecting and studying data from a sample as opposed to a population.
23. Which sampling method involves drawing respondents from a random sample of senior centers?
24. Which sampling method is useful if you want to ensure the presence of a particular subgroup within the sample?
25. Can you think of a situation in which a systematic sample would be inappropriate?
26. Convenience sampling is susceptible to what type of bias?
27. Suppose you have a sampling frame of 500 from which you want to select a random sample of 100. Use Excel to obtain your 100 random numbers.

References

1. Coronavirus. Worldometer. https://www.worldometers.info/coronavirus/?utm_campaign=instagramcoach1? Updated April 26, 2021. Accessed August 10, 2020.
2. Compressed Mortality File 1999–2016. Centers for Disease Control and Prevention. http://wonder.cdc.gov/cmf-icd10.html. Accessed August 10, 2020.
3. Stanford Blood Center. Blood Types: What's Your Type? https://stanfordbloodcenter.org/donate-blood/blood-donation-facts/blood-types/. Accessed July 11, 2020.
4. Ebell MH, Barry HC. Beware of false-positive results with SARS-COV-2 antibody tests. *Am Fam Physician.* 2020;*102*(1):5–6.
5. qSARS-CoV-2 IgG/IgM Rapid Test. Cellex. https://cellexcovid.com/. Accessed April 19, 2020.

6. Dawson B, Trapp RG. *Basic and Clinical Biostatistics*. 4th ed. New York, NY: Lange Medical Books/McGraw-Hill; 2004.
7. Sarndal CE, Swenson B, Wreman JH. *Model Assisted Survey Sampling*. New York, NY: Springer-Verlag; 1992.
8. Merrill RM, Anderson AE, Sloan A. Quality of life indicators according to voice disorders and voice-related conditions. *Laryngoscope*. 2011;*121*:2004–2011.
9. Martin JA, Hamilton BE, Osterman MJK, Driscoll AK. Births: final data for 2018. *National Statistics Reports*. 2019;68(13):Table 25. https://www.cdc.gov/nchs/data/nvsr/nvsr68/nvsr68_13-508.pdf. Accessed July 12, 2020.

CHAPTER 4

Probability and Sampling Distributions

KEY CONCEPTS

- A random variable is a variable whose numerical value is determined by a chance mechanism.
- A discrete random variable can assume only a finite or countable number of values.
- A continuous random variable is able to take on any value in an interval.
- A probability distribution for a random variable describes probabilities that are associated with the values of a discrete or continuous random variable.
- For discrete random variables, the binomial probability distribution is appropriate for determining the probability of *r* successes in a sequence of *n* independent trials, and the Poisson probability distribution is used to determine the probability of rare events.
- A probability distribution for a continuous random variable is specified by a probability density curve (also called a frequency curve), with areas under the probability density curve reflecting probabilities.
- The standard normal probability distribution is symmetric, with a single peak, a mean of 0, a variance of 1, and ranges from negative to positive infinity.
- The standard normal distribution is also called the *Z* distribution.
- The equation for the *Z* statistic assumes that the value of the population standard deviation σ is known.
- When the number of trials *n* is large and *p* (probability of success for each trial) is near 0.5, the binomial distribution is approximately equal to a normal distribution.
- Probability distributions that involve sample statistics are called sampling distributions.
- A sampling distribution is the probability distribution of a statistic for all possible samples of a given size from a population.
- The central limit theorem says the distribution of sample means approximates a normal distribution.
- A related distribution to the standard normal distribution is the *t* distribution, which resembles a normal distribution.
- The variability in the sampling distribution of *t* depends on the sample size *n*.
- Two other continuous probability distributions introduced in this chapter, which will be utilized in this text, are the chi-square and *F* distributions.

Probability is extended in this chapter to probability distributions for random variables. A probability distribution for a random variable describes probabilities as they are associated with the values of a random variable. Two types of random variables will be considered: discrete and continuous. Standard probability distributions will be presented for the discrete and continuous random variables, along with their expected values, variances, and standard deviations.

These distributions are appropriate for answering many important questions in biostatistics.

Probability distributions that involve sample statistics are called sampling distributions. A sample statistic is a random variable because its values change randomly from one random sample to the next. A parameter is not a random variable, but a mathematical constant. Sampling distributions play a primary role in statistical inference.

An important part of biostatistics involves drawing reliable conclusions about the population based on what is discovered in a sample. If the sample is random and sufficiently large, we can expect that any deviation from the truth it is intended to measure is a result of chance. Not all random samples are accurate in their representation of the population. A random sample is random, which means that no random sample will be exactly the same as another. Although we will never know how much what is represented by a random sample differs from the population, probability can be used to evaluate how much we expect random samples to vary. Probability allows us to indicate how likely a sample estimate is no more than a certain amount from the truth. Incorporating probability allows us to say something about the confidence we associate with our inference. For example, to learn and draw conclusions about how the U.S. population feels about wearing protective cloth masks during this time of COVID-19, we take a random sample of 1000 adults. Suppose 80% say they regularly wear a mask while in social gatherings. If we took another sample, it could give a different result. The uncertainty in our estimate is due to chance. We can use probability and estimate the likelihood that our sample will be no more than 5%, for instance, from the true percentage of adults who regularly wear a mask while in social gatherings.

4.1 Probability Distributions for Addressing Questions in Biostatistics

Some research questions in biostatistics can be answered when the probability distribution for the random variable is known. For example, by knowing the probability of occurrence for each level of a random variable, we can answer questions about the expected value and variance of the random variable. If the random variable has a binomial distribution, we can answer questions like, "What is the probability of no more than 2 deaths from COVID-19 out of 20 patients on mechanical ventilation?" or "What is the probability of no more than 5 hospitalized COVID-19 patients requiring mechanical ventilation out of 30 hospitalized patients?" If a Poisson probability distribution exists for a random variable, then we can answer research questions like, "What is the number of arrivals at a testing center for SARS-CoV-2 during a 30-minute period?" or "What is the rate of COVID-19 in California during July?" or "What is the number of false positive tests for SARS-CoV-2 out of 1000 performed?" or "What is the number of COVID-19 cases in a given city block in New York City?" Both the binomial and the Poisson distributions are discrete.

Certain research questions involve continuous random variables. If the random variable has a normal distribution, then we can answer a research question like, "What is the probability that body mass index for COVID-19 patients is at least 30?" If the research question being asked involves the binomial distribution, and if n is large, we can assess it more easily using the standard normal distribution. A question in this context may be, "Among 100 people treated for

COVID-19 using mechanical ventilation, what is the probability that the number who will die is between 20 and 30?" The standard normal distribution is also an effective way to evaluate questions involving the fraction of success, such as, "What is the probability of 10% or more SARS-CoV-2 antibody tests being false positives?"

In order to answer a question about a sample statistic like the mean value of a continuous random variable, if the population distribution is normal we can use the **t statistic**. If the distribution is not normal, we can still use the t statistic if the sample size is sufficiently large. For almost any non-normal population distribution, a sample size of at least 30 is enough to obtain an approximately normal distribution of sample means, such that the t distribution can be used to answer the question. A possible research question that can be addressed using the t distribution is, "What is the probability the mean age of people dying from COVID-19 is at least 65 years of age?"

Some research questions involve proportions, in which the chi-square distribution can be applied to assess the question. For example, "Is the proportion of COVID-19 cases who require hospitalization greater for those with a comorbid condition?"

A research question may ask whether two estimates of the variance are equal. The probability distribution used to test the equality of two estimates of the variance is the ***F* distribution**. For example, a research question may be, "Is the variance of body mass index for one population equal to that of another population?" or "Is the variance between groups greater than the variance within groups?"

4.2 Random Variables

In the first chapter of this text, data were described as the individual observations made on variables. In that sense, a variable is something that yields a data item, containing what is being studied in a sample or population.

The numerical values of a random variable are obtained through a process in which the possible outcomes are characterized by numbers. For example, we can count the number requiring intensive care among the number of patients admitted to a hospital with complications related to COVID-19 during a given time period.

A **random variable** is a variable whose numerical value is determined by a chance mechanism, a numerical result from a random experiment. Random variables are generally denoted by X, Y, and Z.

If X is the outcome of a COVID-19 patient in terms of requiring intensive care, two outcomes are possible per patient: 1 (yes) or 0 (no). The numerical value of X is determined by chance. Once the experiment is completed, the random variable becomes a given number.

In the previous chapter, we talked about a random sample taken from a population. Each member in a population is chosen randomly, having an equal chance of being selected. In addition, each subset of members from the population has the same chance of selection as any other subset of members of the same size. This process of random sampling is called a simple random sample. Many of the random variables we work with arise from random samples.

We classify random variables according to the values they can take: discrete and continuous. A discrete random variable can only take a countable number of values, such as the number of patients having a negative reaction to a drug during the course of a study or the number of patients with COVID-19 being admitted to the hospital on a given day.

A **discrete random variable** can assume only a finite or countable number of values.

A continuous random variable can take on any positive value, such as height, weight, temperature, and time. However, in practice we are sometimes limited in the level of precision of the measure, like a person's weight, which is rounded to the nearest pound.

A **continuous random variable** is able to take on any value in an interval.

4.3 Probability Distributions for Discrete Random Variables

A discrete random variable is described as the probability associated with each of its mutually exclusive, discrete values obtained from an experiment. We often present probability distributions for discrete random variables using tables or graphs. For example, suppose X assumes the values 1, 2, 3, 4, and 5 and has the following distribution, as expressed in the following table.

X	1	2	3	4	5
$P(X = x)$	0.1	0.2	0.3	0.25	0.15

The distribution might be the number of deaths among hospitalized COVID-19 patients during a given time period. The same distribution presented graphically is as follows:

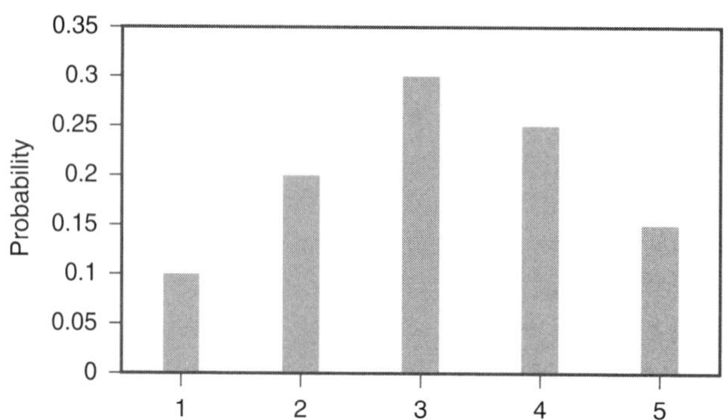

A **probability distribution for a discrete random variable** is a collection of probabilities along with their associated values that the distribution can take.

The expected value of a discrete random variable is denoted by $E(X)$. The word "expected" means "on average." The expected value of X is also called the mean of X or μ (Greek mu). As seen here, the expected value of X is the weighted mean of the possible values of X, where the weights are the probabilities of these values. The equation for the expected value of X is

$$E(X) = \mu = \sum rP(X = r).$$

Extending the previous example gives the expected number of deaths as

$$E(X) = \mu = 1 \times 0.1 + 2 \times 0.2 + 3 \times 0.3 + 4 \times 0.25 + 5 \times 0.15 = 3.15.$$

The equation of the variance of a discrete random variable is

$$\text{Variance}(X) = E(X - \mu)^2 = \sum (r - \mu)^2 P(X = r).$$

Note that if X is a random variable, then a function of X is also a random variable. $E(X - \mu)^2$ measures the extent to which the distribution varies about the mean μ. Since the value of the distance from X to μ is squared, *Variance*(X) is always greater than or equal to 0. Only if the value of X equals μ every time will the variance equal 0.

The standard deviation is simply the square root of the variance. The equation for the standard deviation of a discrete random variable is

$$\begin{aligned}\text{Standard Deviation}(X) &= \sqrt{\text{Variance}(X)} = \sqrt{E(X - \mu)^2} \\ &= \sqrt{\sum (r - \mu)^2 P(X = r)}.\end{aligned}$$

For the distribution of data just presented, with a mean of 3.15, the variance of the discrete random variable X is as follows:

$$\begin{aligned}\text{Variance}(X) = {} & (1 - 3.15)^2 \times 0.1 + (2 - 3.15)^2 \times 0.2 + (3 - 3.15)^2 \\ & \times 0.3 + (4 - 3.15)^2 \times 0.25 + (5 - 3.15)^2 \times 0.15 = 1.43\end{aligned}$$

The standard deviation is

$$\text{Standard Deviation}(X) = \sqrt{1.43} = 1.19.$$

Sometimes the mean, variance, and standard deviation of the random variable X is denoted as μ_X, σ_X^2, and σ_X respectively.

As you can see, these measures for the random variable X are related to the measures for a numerical data set presented in Chapter 2. A random variable is a numerical measure that results from each random experiment, and a series of observations will yield a numerical data set. The mean, variance, and standard deviation for the random variable X are the same as the mean, variance, and standard deviation that would be obtained for the numerical data set if the experiment theoretically consisted of infinitely many observations.[1]

Sometimes our research questions can be addressed by applying a specific probability formula to generate our probability distribution of interest. The formulas for two commonly used discrete probability distributions will be presented. The conditions in which these formulas may be used will be discussed, and probability tables will be presented. Use of the tables can be helpful in saving us some computational work.

4.3.1 Binomial Probability Distributions

The binomial probability distribution is the probability that an outcome will take on one of two values ("success" or "failure") in an experiment that is repeated multiple times. This distribution can be used to answer questions such as:

1. The next 10 customers coming into the grocery store are observed. What is the probability that all 10 will wear a protective face mask given that from experience only 0.5 wear a mask?
2. While checking out at the grocery store, customers are to stand approximately six feet apart, on identified marks on the floor, waiting for the customer in front of them to proceed before advancing themselves. It has been observed that the probability of observing this rule is approximately 0.75. What is the probability that at least 8 of the next 10 customers will adhere to the spacing rule?
3. Aisles at the grocery store are marked as one-way. It is thought that the probability of adhering to this rule is 0.5. What is the probability that out of the next 10 customers going down an isle, at least 2 will go the wrong way?

Trials of an experiment that meet the conditions of a binomial are called Bernoulli trials, named after Jacob Bernoulli, a mathematician who lived from 1654 to 1705. These conditions are:

1. There are a fixed number of trials, n, of an experiment with only two possible mutually exclusive outcomes for each trial: "success" or "failure."
2. The probability of a success for any given trial, designated as p, remains constant from trial to trial. Therefore, the probability of failure is $1 - p$.
3. Each trial is independent of the others.

To illustrate the binomial distribution formula, let p = probability of a success for a single trial; $1 - p$ = the probability of a failure for a single trial; n = number of trials, and X = number of successes. We are interested in finding the probability that a random variable for a number of successes, X, takes on a value r; the probability of a success occurring exactly r times in n trials at chance p. The equation for the binomial probability of r successes given n trials, where the chance of success for each trial is p, is as follows:

$$P(X = r \mid n, p) = \binom{n}{r} p^r (1-p)^{n-r} \qquad r = 0, 1, 2, \ldots, n$$

The number of different sequences that contain r success and $n - r$ failures (i.e., combinations of n things taken r at a time) is denoted by

$$\binom{n}{r} = \frac{n!}{r!(n-r)!}$$

The factorial is symbolized by an exclamation mark (!) and represents the product of all positive integers less than or equal to n.

$$n! = n(n-1)(n-2)\ldots(2)(1)$$

The value of $0! = 1$.

The mean, variance, and standard deviation of a binomial-distributed random variable are as follows:

$$E(X) = np$$
$$\text{Variance}(X) = np(1-p)$$
$$\text{Standard Deviation}(X) = \sqrt{np(1-p)}$$

Now we will apply the binomial formula to our three questions.

- The next 10 customers coming into the grocery store are observed. What is the probability that all 10 will wear a protective face mask given that from experience, only 0.5 wear a mask?

$$P(X = 10 \mid 10, 0.5) = \binom{10}{10} 0.5^{10}(1-0.5)^{10-10} = 0.0010$$

Using Excel, we can obtain an answer to $P(X = r \mid n, p)$ by using the formula BINOMDIST(number, trials, probability, cumulative). For example, in the spreadsheet type =BINOMDIST(10,10,0.5,FALSE). This answer can also be obtained from the Binomial probability table in Appendix B, Table 1.

If we were interested in the probability of 5 successes in 10 trials with $p = 0.25$, we can calculate the answer from the table by subtracting 0.9219 from 0.9803, which equals 0.0584. If we were interested in the probability of no more than 3 successes in 10 trials with $P = 0.4$, the answer is shown in the table as 0.3823.

$$E(X) = np = 10 \times 0.5 = 5$$
$$\text{Variance}(X) = np(1-p) = 10 \times 0.5(1-0.5) = 2.5$$
$$\text{Standard Deviation}(X) = \sqrt{np(1-p)} = \sqrt{10 \times 0.5(1-0.5)} = \sqrt{2.5} = 1.58$$

- While checking out at the grocery store, customers are to stand approximately six feet apart, on identified marks on the floor, waiting for the customer in front of them to proceed before proceeding themselves. It has been observed that the probability of observing this rule is approximately 0.75. What is the probability that at least 8 of the next 10 customers will adhere to the spacing rule?

$$P(X \geq 8 \mid 10, 0.75) = \binom{10}{8} 0.75^{8}(1-0.75)^{10-8} + \binom{10}{9} 0.75^{9}(1-0.75)^{10-9} + \binom{10}{10} 0.75^{10}(1-0.75)^{10-10}$$
$$= 0.2816 + 0.1877 + 0.0563 = 0.5256$$

$$E(X) = np = 10 \times 0.75 = 7.5$$
$$\text{Variance}(X) = np(1-p) = 10 \times 0.75(1-0.75) = 1.875$$
$$\text{Standard Deviation}(X) = \sqrt{np(1-p)} = \sqrt{10 \times 0.75(1-0.75)} = \sqrt{1.875} = 1.37$$

- Aisles at the grocery store are marked as one-way. It is thought that the probability of adhering to this rule is 0.5. What is the probability that for the next 10 customers going down an aisle, at least 2 will go the wrong way?

$$P(X \geq 2 \mid 10,0.5) = 1 - \left[\binom{10}{0} 0.5^0 (1-0.5)^{10-0} + \binom{10}{1} 0.5^1 (1-0.5)^{10-1}\right]$$
$$= 1 - [0.00098 + 0.00977] = 0.9893$$

Using Excel, we can obtain this answer by using the formula = 1-BINOMDIST (1,10,0.5,TRUE).

4.3.2 Poisson Probability Distributions

The Poisson probability distribution is very useful when determining the probability of rare events over a continuum, such as the occurrence of selected exposures or diseases in a specific time frame. It can be used to model things like the emission of radioactive particles from a specified source, the number of arrivals at an emergency room during a specific period, the number of cells in a given volume of fluid, or the number of bacterial colonies growing in a certain amount of medium.

Each of these questions satisfy the conditions that must be met to use the Poisson probability equation. The Poisson probability distribution is named after the man who developed it, Simeon Poisson (1781–1840). The Poisson probability distribution has the following conditions:

1. The experiment consists of a countable number of events occurring during a given time interval, area, or volume.
2. The rate that an event occurs remains constant.
3. Events occur independently.
4. The probability that an event occurs is proportional to the length of the time interval, area, or volume.

The equation for the probability is

$$P(X = r \mid \lambda) = \frac{e^{-\lambda} \lambda^r}{r!} \qquad r = 0, 1, 2, \ldots$$

where λ is the mean number of Poisson-distributed events over the sampling medium under examination (λ is also the variance) and e is a mathematical constant equal to 2.71828.

The Poisson distribution is bounded at 0, with its basic shape changing, becoming less skewed as the mean increases. When the number of trials n is large and the chance of success p for each trial is small, then the binomial probability is approximately equal to the Poisson probability. More specifically, if $n > 20$ and $np < 5$ or $n(1 - p) < 5$, then the Poisson is a good approximation. Under these conditions, $\lambda = np$, the mean for the binomial distribution.

For example, suppose the positive test rate for COVID-19 is 4.8%. The expected number of COVID-19 cases for 100 people tested is $\lambda = np = 100 \times 0.048 = 4.8$. What is the probability that 0, 1, 2, 3, or 4 people will test positive?

$$P(X = 0 \mid \lambda = 4.8) = \frac{(2.718)^{-4.8} 4.8^0}{0!} = 0.0082$$

$$P(X=1 \mid \lambda=4.8)=\frac{(2.718)^{-4.8}4.8^{1}}{1!}=0.0395$$

$$P(X=2 \mid \lambda=4.8)=\frac{(2.718)^{-4.8}4.8^{2}}{2!}=0.0948$$

$$P(X=3 \mid \lambda=4.8)=\frac{(2.718)^{-4.8}4.8^{3}}{3!}=0.1517$$

$$P(X=4 \mid \lambda=4.8)=\frac{(2.718)^{-4.8}4.8^{4}}{4!}=0.1820$$

Using Excel, the $P(X=r \mid \lambda=4.8)$ can be obtained by using the formula POISSON(r, mean, cumulative). For example, $P(X=4 \mid \lambda=4.8)$ can be obtained as follows: =POISSON(4,4.8,FALSE)

The probability that fewer than 5 people will test positive is

$$P(X \le 4 \mid \lambda=4.8)=0.0082+0.0395+0.0948+0.1517+0.1820=0.4763$$

To obtain $P(X \le 4 \mid \lambda=4.8)$ we use the Excel formula =POISSON(4,4.8, TRUE).

These answers can also be found in the Poisson probability table in Appendix B, Table 2. The table gives cumulative values, so $P(X \le 4 \mid \lambda=4.8)$ can be seen directly on the table. To get $P(X=4 \mid \lambda=4.8)$ subtract 0.2942 from 0.4763, which equals 0.1821.

News File

Opioids are a widely used class of drugs that help reduce pain. Endorphins block pain through a natural process by binding to opioid receptors in parts of the nervous system. Endorphins also prompt the release of dopamine, which causes feelings of pleasure and well-being. Opioid drugs mimic endorphins but have a much stronger signal for blocking pain and prompting a greater release of dopamine. With an altered dopamine response from repeated opioid abuse, the brain begins to crave greater feelings of pleasure and well-being.[2]

Opioid receptors also regulate breathing. Although appropriate doses of opioid drugs slow breathing and help a person relax, too much of the drug can stop breathing altogether and cause death.[2]

In 2018, the United States had 67,367 drug overdose deaths. Opioids were involved in the majority of these deaths (46,802 or 69.5% of all overdose deaths).[3] Only 32% of the opioid deaths involved opioids that had been prescribed.[4] The probability distribution of opioid deaths according to prescription status and age group are presented in **Table 4.1**.

The highest proportion of deaths occur in ages 25 through 54. Nonprescription opioid deaths are most common in the 25–34 age group, and prescription opioid deaths are most common in the 45–54 age group.

The rate (per 100,000) of all opioid deaths is 20.1 for males and 9.0 for females. The rate ratio says opioid death is 2.23 times greater in males than females (2.64 for nonprescription and 1.43 for prescription opioid deaths).[3]

A primary concern is whether the coronavirus pandemic may increase opioid abuse, as a larger proportion of the population is struggling with isolation, job loss, and economic concerns. A recent report confirms this to be the case. In a January–April 2019 and 2020 comparison, the number of opioid-related fatal overdoses increased 11.4%, and the number of nonfatal overdoses increased 18.6%.[5]

Table 4.1 Probability Distribution of Opioid Deaths by Prescription Status and Age

x	0–14	15–24	25–34	35–44	45–54	55–64	≥65
P(Opioid Death = x)	0.001	0.077	0.274	0.244	0.204	0.156	0.043
P(No Presc Opioid Death = x)	0.001	0.089	0.313	0.253	0.191	0.125	0.027
P(Prescription Opioid Death = x)	0.002	0.053	0.191	0.224	0.233	0.220	0.077

4.4 Probability Distributions for Continuous Random Variables

For discrete random variables, probabilities are available for their various possible values. For continuous random variables, infinitely many values are possible, such that we cannot list all of those values in a table as we have with probability distributions for discrete random variables. For example, if we found that a person had a body mass index (BMI) of 25, on a finer scale, we might find the BMI was not 25, but 25 and infinitely many places after the decimal. In the extreme, it would be impossible to find a BMI of exactly 25; $P(X = 25) = 0$. In practice, the distribution of a continuous random variable X is represented by a continuous curve called a frequency curve or a probability density curve. The area under the curve between two values on the horizontal axis is the probability of the random variable being between those two limits. The relative probability (i.e., the relevant area under the curve) is determined by integral calculus.

A **probability distribution for a continuous random variable** is specified by a probability density curve (also called a frequency curve). Areas under the probability density curve are probabilities.

Consider the theoretical probability distribution for the continuous random variable BMI (**Figure 4.1**). The curve lies above the horizontal axis, and the area under the curve equals 1. The probability that BMI will assume a value in a given interval equals the area under the curve and over the interval. Because the probability of an individual point is 0, $P(29 < X < 33) = P(29 \leq X \leq 33)$. This condition does not exist for discrete probability distributions.

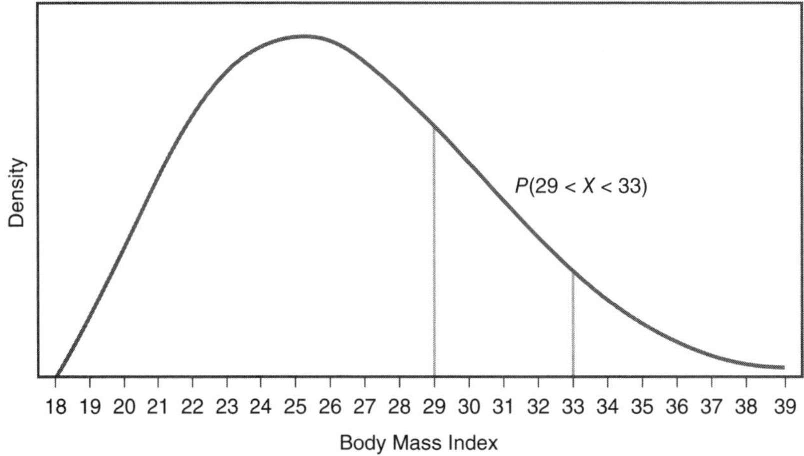

Figure 4.1 Theoretical Distribution of Body Mass Index

4.4.1 Normal Probability Distribution

The probability that a continuous measure, such as BMI, lies within a particular interval can be determined using the normal distribution. Probabilities for variables that are normally distributed can be found by converting to the standard normal distribution. Before we talk about the standard normal distribution, consider that normal distributions in general are symmetric, bell-shaped curves, with 50% of the scores above and 50% below the midpoint of the distribution. The curve of a normal distribution is asymptotic to the *x*-axis, and the mean, median, and mode are located at the midpoint of the *x*-axis.

The equation for the normal distribution is shown as follows:

$$\frac{1}{\sqrt{2\pi\sigma^2}}\exp\left[-\frac{1}{2}\left(\frac{x-\mu}{\sigma}\right)^2\right]$$

In the equation, π is a mathematical constant, 3.14159. The values of μ and σ are parameter values. There is a normal distribution for each pair of mean μ and standard deviation σ. For example, normal curves with the same mean μ but different variances may look like those in **Figure 4.2**. Normal curves with different means but the same variance may look like those in **Figure 4.3**. There are many continuous random variables in epidemiology and clinical medicine with distributions in which the normal distribution is a good approximation. For example, biometric measures such as blood pressure, cholesterol, and blood sugar tend to be normally distributed.

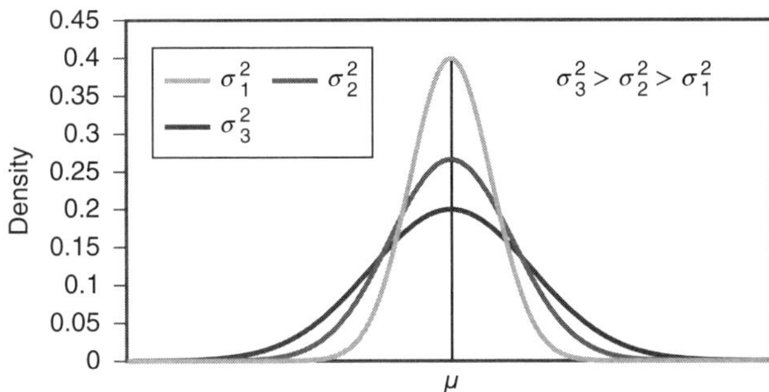

Figure 4.2 Normal Distribution: Same Means and Different Variances

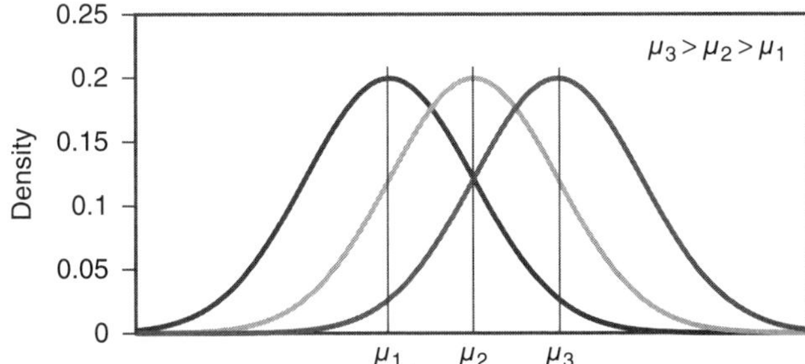

Figure 4.3 Normal Distributions: Same Variance and Different Means

The normal distribution is also sometimes called the Gaussian distribution.

To determine the probability that the BMI for a certain population lies between 29 and 33, we can integrate the normal distribution equation over this range. Yet, there is a simpler way. Rather than applying integral calculus to answer questions about probabilities for each specific variable, we can find probabilities for normally distributed variables by converting to the standard normal distribution. Of course, it would be impossible to construct a table for each possible pair of μ and σ. We can use the standard normal table to estimate probabilities by transforming any normally distributed variable.

The standard normal distribution is symmetric, has a single peak, has a mean of 0 and variance of 1, and ranges from $-\infty$ to $+\infty$.

By convention, Z is called the standard normal variable. The z transformation allows us to use the standard normal table (see Appendix B Table 3), which is a table of areas computed for the standard normal curve to estimate probabilities that correspond with X. If X is a random variable with a mean of μ and a variance of σ^2, then the standard normal variable has a mean of 0 and a variance of 1.

Standardized Variable

$$z = \frac{x - \mu}{\sigma}$$

The total area under the standard normal curve is equal to 1, as shown in the following figure.

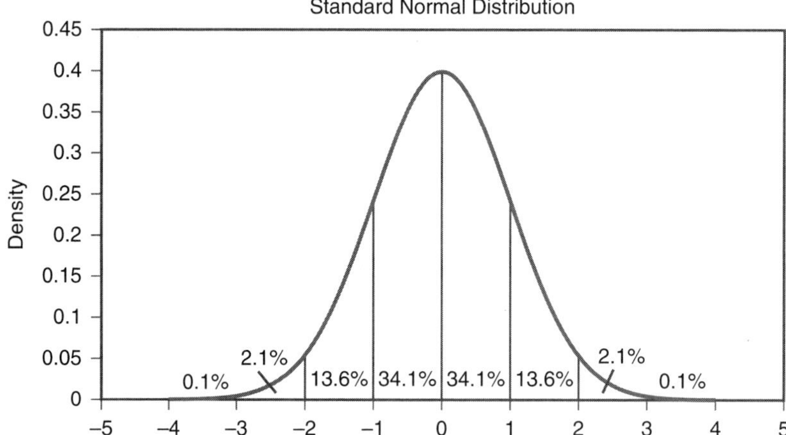

An outcome of the random variable Z is denoted as z, which is called a z-score.

To answer questions about probability for continuous random variables, we are interested in determining the area under the curve, not the height of the curve. For example, assume that the BMI in a healthy population is normally distributed with $\mu = 25$ and $\sigma^2 = 9$ kg/m². What is the area under the curve above 29?

$$P(X > 29) = P\left(Z > \frac{29 - 25}{3}\right) = P(Z > 1.33) = 0.0912$$

This answer can be obtained from Appendix B, Table 3. We can also use Excel with the formula NORMDIST(X,mean,standard deviation,cumulative).

For this problem, enter the formula =1–NORMDIST(29,25,3,TRUE) into the spreadsheet.

What is the area under the curve above 33?

$$P(X > 33) = P\left(Z > \frac{33-25}{3}\right) = P(Z > 2.67) = 0.0038$$

Use the Excel formula =1–NORMDIST(33,25,3,TRUE) to obtain the answer.

What is the area under the curve between 29 and 33?

$$P(33 > X > 29) = P\left(\frac{33-25}{3} > Z > \frac{29-25}{3}\right) = P(2.67 > Z > 1.33) = 0.088$$

Use the Excel formula =NORMDIST(33,25,3,TRUE)–NORMDIST(29,25,3,TRUE) to obtain the answer.

4.4.2 Normal Approximation to the Binomial

As discussed earlier, the equation for the binomial probability distribution is a way to compute the binomial probability of r successes in n trials, with p representing the probability of a success for each trial. However, the binomial equation is cumbersome to compute when n is large. Before modern statistical software, calculations were done manually. Hence, a normal approximation to the binomial was used with a continuity correction.

Briefly, when the number of trials n is large and p is near 0.5, the binomial distribution is approximately equal (denoted by the symbol $\approx$) to a normal distribution. However, if n is very large and the probability of success is close to 0 or 1, the binomial distribution still approximates the normal distribution. We may then ask how large n needs to be and how far can p depart from 0.5 before the normal approximation fails to approximate binomial probabilities. It is appropriate to use the normal approximation to the binomial when $np > 5$ and $n(1 - p) > 5$.

Since the **Z distribution** is continuous and the binomial distribution is discrete, a small correction to the test statistic creates a more accurate approximation. This is called the continuity correction and involves adding or subtracting $\frac{1}{2}$ to a discrete X value. To make this clearer, consider the case where $X = 10$ and then we add or subtract $\frac{1}{2}$, as shown in the following table:

Discrete	Continuous
$X = 20$	$19.5 < X < 20.5$
$X > 20$	$X > 20.5$
$X \leq 20$	$X < 20.5$
$X < 20$	$X < 19.5$
$X \geq 20$	$X > 19.5$

Suppose that the positive test rate for SARS-CoV-2 is 17%. We want to know the probability that for 100 tests performed at a certain location, at least

20 cases are identified. To approximate the binomial distribution by a continuity correction to the normal distribution, the following steps are taken:

Step 1. Verify that $np > 5$ and $n(1-p) > 5$.

$np = 100 \times 0.17 = 17$ and $n(1-p) = 100(1-0.17) = 83$, so we can proceed.

Step 2. Determine whether to add or subtract $\frac{1}{2}$.

We are working with the probability, $P(X \geq 20)$. To use the normal approximation to the binomial, we would instead find $P(X \geq 19.5)$.

Step 3. Find the mean and standard deviation of the binomial distribution:

$$\mu = np = 100 \times 0.17 = 17$$
$$\sigma = \sqrt{np(1-p)} = \sqrt{100 \times 0.17(1-0.17)} = 3.76$$

Step 4. Find the z-score:

$$z = \frac{19.5 - 17}{3.76} = 0.67$$

Step 5. Find the probability associated with the z-score.

From the Z table, the area under the curve up to $z = 0.67$ is 0.7486. Then, the area under the curve above this value is $1 - 0.7486 = 0.2514$.

The exact probability found using the binomial distribution is 0.2477. This value was obtained in Excel using the formula =1-BINOMDIST(19,100, 0.17,TRUE).

4.5 Sampling Distribution

To complete the topic of probability, we will address an important concept in statistics called sampling distributions. Probability distributions for sample statistics are called sampling distributions. The **central limit theorem** will also be presented in this section.

As seen, the binomial, Poisson, and normal distributions can be used to determine the likelihood that a specific measurement is in the population. The sampling distribution is a theoretical distribution of all possible values of a statistic taken from all possible samples of a given size from a population. This distribution is distinct from the distribution of individual observations.

> A **sampling distribution** is the probability distribution of a given statistic based on a random sample of size n, the distribution of the statistic for all possible samples of a given size.

Four features characterize the sampling distribution: (1) the statistic of interest (e.g., mean, standard deviation, or proportion), (2) random selection of the sample, (3) size of the random sample, and (4) specification of the population being sampled. The sampling distribution of the mean plays a very important role in statistics and will be used as the statistic of interest in our discussion.

4.5.1 Sampling Distribution of the Mean

Let $\bar{x}$ be the sample mean for an independent sample of size n. As previously seen, the population mean and variance are μ and σ^2. In addition,

$$E(\overline{x}) = \mu,$$
$$\text{Variance}(\overline{x}) = \sigma^2/n.$$

The sampling distribution of the sample mean is normally distributed if the population distribution is normal; that is, if the parent population is normal, then $\overline{x}$ is normally distributed with mean μ and variance σ^2/n. The variances of sampling distributions are smaller than the variance of the population distribution and decreases as the sample size increases. For example, the normal probability distribution where the mean is 30 and the standard deviation is 10 is shown in **Figure 4.4**.

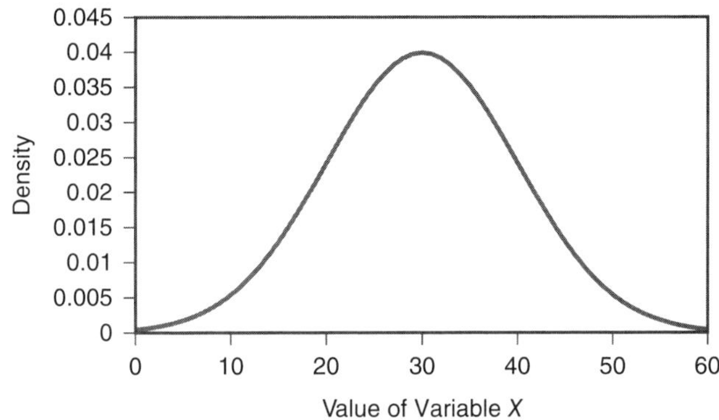

Figure 4.4 An Example of a Normal Probability Distribution

If a sample was taken from this population and the mean calculated, and the process repeated many times, the distribution of means would look something like the following for sample sizes of 10 and 20, respectively.

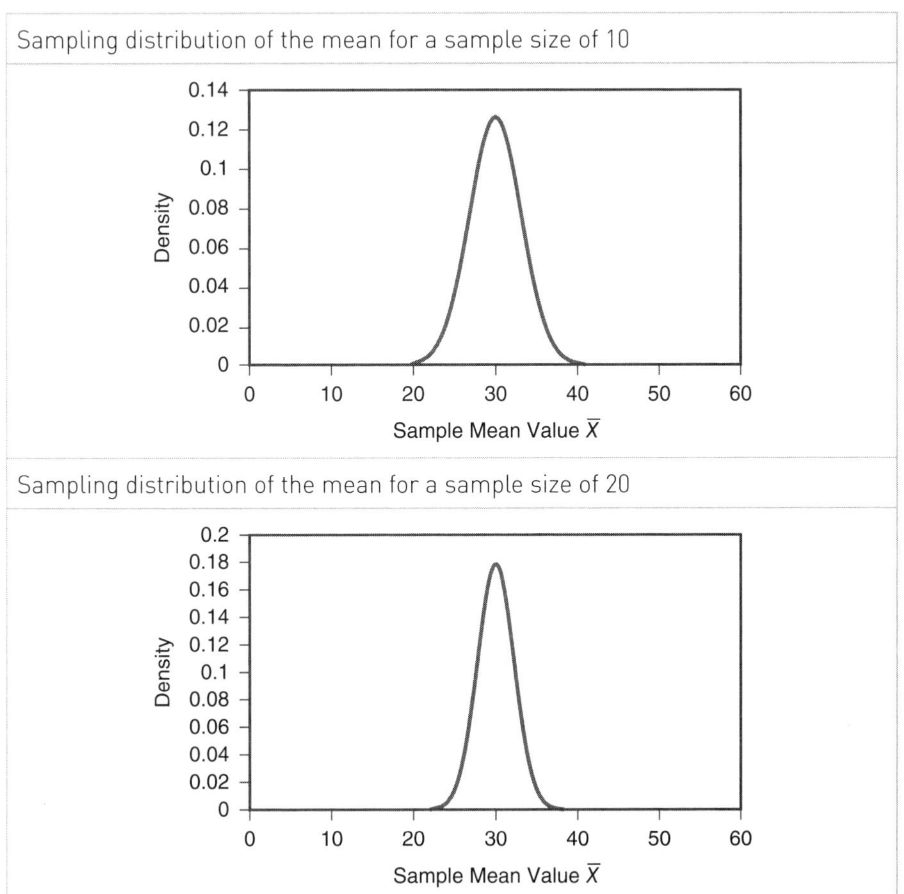

Sample Means from Normal Populations

If the population for X is normally distributed with mean μ and variance σ^2, the sample mean $\bar{x}$ is normally distributed with mean μ and variance σ^2/n.

The following equation is used to standardize a sample mean $\bar{x}$ for a sampling distribution.

Equation for the Standardized Sample Mean

Since $\bar{x}$ has mean μ and standard deviation $\sigma/\sqrt{n}$, the standardized sample mean is

$$z = \frac{\bar{x} - \mu}{\sigma/\sqrt{n}}.$$

The mean of the standardized sample mean is 0, and the variance is 1. If the population is normal, then z is a standard normal variable. In this case, we may use the standard normal distribution table to calculate probabilities for the sample mean (Appendix B, Table 3).

In Excel, we can use the formula NORMDIST(r,mean,standard error, cumulative).

It would be very tedious to take many samples in order to estimate the variability of the mean. Luckily, in reality, we only take one sample. Therefore, among the several desirable characteristics of the sampling distribution is that it allows us to answer questions about the mean based on only one sample.

For example, in the United States in 2017, the percentage of adults in the 50 states and the District of Columbia who participated in enough aerobic and muscle strengthening exercises to meet guidelines was normally distributed around a mean of $\mu = 20.26$. The standard deviation around the mean was $\sigma = 2.46$.[6] A random sample of $n = 10$ was taken, and the mean for this sample was $\bar{x} = 21.17$. What is the probability of getting a sample mean that is as high or higher if the true mean is $\mu = 20.26$?

$$P(\bar{X} \geq 21.17) = P\left(Z \geq \frac{21.17 - 20.26}{2.46/\sqrt{10}}\right) = P(Z \geq 1.17) = 0.121$$

This probability can be obtained from Appendix B, Table 3, or the Excel formulas NORMDIST(x-bar,mean,standard error,cumulative) or NORM.S.DIST (z,cumulative). Specifically,

=1–NORMDIST(21.17,20.26,0.77792,TRUE)
= 0.121.

4.5.2 The Central Limit Theorem

In probability theory, the central limit theorem says the distribution of sample means approximates a normal distribution. The approximation improves as the sample size increases, assuming all samples are of the same size and regardless of the shape of the population distribution. A mathematical proof of the central limit theorem will not be presented here, but some empirical arguments will be given. For a population with mean μ and standard deviation σ, the sampling distribution of the mean with repeated random samples of size n has the following properties:

1. The mean of the sampling distribution of $\overline{x}$ equals the mean of the population μ from which the sample is taken.
2. The standard deviation in the sampling distribution of $\overline{x}$ equals the standard deviation of the sampled population divided by the square root of the sample size. That is, $\sigma/\sqrt{n}$ is called the standard error of the mean.
3. If the distribution in the population is normal, then the sampling distribution of the mean is also normal. However, regardless of the shape of the original population distribution, if the sample size is sufficiently large, the sampling distribution of the mean is approximately normally distributed.

Central Limit Theorem

If n is large, then

$$z = \frac{\overline{x} - \mu}{\sigma/\sqrt{n}}$$

has an approximately standard normal distribution; that is, $\overline{x}$ has an approximately normal distribution with mean μ and variance σ^2/n.

A sample size of 30 is almost always sufficiently large so that regardless of the original population distribution, the sampling distributions of the mean will be approximately normally distributed. However, a sample size smaller than this is sufficient to obtain an approximately normal distribution if the original population distribution is close to being normal.

To summarize, the central limit theorem indicates that we can use normal theory for inferences about the population mean, regardless of the form of the population, if the sample size is large enough. A sample size of 30 or more is sufficiently large in almost all cases, but we may get by with a sample size smaller than 30, depending on how close the population is to being normal.

4.6 *t* Distribution

The equation for the **z statistic** assumes that the value of the population standard deviation σ is known. In reality, we rarely know this value but estimate its value by the sample standard deviation s. When s is used, the sampling distribution of the mean instead follows a t distribution. The t distribution resembles a normal distribution.

The t distribution is a theoretical probability distribution that is symmetric, bell-shaped, has a mean of 0, is similar to the standard normal curve but with more area in the tails, and is not as high in the middle. The primary difference between the t and z is that the t distribution is more variable because s will vary more from sample to sample for small samples. However, s varies little for large samples. The variability in the sampling distribution of t depends on the sample size n. A convenient way of expressing this dependence is to say that the t statistic has $n - 1$ degrees of freedom. The smaller the number of degrees of freedom associated with the t statistic, the more variable its sampling distribution will be.

To ensure the validity of a small sample test of hypothesis about the population mean μ, or to calculate a confidence interval for μ, two conditions must be met. First, a random sample is taken from the population. Second, the population is approximately normally distributed. Nevertheless, it has been shown that the t distribution is somewhat insensitive to moderate departures from normality. For small sample sizes and large deviations from normality, a nonparametric statistic is preferred.

4.7 Other Sampling Distributions

There are sampling distributions for more than just the mean. Statistics such as the proportion, standard deviation, median, and correlation coefficient also have sampling distributions. Although the sampling distribution for the mean is approximately normal, the sampling distributions for these other statistics are not. The mean has a standard normal distribution when the variance σ^2 is known. When it is not known, we saw that it follows a t distribution. We also saw that the proportion based on the binomial distribution is approximately normal if the number of trials n is large and p is near 0.5. In the next chapter, we will see that to test the hypothesis of independence between two categorical variables in a contingency table a statistic called the chi-square will be used. In addition, we will talk more about the sampling distribution of the ratio of two variances, which follows the F distribution.

One common property of all sampling distributions is that they each have a standard error. The variation of the statistic with respect to its sampling distribution is the standard error. We have already discussed the standard error of the mean, which is the most common standard error. Standard errors for other statistics will be presented in this text.

In addition to the Z distribution and the t distribution, two other continuous distributions will be briefly discussed in this chapter, but developed more fully later in this text, are the chi-square distribution and the F distribution.

4.7.1 Chi-Square Distribution

In probability theory, the **chi-square** (χ^2) **distribution** is a continuous probability distribution typically derived as the sampling distribution of a sum of squares of independent standard normal variables. Chi is the Greek letter χ and sounds like "Hi" only with a K, thus pronounced as "Ki." The distribution is bounded at 0 and its shape depends on the degrees of freedom. Specifically, the skewness of the distribution decreases as the degrees of freedom increases. As the degrees of freedom increase without limit, the χ^2 distribution approaches the normal distribution.

The mean of the χ^2 distribution is equal to the number of degrees of freedom. The variance of the χ^2 distribution is equal to two times the number of degrees of freedom. In the next chapter, we will consider the χ^2 distribution for testing specific types of hypotheses.

4.7.2 *F* Distribution

In probability theory, the *F* distribution is a continuous probability distribution that depends on two parameters or degrees of freedom, v_1 and v_2. It is derived from a ratio of the variances of two χ^2 random variables, each divided by their degrees of freedom. The first degree of freedom, v_1 is associated with the numerator, and the second degree of freedom, v_2 is associated with the denominator in the *F* ratio.

The *F* distribution has specific properties. First, the mean of the distribution is $v_2 / v_2 - 2$. Second, the variance of the distribution is equal to $2v_2^2(v_1 + v_2 - 2) / v_1(v_2 - 2)^2(v_2 - 4)$. Third, the curve is bounded by 0 on the left, has a single peak, and approaches but never touches the horizontal axis on the right. Fourth, the curve peaks not far to the right of 0 but approaches symmetry as the degrees of freedom increase. In the next couple chapters, we will talk about using an *F* test for evaluating the equality of variances.

4.8 Finite Population Correction

When a population size has a fixed upper bound, it is finite. For a finite population, where the total number of observations is *N* and the size of the sample is *n*, it is sometimes appropriate to correct the standard errors of the sample means. However, this correction is only necessary if the ratio of the sample size *n* to the population size *N* is greater than 0.05. The general formula for the **finite population correction factor** is $\sqrt{((N-n)/(N-1))}$. The correction is combined in the formula for the *z* as follows:

$$z = \frac{\overline{x} - \mu}{\frac{\sigma}{\sqrt{n}}\sqrt{\frac{N-n}{N-1}}}$$

Thus, we can see how the standard error is modified accordingly in the *z* formula.

4.9 Summary

A probability distribution is a table or an equation that represents each outcome of the random variable with its probability of occurrence. If a variable can assume any value between two specified values, it is a continuous variable; if it cannot, it is a discrete variable. If a variable is continuous, its probability distribution is continuous. Similarly, if a variable is discrete, its probability distribution is discrete. There are several discrete and continuous probability distributions. In this chapter, we presented two discrete probability distributions: the binomial and Poisson distributions. The binomial probability distribution is appropriate for determining the probability of *r* successes in a sequence of *n* independent trials. The Poisson probability distribution is used to determine the probability of the number of occurrences in a time interval, area, or volume.

A probability distribution for a continuous random variable is specified by a probability density curve. The area under the probability density curve represents probabilities. The standard normal probability distribution, represented by the letter z, is symmetric and has a single peak, a mean of 0, and variance of 1. It ranges from negative to positive infinity. When the number of trials, n, is large and p is near 0.5, the binomial distribution is approximately equal to a normal distribution.

The equation for the z statistic assumes that the value of the population standard deviation σ is known. A related distribution to the standard normal distribution is the t distribution. It resembles a normal distribution. When the population standard deviation is not known, the t distribution is a theoretical probability distribution that is symmetric, bell-shaped, has mean 0, and is similar to the Z distribution, only there is more area in the tails and it is not as high in the middle.

A sampling distribution is a probability distribution of a statistic for all possible samples of a given size from a population. The central limit theorem says the distribution of sample means approximates a normal distribution. The variability in the sampling distribution of t depends on the sample size n. Two other important continuous probability distributions, the χ^2 and F distributions, were introduced and will be applied in the coming chapters.

The primary equations in this chapter are summarized in **Table 4.2**.

Table 4.2 Equations for Random Variables and Probability Distributions

Description	Equation
Expected value of a discrete random variable	$E(X) = \mu = \sum rP(X = r)$
Variance of a discrete random variable	$\text{Variance}(X) = E(X - \mu)^2 = \sum(r - \mu)^2 P(X = r)$
Standard deviation of a discrete random variable	$\text{Standard Deviation}(X) = \sqrt{\text{Variance}(X)} = \sqrt{E(X - \mu)^2} = \sqrt{\sum(r - \mu)^2 P(X = r)}$
Binomial probability distribution	$P(X = r \mid n, p) = \binom{n}{r} p^r (1 - p)^{n-r} \quad r = 0, 1, 2, \ldots, n$
Mean of a binomial distribution	$E(X) = np$
Variance of a binomial distribution	$\text{Variance}(X) = np(1 - p)$
Standard deviation of a binomial distribution	$\text{Standard Deviation}(X) = \sqrt{np(1 - p)}$
Poisson probability distribution	$P(X = r \mid \lambda) = \dfrac{e^{-\lambda}\lambda^r}{r!}$ $r = 0, 1, 2, \ldots$
Mean of a Poisson distribution	$\lambda = np$
Standardized variable	$z = \dfrac{x - \mu}{\sigma}$
Normal approximation to the binomial	$z = \dfrac{x - np}{\sqrt{np(1 - np)}}$

Table 4.2 Equations for Random Variables and Probability Distributions *(Continued)*

Description	Equation
Standardized binomial fraction of success $f = x/n$	$z = \dfrac{f - p}{\sqrt{p(1-p)/n}}$
Mean of the binomial fraction of success	$E(f) = p$
Variance of the binomial fraction of success	$\text{Variance}(f) = \dfrac{p(1-p)}{n}$
Standard deviation of the binomial fraction of success	$\text{Standard Deviation}(f) = \sqrt{\dfrac{p(1-p)}{n}}$
Standardized sample mean	$z = \dfrac{\overline{x} - \mu}{\sigma/\sqrt{n}}$
Finite population correction factor	$\sqrt{\dfrac{N-n}{N-1}}$

Exercises

1. What is a random variable?
2. Compare and contrast discrete and continuous random variables.
3. How is a probability distribution related to a random variable?
4. What are three properties of the binomial probability distribution?
5. What are four characteristics of the Poisson probability distribution?
6. Under which two conditions will the binomial probability be approximately equal to the Poisson probability?
7. Describe the properties of the normal distribution.
8. Describe the standard normal random variable Z.
9. What is the practical value of the z-score?
10. What are the properties of the sampling distribution?
11. Consider 110 single students in a college class as the population of interest. The mean number of different individuals dated in the past month for these students is 2.0. A simple random sample of 10 students was selected, and their mean was 1.5. The values 1.5 and 2.0 are __________ and ___________, respectively.
    a. parameter, statistic
    b. statistic, parameter
    c. parameter, parameter
    d. statistic, statistic
12. If all possible simple random samples of size 10 were taken from the 110 values described in the previous exercise, and the mean calculated for each of these samples, what would be the mean of all these sample means?

13. Tolerability to two drugs were evaluated among several patients on a scale from 1 (low) to 5 (high). The results are shown in the following table:

Tolerability score (x)	1	2	3	4	5
Drug A $P(X = x)$	0.15	0.20	0.25	0.25	0.15
Drug B $P(X = x)$	0.05	0.15	0.20	0.30	0.30

Calculate μ_x, σ_x^2, and σ_x for Drug A and Drug B. Which drug do you prefer?

14. Five patients receive a treatment that is successful 70% of the time. The random number of success is a binomial random variable with $n = 5$ and $p = 0.70$. Complete the following table.

No. of successes (r)	0	1	2	3	4	5
$P(X = r)$						
$P(X \leq r)$						

In one study, cancer-related claims were presented according to type of service rendered. Let X be a discrete random variable that represents the number of three specific combinations of services. The probability distribution for X appears as follows:[7]

Non-Skin-Cancer-Related Claims*

Physician Services	Nonphysician Professional Health Services	Hospital Services	No.	$P(X = r)$
Yes	Yes	Yes	698	0.310
Yes	Yes	No	151	0.067
Yes	No	Yes	788	0.349
Yes	No	No	526	0.233
No	Yes	Yes	10	0.004
No	Yes	No	13	0.006
No	No	Yes	69	0.031
No	No	No	0	0.000

Data source: DMBA enrollees during 1998–2006, aged 15–64.
* First ICD-9-CM cancer code assigned 140–208, excluding 172.0–173.9 (skin cancer).

For exercises 15–19, refer to the table of cancer-related claims according to type of service rendered.

15. Construct a graph of the probability distribution.

16. What is the probability that a cancer patient receives all three types of services?

17. What is the probability that the cancer patient received both physician and hospital services only?

18. What is the probability of receiving nonphysician professional health services?

19. Thirty percent of psychiatric patients being taken to the hospital require police assistance. If 10 patients are admitted to the hospital on a given day, what is the probability that none will involve the police? What is the probability less than five will involve the police?

20. The rate of COVID-19 in Massachusetts as of July 6, 2020, was 1596 per 100,000. Approximately 692,600 people live in Boston. What is the expected number of cases in Boston?

21. Continuing with the previous exercise, suppose we take a random sample of 100 residents in Boston. What is the probability of finding two to five cases of COVID-19? Use both the binomial and the Poisson to calculate your answer. Note that because the number of trials is large and the chance of success is small, the binomial probability is approximately equal to the Poisson.

22. In the United States, the case fatality rate for COVID-19 on December 28, 2020, was 1.74%.[8] Find the probability of at least 20 cases in a population of 1000. Show that the normal approximation to the binomial is close to the exact binomial probability.

23. In a sampling distribution of the mean, what is the expected value and standard deviation of the sample mean?

24. The number of people that an emergency room doctor sees on her shift each week averages 35. The number of people the doctor sees varies from week to week, with a standard deviation of 12. What is the probability that during a sample of $n = 30$ shifts, the mean number of people the doctor sees will be at least 30?

25. Assume that minutes engaged in aerobic activity in a population is normally distributed with $\mu = 20$ and $\sigma^2 = 20$ kg/m². What is the area under the curve below 15?

26. Continuing with the previous exercise, what is the probability of between 15 and 30 minutes of aerobic exercise?

27. The mean number of children under 18 years of age in families in the United States is 1.9, and the standard deviation is 1.1.[9] Assuming a standard normal distribution, what is the probability of three or more children?

28. When is it appropriate to use the finite population correction?

29. The distribution of the age in which male students at a large university got married is right skewed with $\mu = 23$ years and $\sigma = 8$ years. What is the probability that a random sample of 50 married male students would have a sample mean age at marriage of between 22 and 24?

30. Continuing with the previous exercise, what is the probability that a random sample of 50 male students would have a sample mean age at marriage of less than 22?

31. Continuing with exercise 29, suppose the total number of married male students at the university is only 500. Then, applying the finite

population correction factor, what is the probability that a simple random sample of 50 male students would have a sample mean age at marriage of less than 22?

32. In the United States, men marry women about 2.5 years younger than them, on average, with a standard deviation of 2.8 years. In approximately what percentage of married couples is the wife older than the husband (i.e., what percentage of married couples have a difference in age less than 0)?

33. Referring to the previous exercise, what is the value of a difference such that 60% of the age differences are less than it?

34. Compare and contrast the *Z* and *t* distributions.

35. The sampling distribution of the ratio of two variances follows which of the following?
    a. *Z* distribution
    b. *t* distribution
    c. χ^2 distribution
    d. *F* distribution

References

1. Watson CJ, Billingsley P, Croft DJ, Huntsberger DV. *Brief Business Statistics*. Needham Heights, MA: Allyn and Bacon, Inc.; 1988.
2. Scholastic. Prescription pain medications: What you need to know. http://headsup.scholastic.com/students/prescription-pain-medications-what-you-need-to-know#:~:text=Opioids%20and%20Addiction%20Opioid%20receptors%20are%20also%20found,release%20of%20dopamine%2C%20known%20as%20a%20%E2%80%9Crunner%E2%80%99s%20high.%E2%80%9D. Published 2016. Accessed July 10, 2020.
3. Hedegaard H, Miniño AM, Warner M. Drug Overdose Deaths in the United States, 1999–2018. *NCHS Data Brief*, no *356*. Hyattsville, MD: National Center for Health Statistics; 2020.
4. Wilson N, Kariisa M, Seth P, et al. Drug and opioid-involved overdose deaths—United States, 2017–2018. *MMWR*. 2020;*69*:290–297.
5. Alter A, Yeager C. The consequences of COVID-19 on the overdose epidemic: overdoses are increasing. https://files.constantcontact.com/a923b952701/dbf0b5a5-f730-4a6f-a786-47097f1eea78.pdf. Published 2020. Accessed July 20, 2020.
6. Center for Disease Control and Prevention. BRFSS Prevalence & Trends Data. https://www.cdc.gov/brfss/brfssprevalence/index.html. Accessed July 24, 2020.
7. Merrill RM, Baker RK, Lyon JL, Gren LH. Healthcare claims for identifying the level of diagnostic investigation and treatment of cancer. *Med Sci Monit*. 2009;*15*(5):PH25–31.
8. Center for Disease Control and Prevention. Coronavirus (COVID-19) statistics. https://www.bing.com/search?q=covid+19+stats+global+country&form=EDGEAR&qs=PF&cvid=ea2f3c8f05cd488d8bf6244975e32300&cc=US&setlang=en-US&plvar=0. Accessed December 28, 2020.
9. US Census Bureau, America's Families and Living Arrangements: 2019, Average Number of People per Family Household. Table AGV3. https://www.census.gov/data/tables/2017/demo/families/cps-2017.html. Updated March 22, 2019. Accessed December 28, 2020.

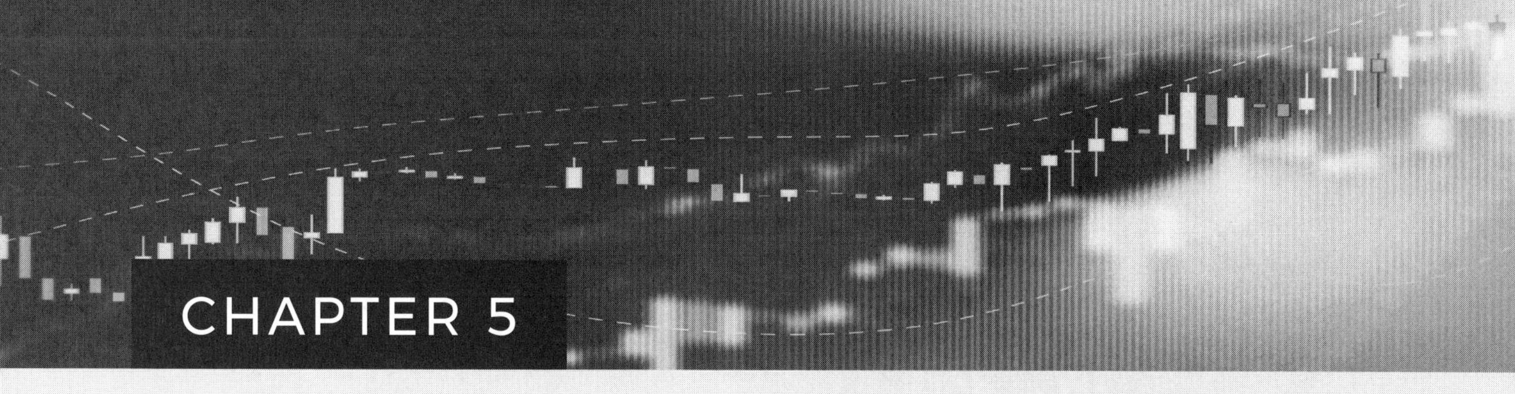

Estimation and Hypothesis Testing

KEY CONCEPTS

- Estimation is a process by which we make inferences about a population using information from a sample.
- An estimator is a sample statistic that estimates a population parameter.
- An estimate (or point estimate) is the numerical value of an estimator.
- An unbiased estimator is a sample estimator whose expected value equals the population parameter.
- A minimum-variance unbiased estimator is termed a best estimator because, in addition to being unbiased, it has the smallest variance among all unbiased estimators.
- A confidence interval is a range of values associated with the probability that the value of an unknown parameter lies within its limits.
- The width of the confidence interval is influenced by the confidence level, standard deviation, and sample size.
- Confidence intervals provide information about statistical precision and significance.
- The *t* distribution is similar to the *Z* distribution, in that both are bell-shaped, symmetric and unimodal, but the *t* distribution has thicker tails. The *t* distribution approaches the *Z* distribution as the sample size increases.
- A statistical hypothesis is a statement about one or more parameters of a population that requires verification.
- Hypothesis testing is the process of selecting between the null and alternative hypothesis and involves six recommended steps.
- Hypothesis testing involves specific assumptions, which depend on the measurement scale of the variable, the shape of the population distribution, and the sample size.
- Hypothesis testing assumes random sampling.
- Hypothesis testing can result in error if we reject the null hypothesis when it is true (Type I error) or accept the null hypothesis when it is false (Type II error). The probability of committing these errors is denoted by the symbols α and β, respectively.
- Power is the probability that a statistical test will reject the null hypothesis when H_0 is false. It is the complement of β (i.e., $1-\beta$) and is directly related to sample size.
- The *p*-value is the probability of obtaining a result at least as large as the one observed, given the null hypothesis is true; the smaller the *p*-value, the greater the evidence against the null hypothesis.
- The *Z* approximates the binomial when the sample size is sufficiently large. It is used to construct confidence intervals and test hypotheses involving proportions.
- With paired data, subjects serve as their own controls.
- Paired studies involving numerical data are evaluated using the *t* test. Paired studies using categorical data use the McNemar test or Cohen's kappa *k*.
- The χ^2 test is particularly useful for evaluating goodness of fit, independence between categorical variables, and for determining whether the variance of a population is equal to a specified value.

People are inquisitive by nature, asking questions and sometimes putting those questions to the test. In the year 1600, Sir Francis Bacon (1561–1626), an English philosopher, created the Scientific Method. This method involves systematically observing and describing a phenomenon, asking questions, formulating hypotheses, testing the hypotheses, and developing theories and laws based on validated results.[1]

The form of reasoning in which rational decisions about certain phenomena are made on the basis of incomplete information is called statistical inference. Classical statistical inference encompasses estimation, interval estimation, and hypothesis testing. With statistical inference, conclusions are made about the underlying population of interest, usually based on data from a random sample. The data may be used for estimation of the value of an unknown parameter or for a test of hypothesis regarding the value. For example, an investigator may take a random sample from a population of hospital patients with COVID-19 and consider whether they require mechanical ventilation or not. The unknown parameter is the proportion p of patients who require this form of treatment. We may estimate the population parameter p, estimate an interval that is likely to contain p, or test a hypothesis about p. In each situation, we infer something about p.

The purpose of this chapter is to introduce methods of estimation, interval estimation, and how to establish and test hypotheses. Steps of hypothesis testing, hypothesis tests, and test assumptions will be covered. Hypotheses will be presented for assessing several different situations.

5.1 Questions and Hypotheses

Researchers sometimes ask questions about a population proportion or mean. A few questions that are currently receiving attention in the literature are:

- "What is the proportion of COVID-19 patients undergoing echocardiography who have cardiac abnormalities?"[2]
- "What is the gestational age of newborns whose mothers had COVID-19?"[3]
- "What is the mean birth weight of infants born to women with COVID-19?"[3]
- "Does severity of COVID-19 relate to blood type?"[4]

It is often of interest to not just obtain a simple point estimate of a parameter, but to also identify the variability that the estimate would have in other samples. To identify this variability, we use interval estimates. As we will discuss, interval estimates are called confidence intervals. For example, investigators in one study were 95% confident that the interval 15.5% to 20.2% contained the true proportion of COVID-19 cases who were asymptomatic.[5] A research question could be, "What is the 95% confidence interval for the death-to-case ratio of COVID-19 in the United Kingdom?"

A focus of this chapter is on hypothesis testing. Research questions are made precise using hypothesis testing. In other words, while the research question is inquisitive in nature and sets to answer something, the hypothesis is predictive in nature and presents a tentative prediction about the value of a variable or an association between two or more variables. The research question could be, "Is there an effective vaccine for COVID-19?" We might have a research hypothesis that evaluates whether at least 90% of subjects have a neutralizing antibody response against SARS-COV-2 after taking a single dose of a vaccine.

5.2 Estimators

Estimation is the process that we use to make inferences about a population, based on information that is obtained from a sample. A sample quantity used to estimate an unknown parameter is called an estimator. An estimator is a random variable or statistic that is used to estimate the numerical value of an unknown parameter. The estimate is also called a point estimate. A point estimate of a parameter is a single value of a statistic, such as the sample mean.

An **estimator** is a random variable or a sample statistic that is used to estimate an unknown population parameter.

An **estimate** or **point estimate** is the actual numerical value of an estimator.

An estimator of a parameter is an unbiased estimator if its expected value equals the parameter. Common measures in statistics, the sample probability of success f, the sample mean $\bar{X}$, and the sample variance s^2 are each unbiased estimators because the distribution of these sample statistics center around their population values. An unbiased estimator is defined as follows:

An **unbiased estimator** is one in which the expected value of a sample estimator equals the population parameter:

$$E(\text{Sample estimator}) = \text{Population parameter}.$$

To illustrate, if X_i is a Bernoulli random variable with parameter p, $E(X_i) = p$. The estimator of p is $f = \frac{1}{n}\sum_{i=1}^{n} X_i$. The expected value of this estimator is

$$E(f) = E\left(\frac{1}{n}\sum_{i=1}^{n} X_i\right) = \frac{1}{n}\sum_{i=1}^{n} E(X_i) = \frac{1}{n}\sum_{i=1}^{n} p = \frac{1}{n}np = p.$$

Therefore, f is an unbiased estimator of p.

If X_i is a normally distributed random variable with mean μ and variance σ^2, then $E(X_i) = \mu$.

$$E(\bar{X}) = E\left(\frac{1}{n}\sum_{i=1}^{n} X_i\right) = \frac{1}{n}\sum_{i=1}^{n} E(X_i) = \frac{1}{n}\sum_{i=1}^{n} \mu = \frac{1}{n}n\mu = \mu$$

Therefore, $\bar{X}$ is an unbiased estimator of μ.

If X_i is a normally distributed random variable with mean μ and variance σ^2, then $\frac{(n-1)s^2}{\sigma^2} \sim \chi^2_{n-1}$. The expression is distributed as a chi-square (χ^2) with $n-1$ degrees of freedom. The expected value of a χ^2 random variable is its degrees of freedom; that is, $E\left[\frac{(n-1)s^2}{\sigma^2}\right] = n-1$. Then,

$$E(s^2) = E\left[\frac{\sigma^2}{n-1} \times \frac{(n-1)s^2}{\sigma^2}\right] = \frac{\sigma^2}{n-1}E\left[\frac{(n-1)s^2}{\sigma^2}\right] = \frac{\sigma^2}{n-1} \times (n-1) = \sigma^2.$$

Therefore, s^2 is an unbiased estimator of σ^2.

When an unbiased estimator also has smaller variances than any other unbiased estimator, it is termed a best estimator.

A **minimum-variance unbiased estimator** is termed a best estimator because in addition to being unbiased, it has the smallest variance among all unbiased estimators.

5.3 Interval Estimates

A limitation of point estimates is that they do not have an associated probability showing the likelihood of the value. In contrast, we can show associated probability with interval estimates. Hence, in addition to estimating a parameter using a point estimate, we are also interested in estimating an interval in which we think the anticipated parameter will lie. An interval estimate is an interval of probable values of an unknown population parameter based on sample data. An interval estimate is a confidence interval. The next section will show how confidence intervals are derived.

5.3.1 Confidence Intervals for Normal Means and Known Variance

In this section, we will assume we do not know μ but we do know σ^2. It is unlikely that we would not know the population mean but would know the population variance. However, this situation allows us to present the reasoning for confidence interval estimation. We will then build on this to the more realistic situation in which neither the population mean nor the population variance are known.

Confidence intervals define an upper limit and a lower limit with an associated probability. The ends of the confidence interval are called the **confidence limits.**

A **confidence interval** is an interval, bounded on the left by L and on the right by R, used to estimate an unknown population parameter. L and R are referred to as confidence limits. Reliability of the estimate may be evaluated objectively by the use of a confidence statement.

A confidence interval can be calculated for any population parameter, such as the mean or proportion. Confidence intervals for various types of measures will be presented throughout this text. For now, we will present the confidence interval for the population mean μ when the population variance σ^2 is known.

The $100(1 - \alpha)\%$ confidence interval for the population mean μ when the population is normally distributed and the variance σ^2 is known is the interval with the confidence limits

$$L = \overline{x} - z_{1-\alpha/2}\frac{\sigma}{\sqrt{n}} \text{ and } R = \overline{x} + z_{1-\alpha/2}\frac{\sigma}{\sqrt{n}}.$$

The value of z is obtained from Appendix B, Table 3.

Some related terms are presented as follows:

The value $1 - \alpha$ is called the confidence coefficient, and $100(1 - \alpha)\%$ is referred to as the confidence level.

If the level of significance $\alpha = 0.05$, then the confidence level is 95%. The margin of error for a sample mean is the z-score multiplied by the standard error. We will see that all confidence intervals have the same general form: estimate ± the margin of error.

EXAMPLE 5.1

The 95% confidence interval for the exercise example presented in the previous chapter is

$$L = 21.17 - 1.96\frac{2.46}{\sqrt{10}} = 19.65 \text{ and } R = 21.17 + 1.96\frac{2.46}{\sqrt{10}} = 22.69.$$

Thus we can feel 95% confident that the mean percentage of the adult population who participate in enough aerobic and muscle strengthening exercises to meet guidelines in the United States lies between 19.65% and 22.69%.

The reason why we are 95% confident is because if we were to take 100 different samples from the sample population and calculate the confidence limits for each sample, we would expect that about 95 out of these 100 intervals would contain the true value of μ. We would also expect that 5 of the 100 intervals would not contain the true value of μ. Because we only have one confidence interval based on a single sample, we do not know whether the interval is one of the 95 or of the 5. It is in this sense that we are 95% confident.

5.3.2 Confidence Intervals for Normal Means and Unknown Variance

In this section, in addition to not knowing the population mean μ, we do not know the population variance σ^2. To calculate the confidence interval when the population variance σ^2 is unknown, we replace σ^2 by its estimator s^2 in the equation. In addition, assuming the sample is taken from a normal population, the t is used instead of the z. As the sample size increases, the confidence interval narrows and the t value approaches the z value.

The $100(1 - \alpha)\%$ confidence interval for the population mean μ when the population is approximately normally distributed and the variance σ^2 is not known is the interval with the confidence limits

$$L = \bar{x} - t_{1-\alpha/2,n-1}\frac{s}{\sqrt{n}} \text{ and } R = \bar{x} + t_{1-\alpha/2,n-1}\frac{s}{\sqrt{n}}.$$

The value of t is obtained from Appendix B, Table 4, using $n-1$ degrees of freedom.

EXAMPLE 5.2

Returning to the exercise example, the sample mean was 21.17. In addition, the sample standard deviation was 2.46. Assuming we do not know the population standard deviation, we could use the sample standard deviation to calculate a 95% confidence interval, as follows:

$$L = 21.17 - 2.262\frac{2.46}{\sqrt{10}} = 19.41 \text{ and } R = 21.17 + 2.262\frac{2.46}{\sqrt{10}} = 22.93$$

Thus we can feel 95% confident that the mean percentage of the adult population who participate in enough aerobic and muscle strengthening exercises to meet guidelines in the United States lies between 19.41% and 22.93%.

EXAMPLE 5.3

On July 8, 2020, the cumulative number of COVID-19 cases and deaths were reported by each state and the District of Columbia. A random sample of 30 was taken and a mean death-to-case ratio of 0.0365 was obtained, with a standard deviation of 0.0229. The 95% confidence interval is as follows:

$$L = 0.0365 - 2.045\frac{0.0229}{\sqrt{30}} = 0.0279 \text{ and}$$

$$R = 0.0365 + 2.045\frac{0.0229}{\sqrt{30}} = 0.0451$$

Hence, we are 95% confident that the true death-to-case ratio among the 50 states and the District of Columbia is in the interval 2.80% to 4.51%.

The t distribution is similar to the normal distribution. Small sample sizes require that the distribution for the random variable be approximately normal to employ the t statistic. However, because of the central limit theorem, if the population has a distribution that is not normal, the t can still be used if the sample size is sufficiently large. For the sample size to be sufficiently large, it depends on how far the population distribution deviates from normality. With extreme deviation, a sample size of at least 30 is required. If the population distribution does not deviate much from normality, a sample size of less than 30 is sufficient.

5.3.3 Confidence Intervals for the Binomial with Large Sample Sizes

We previously defined a binomial population as one in which its elements fall into two classes: success and failure. The fraction of success is $f = \frac{x}{n}$ and the expected value of f is p; $E(f) = p$. The normal approximation to the binomial provides a method of finding fairly accurate confidence limits for large sample sizes. To apply this, the formula requires $nf > 10$ and $n(1-f) > 10$.

Confidence Interval for *p*

The $100(1 - \alpha)\%$ confidence interval for the binomial proportion of success p is the interval with the confidence limits

$$L = f - z_{1-\alpha/2}\sqrt{\frac{f(1-f)}{n}} \text{ and } R = f + z_{1-\alpha/2}\sqrt{\frac{f(1-f)}{n}}$$

EXAMPLE 5.4

A state survey of adults asks about selected behaviors during the COVID-19 crisis. One question is, "If I had exhibited symptoms of sickness, I would have immediately informed the people around me." Suppose that 25 people were randomly surveyed, of which 20 indicated that they would immediately inform the people around them of their possible illness. Is the sample size large enough to apply the confidence interval formula according to the requirement $nf > 10$ and $n(1-f) > 10$? The answer is No.

Now suppose the sample size was 250, of which 200 indicated that they would immediately inform people around them if they showed symptoms of sickness. In this case, it is appropriate to apply the confidence interval formula because $nf > 10$ and $n(1-f) > 10$ is satisfied. The 95% confidence interval is

$$L = 0.80 - 1.96\sqrt{\frac{0.80(1-0.80)}{250}} = 0.75 \text{ and}$$

$$R = 0.80 + 1.96\sqrt{\frac{0.80(1-0.80)}{250}} = 0.85.$$

Thus we can feel 95% confident that the proportion who would immediately inform people around them if they showed any signs of COVID-19 is from 0.75 to 0.85.

News File

The 2020 COVID-19 pandemic, resulting from severe acute respiratory syndrome coronavirus 2 (SARS-COV-2) has reached levels not experienced since the 1918 influenza pandemic. As the pandemic progresses, researchers are finding it to be associated with lung scarring,[6,7] cerebrovascular events,[8,9,10] and kidney failure.[11] There is also an increasing number of case reports and series of neurological manifestations being reported.[12] One study investigated the extent of complications in COVID-19 patients in the United Kingdom.[13] Median age of patients was 71 years, ranging from 23 to 94. Of 125 patients, 39 (31%, 95% CI = 16.5–45.5%) experienced altered mental status. Data on age were available for 37 of the 39 patients, of which 18 (49%, 25.9–72.1%) were younger than 60. In contrast, only 18% (9.4–26.6%) of 77 patients with cerebrovascular events were younger than 60 years. In another study, 55% (42.4–67.6%) of 60 COVID-19 patients were manifesting neurological symptoms three months after testing. In addition, brain scans for these patients compared with a control group not infected with SARS-COV-2 found that the brains of the patients had more structural changes related to loss of memory and smell.[14] Finally, a case series investigation of four children linked COVID-19 with multisystem inflammatory syndrome.[15] Neurological symptoms such as confusion and disorientation, muscle weakness, and headaches developed in these children. Two of the children continued to show symptoms.

5.4 Tests of Hypotheses

A scientific hypothesis is a testable statement about a phenomenon or relationship that requires verification. Some examples of scientific hypotheses are people with comorbid illness who contract SARS-CoV-2 are more likely to require hospitalization; age is positively associated with a person wearing a protective face covering to guard against the virus; and rates of COVID-19 are greater in lower income communities. Evidence to support whether these hypotheses are true is determined by observation or experimentation.

As with the confidence interval, a hypothesis test is a way to generalize results to the population, based on sample information. A hypothesis test makes an assumption about the population. Then, probability is used to estimate the likelihood of the result obtained from the sample under the assumption about the population.

In this section, we assess how to establish and test hypotheses. A six-step process for testing hypotheses will be introduced. In testing hypotheses, there is potential for reaching a wrong conclusion. There are two types of errors possible. The probability of committing these types of errors will be discussed. We will focus on hypotheses about means, proportions, and variances in one or two populations. Finally, we will formulate hypotheses as one-sided or two-sided.

The first step in evaluating a scientific hypothesis is to express it as a statistical hypothesis. Movement from a scientific hypothesis to a statistical hypothesis is a deductive process. An example of a statistical hypothesis is that the population mean body mass index (BMI) is at least 25, denoted as $\mu \geq 25$. Another statistical hypothesis can be formulated that states that the mean BMI is less than 25; $\mu < 25$. These hypotheses $\mu \geq 25$ and $\mu < 25$ are mutually exclusive and exhaustive. If one is true, the other is false. They are examples of the null hypothesis and the **alternative hypothesis**. The null hypothesis is the one whose tenability is being tested. If sufficient evidence is found to reject the null hypothesis, the alternative hypothesis is tenable. By convention, the alternative hypothesis is formulated to reflect the investigator's scientific premonition. Choosing between the null and alternative hypotheses is the process called hypothesis testing.

A **statistical hypothesis** is a statement about one or more parameters of a population that require verification.

Hypothesis testing may apply to a single variable or involve relationships between or among variables. Hypotheses are shown to be consistent or inconsistent with the facts. If established information or facts are lacking to substantiate a research hypothesis, then additional information is needed or we fail to support the hypothesis.

Hypothesis testing is the process of selecting between the null and alternative hypothesis.

The standard framework in hypothesis testing is to begin by presenting two hypotheses. The first is the null hypothesis, which usually states what is currently believed, expected, claimed, or has been in the past. The null hypothesis is assumed to be correct unless enough evidence can be found to show otherwise. The second is the alternative hypothesis, also called the research hypothesis. The aim of the investigator is to provide support for this hypothesis.

Example 5.5

Suppose the mean death-to-case ratio among COVID-19 patients in the United States is believed to be 3.65%. However, in Utah, the average age of the population is younger than anywhere else in the country. Given that the deaths among

COVID-19 patients increase with age, you believe the death-to-case ratio will be significantly lower in Utah than in the country as a whole. The two hypotheses for this problem can be expressed as follows:

$$\text{Null Hypothesis } H_0\text{: } \mu \geq 3.65$$

$$\text{Alternative Hypothesis } H_a\text{: } \mu < 3.65$$

By convention, the null hypothesis is assumed to be correct unless sufficient evidence can show otherwise. If we no longer believe the null hypothesis to be true, we accept the alternative hypothesis. This is an example of a one-sided test, as indicated by looking at the sign of the alternative hypothesis. In Florida, which has the oldest average age in the population, we may formulate the hypotheses as:

$$\text{Null Hypothesis } H_0\text{: } \mu \leq 3.65$$

$$\text{Alternative Hypothesis } H_a\text{: } \mu > 3.65$$

We also may be interested in whether a given state differs from the national average death-to-case ratio, such that we formulate the hypotheses as:

$$\text{Null Hypothesis } H_0\text{: } \mu = 3.65$$

$$\text{Alternative Hypothesis } H_a\text{: } \mu \neq 3.65$$

Example 5.6

Suppose it is commonly believed that 0.8 of the adult population would immediately inform the people around them if they exhibited symptoms of COVID-19. You would like to test whether this is accurate. Hence, you pursue a study with the hypotheses formulated as:

$$\text{Null Hypothesis } H_0\text{: } p = 0.8$$

$$\text{Alternative Hypothesis } H_a\text{: } p \neq 0.8$$

Perhaps you are also interested in knowing whether this proportion differs according to one's level of education. You may believe that people with a college degree are more likely than those with a high school degree to immediately inform people around them if they exhibit symptoms of the disease. The hypotheses are formulated as follows:

$$\text{Null Hypothesis } H_0\text{: } p_{HS} \geq p_C$$

$$\text{Alternative Hypothesis } H_a\text{: } p_{HS} < p_C$$

Hence, we see that research questions are made precise using hypothesis testing. Formulation of the statistical hypotheses depends on the scientific hypothesis. Following the formulation of the statistical hypotheses comes random sampling and estimation of population parameters. The data are then evaluated using a statistical test, with conclusions drawn from the results.

The process of hypothesis testing can be broken down into six steps:

1. Formulate the null hypothesis in statistical terms.

   The **null hypothesis**, denoted by H_0, specifies the value of a population parameter. We want to show that the null hypothesis is incorrect. The null hypothesis is what is currently believed, the status quo.

2. Formulate the alternative (or research) hypothesis in statistical terms.

   The alternative hypothesis, denoted by H_a, gives an opposing conjecture to that of the null hypothesis. We want to support this hypothesis as being true.

3. Select the sample size and the level of significance. The level of significance α is generally 0.05, but if a more conservative test is desired, 0.01 can be used. In exploratory studies, 0.1 or higher may be used.

   There are several variations in the process of estimating sample size in analytic or experimental studies, which may be referred to in other sources.

4. Select the appropriate test statistic and identify the degrees of freedom and the critical value for rejecting the null hypothesis.

   A **rejection region** specifies the values of the test statistic wherein the null hypothesis is rejected in favor of the alternative hypothesis.

5. Collect the data and calculate the test statistic.

   A **test statistic** is a quantity calculated from the sample that is used when making a decision about the hypotheses of interest.

6. Reject or fail to reject the null hypothesis.

   If we reject the null hypothesis, we accept the alternative hypothesis. However, if we do not reject the null hypothesis we do not necessarily accept the null hypothesis. We simply do not have sufficient evidence to reject it.

5.4.1 Type I and Type II Errors

A hypothesis test may result in an incorrect conclusion. Two types of errors may occur, as shown in **Table 5.1**. The truth is represented in the headings of the table, and the decisions made by the investigator are represented by the rows of the table. For example, if H_0 is true and we fail to reject H_0, we have made the correct decision. If H_a is true and we reject H_0 (accept H_a), we have also made the correct decision. On the other hand, there is always the concern of rejecting H_0 when it is true (**Type I error**) or accepting H_0 when it is not true (**Type II error**). Hence, we should consider the probability of making these two types of errors. The probability of a Type I error is denoted by the Greek letter **alpha** α.

Table 5.1 Possible Decisions and Consequences in Hypothesis Testing

Possible Decisions	True State of the Population	
	H_0 is true	**H_a is true**
Reject H_0	Type I error	Correct decision
Fail to reject H_0	Correct decision	Type II error

The probability of a Type II error is denoted by the Greek letter **beta** β. The chance of error in our conclusion cannot exceed α and β.

$$\alpha = P(\text{Type I error}) = P(\text{Reject } H_0 \mid H_0 \text{ is true})$$

$$\beta = P(\text{Type II error}) = P(\text{Fail to reject } H_0 \mid \text{H}_\text{a} \text{ is true})$$

Although the preference is for α and β to be near 0, this is often not possible. In general, we want it to be unlikely to reject H_0 if it is true. It is important to keep in mind that the investigator is free to choose how rare an observation must be in order to reject H_0.

In order to reject a null hypothesis, we compare the calculated value of a test statistic with a critical value. The test statistic used to evaluate hypotheses depends on the type of parameter being evaluated. The critical value is influenced by α, the level of which is chosen by the investigator (typically 0.05). The investigator also chooses the value of β (typically 0.20). If $\beta = 0.20$, then the investigator is willing to accept a 20% chance of incorrectly accepting H_0.

A **statistical test** is the process in which we decide whether to reject (or fail to reject) the null hypothesis. A **test statistic** is a single numerical summary value derived from a sample used in hypothesis testing. It is used to provide support for either the null or alternative hypothesis. Common statistical tests include the one- and two-sample ***z* test**, one-sample ***t* test**, paired *t* test, two-sample pooled *t* test, two-sample unpooled *t* test, one-proportion *z* test, two proportion *z* test, χ^2 test for goodness of fit, χ^2 test for variance, and two sample *F* tests for equality of variance.

Another probability measure that is related to β, the quantity $(1 - \beta)$, is called power. Power may be thought of as the chance that a given study will detect a deviation from the null hypothesis when one really exists. As power increases, the probability of committing a Type II error decreases.

Power is the probability that a statistical test will reject the null hypothesis when H_0 is false.

Power is directly related to sample size. As the sample size increases, power increases. It is critical for the study sample size to be large enough to identify a difference if it actually exists.

5.4.2 *p*-Value

Once a test statistic is calculated we can determine a ***p*-value**, which is the probability of obtaining a result as or more extreme than the one observed, given the null hypothesis is true. The p-value ranges from 0 to 1, with smaller values corresponding to the data being more incompatible with the null hypothesis. In other words, the smaller the p-value, the greater the evidence against the null hypothesis. In practice, if the p-value is less than our chosen **level of significance** we reject the null hypothesis. To illustrate, suppose we want to evaluate whether men and women are equally likely to wear a mask while in public, prior to the availability of a vaccine. Let's assume a null hypothesis that the proportion who wear a mask in public is the same for men and women. The alternative hypothesis is otherwise. Let $\alpha = 0.05$ and the sample size be 300 men and 300 women. A **chi-square test** is appropriate. The following data were collected:

	Mask	No Mask
Men	225	75
Women	250	50

From this data we can calculate a chi-square statistic, which is 6.316, and get a corresponding p-value. This process will be shown later. For now, note that the p-value is 0.0120. Since the p-value < 0.05, we reject the null hypothesis that men and women are equally likely to wear a mask while in public. The estimated proportion is 75% for men and 83% for women.

When statistical tests are used to draw conclusions about a population, a corresponding p-value is obtained and typically reported alongside the value of the statistical test.

The p-value is the probability that the test statistic used to evaluate a hypothesis has a value as extreme as or more extreme than the sample statistic, given the null hypothesis is true.

If the p-value is lower than the level of significance chosen by the investigator, then we can say that there is sufficient evidence to reject the null hypothesis. There is still a **chance** that a Type I error is committed, but it is small enough that we are willing to take the risk. However, if committing a Type I error is quite serious, for example resulting in deaths, we may choose to lower our level of significance to 0.01.

Criteria for Evaluating Hypotheses Based on the p-value

If p-value $< \alpha$, then reject H_0.
If p-value $\geq \alpha$, then do not reject H_0.

5.5 Hypotheses Involving a Parameter in One Group

Hypotheses involving one group may involve the mean, the mean of differences between paired data, a proportion, and the change in a proportion.

5.5.1 Hypotheses Involving the Mean in One Group

Consider a population that is normally distributed with the variance σ^2 unknown. There are three possible formulations of hypotheses on normal mean and rejections regions:

Null Hypothesis	Alternative Hypothesis	Rejection Region
H_0: $\mu \leq \mu_0$	H_a: $\mu > \mu_0$	$t > t_{1-\alpha,n-1}$
H_0: $\mu \geq \mu_0$	H_a: $\mu < \mu_0$	$t < -t_{1-\alpha,n-1}$
H_0: $\mu = \mu_0$	H_a: $\mu \neq \mu_0$	$\lvert t \rvert > t_{1-\alpha/2,n-1}$

For these hypotheses, the *t* statistic has a *t* distribution with $n-1$ degrees of freedom. The *t* statistic is used in a *t* test when we are deciding whether to support a null hypothesis. It is the departure of an estimated parameter of a sample from its hypothesized value divided by its standard error. Once we calculate the *t* statistic, we can compare it with a critical value of *t* to determine statistical significance.

Equation for the *t* Statistic

$$t = \frac{\bar{x} - \mu_0}{s/\sqrt{n}}$$

Example 5.7

Suppose that it is commonly believed that the mean death-to-case ratio of COVID-19 in the U.S. adult population who are obese is 5%. However, we believe it is lower. Assuming a normal distribution of death-to-case ratio for each state and the District of Columbia, let us take a **random sample** of 30 states. Applying the steps to hypothesis testing gives the following:

1. H_0: $\mu \geq 5$
2. H_a: $\mu < 5$
3. $\alpha = 0.05$, $n = 30$
4. *t* statistic and 30 – 1 = 29 degrees of freedom. On the basis of the alternative hypothesis, we see that the rejection region is in the lower tail of the *t* distribution. Referring to Appendix B, Table 4, the critical value is –1.70.
5. From our sample, suppose $\bar{x} = 3.65$ and $s = 2.29$, then

$$t = \frac{3.65 - 5}{2.29/\sqrt{30}} = -3.23$$

6. Since $t = -3.23 < t_{0.05,29} = -1.70$, reject H_0 and conclude that the death-to-case ratio in the United States and the District of Columbia is significantly less than 5%. We can also use the *p*-value to evaluate statistical significance. The *p*-value that corresponds with –3.23 and 29 degrees of freedom is 0.0015. Since the *p*-value is smaller than our chosen level of significance, $\alpha = 0.05$, we reject the null hypothesis and accept the alternative. That is, we reject H_0 and conclude that the mean death-to-case ratio in the United States and the District of Columbia is significantly below 5%.

To obtain the p-value from Appendix B, Table 4, we go to the row that corresponds with 29 degrees of freedom and go to the right until we find 3.23. The corresponding p-value at the top of the table is not shown, but we know it is less than 0.0025 (1 – 0.9975). To obtain the exact p-value, use the Excel function T.DIST(x, degrees of freedom, cumulative), which for this example is =T.DIST(–3.23,29,TRUE). Entering this function returns the p-value 0.0015.

5.5.2 Paired Design: Mean

Sometimes a measure is taken twice on the same subject, and we are interested in whether a change occurred. For example, to evaluate whether an intervention significantly lowered cholesterol, we may compare pre- and post-intervention cholesterol scores. In this situation, we use a **paired design** because before and after measurements are taken. A paired t test is used to evaluate whether a significant mean difference ($\bar{d}$) occurred. The paired t statistic involves $n-1$ degrees of freedom, and the denominator is the standard error of the mean differences.

Paired *t* Statistics

$$t = \frac{\bar{d} - 0}{s_d / \sqrt{n}}, \quad s_d = \sqrt{\frac{\sum_{i=1}^{n}(d_i - \bar{d})^2}{n-1}}$$

We assume that the difference score is normally distributed with the variances σ^2 unknown. The statistical hypothesis for a paired design has potential forms of the hypotheses and rejection regions as shown in the following table:

Null Hypothesis	Alternative Hypothesis	Rejection Region
H_0: $\mu_d \le 0$	H_0: $\mu_d > 0$	$t > t_{1-\alpha,n-1}$
H_0: $\mu_d \ge 0$	H_0: $\mu_d < 0$	$t < -t_{1-\alpha,n-1}$
H_0: $\mu_d = 0$	H_0: $\mu_d \ne 0$	$\lvert t \rvert > t_{1-\alpha/2,n-1}$

The confidence interval for the mean difference in paired data can also be used to determine the precision in our estimate. It can also tell us something about statistical significance, as will be discussed in the next example.

Confidence Interval for the Mean Difference in Paired Design

The 100(1 – α)% confidence interval for the population mean difference in paired design when the mean difference in the population is approximately normally distributed and the variance σ_d^2 is not known is the interval bounded by the confidence limits

$$L = \bar{d} - t_{1-\alpha/2,n-1}\frac{s_d}{\sqrt{n}} \text{ and } R = \bar{d} + t_{1-\alpha/2,n-1}\frac{s_d}{\sqrt{n}}.$$

The value of t is obtained from Appendix B, Table 4, using $n-1$ degrees of freedom.

EXAMPLE 5.8

In a study evaluating the efficacy of a coronary heart disease prevention program at improving selected health indicators, researchers wanted to identify whether an increase in these health indicators from baseline to six weeks occurred after beginning the intervention.[16] Of interest is whether the number of steps taken each day increased. Applying the steps to hypothesis testing gives the following:

1. H_0: $\mu_d \le 0$
2. H_a: $\mu_d > 0$
3. $\alpha = 0.05$, $n = 121$
4. t-statistic and (121 − 1) = 120 degrees of freedom. On the basis of the alternative hypothesis, we see that the rejection region is in the upper tail of the t distribution. Referring to Appendix B, Table 4, the critical value is 1.658.
5. From our sample, $\bar{d} = 75$ and $s_d = 250$, then

$$t = \frac{75 - 0}{250/\sqrt{121}} = 3.3.$$

6. The exact p-value is 0.00064, obtained from the Excel formula =1-T.DIST(3.3,120,TRUE). Because the calculated value is in the rejection region (and the p-value is less than 0.05), we reject H_0 and conclude that a significant increase occurred in the average number of steps taken per day.

The 95% confidence interval is as follows:

$$L = 75 - 1.98\frac{250}{\sqrt{121}} = 30 \text{ and } R = 75 - 1.98\frac{250}{\sqrt{121}} = 120$$

Since the 95% confidence interval does not contain 0, this also tells us that at the 0.05 level, a significant change in steps occurred per day. In general, any time the p-value is less than 0.05, the 95% confidence interval will also indicate statistical significance.

Use of the t test requires that the difference scores are normally distributed. This is particularly important when the sample size is less than 30. When the paired difference is not normally distributed and the sample size is small, we can use a nonparametric procedure called the **Wilcoxon signed rank test** (see Chapter 9). There is not much of a disadvantage to using this test in terms of power, even if the difference is normally distributed. Prior to statistical software and computers, this test required considerable computational effort. However, nonparametric tests can now be easily done with the computer.

5.5.3 Hypotheses Involving a Proportion in One Group

We are now interested in testing the hypothesis that the proportion of successes in the population p has a value of p_0. When the sample size n is large, such that $np_0 > 10$ and $n(1 - p_0) > 10$, we can assume an approximate Z distribution, based on the central limit theorem.

Under H_0: $p = p_0$, the following equation has an approximate standard normal distribution if n is large.

$$z = \frac{x - np_0}{\sqrt{np_0(1-p_0)}} = \frac{f - p_0}{\sqrt{p_0(1-p_0)/n}}$$

x is the number of successes obtained in our sample. $f = \dfrac{x}{n}$ is the fraction of success in the sample.

Evaluating hypotheses in this situation is similar to testing for a normal mean where an infinite number of degrees of freedom exist. The rejection region is either one- or two-tailed, depending on whether the alternative hypothesis is one- or two-sided. There are three forms of hypotheses for a specified value of the proportion of success in the population p with a specified value p_0.

Null Hypothesis	Alternative Hypothesis	Rejection Region
H_0: $p \le p_0$	$H_a: p > p_0$	$z > z_{1-\alpha}$
H_0: $p \ge p_0$	$H_a: p < p_0$	$z < -z_{1-\alpha}$
H_0: $p = p_0$	$H_a: p \ne p_0$	$\lvert z \rvert > z_{1-\alpha/2}$

Example 5.9

A researcher is trying to accrue participants into a clinical trial and offers a cash incentive of $25 or a gift card of equal value to a local restaurant. She wants to learn whether the incentives are equally effective at recruiting participation into the study. For the first 100 entering the study, 30 chose the gift card, and 70 chose the cash. Applying the steps to hypothesis testing gives the following:

1. H_0: $p = 0.5$
2. H_a: $p \ne 0.5$
3. $\alpha = 0.05$, $n = 100$
4. z statistic, with critical values of $z_{1-0.05/2} = 1.96$
5. $z = \dfrac{f - p_0}{\sqrt{\dfrac{p_0(1-p_0)}{n}}} = \dfrac{0.3 - 0.5}{\sqrt{\dfrac{0.5(1-0.5)}{100}}} = -4$
6. Because $|z| = 4 > z_{1-0.05/2} = 1.96$, we reject the null hypothesis and conclude that the cash is a better incentive than the gift card.

The 95% CI for the population proportion is $0.3 \pm 1.96\sqrt{0.3(1-0.3)/100}$ $\rightarrow 0.21 - 0.39$, which indicates statistical significance because it does not overlap 0.5.

5.5.4 Paired Design: Proportion

It is sometimes desired to evaluate change in proportions when the same group is measured twice over time. For example, it is often of interest to compare a proportion before and after an intervention or event occurs. It is a test applied to paired data by assessing the marginal homogeneity of two binary (two-level) variables.

Consider the following contingency table, where the letters are placeholders for the data.

	Follow-Up Measure		
Baseline Measure	**Yes**	**No**	**Total**
Yes	a	b	$a+b$
No	c	d	$c+d$
Total	$a+c$	$b+d$	$n=a+b+c+d$

A **contingency table** is a table showing the distribution of one variable in rows and another in columns, used to study the association between the two variables.

The hypotheses are formulated as follows:

$$H_0: p_1 = p_2$$

$$H_a: p_1 \neq p_2$$

In a situation like this where we want to know whether the proportion of subjects with or without the characteristic of interest changes over time, the **McNemar test** is an appropriate method of assessment. The null hypothesis is rejected if the $\text{McNemar} > \chi^2_{\alpha,df}$, where $df = (\text{rows}-1)(\text{columns}-1)$. The McNemar test is written as

$$\text{McNemar} = \frac{(|b-c|)^2}{b+c}.$$

EXAMPLE 5.10

Do you approve of the way your governor is handling the COVID-19 pandemic

$$\text{McNemar} = \frac{(|b-c|-1)^2}{b+c} \text{ with Yates' Continuity Correction}$$

in your state? Assume this question was asked to a random group of 100 adult citizens before and then after a recent upsurge in COVID-19 cases. Consider the following hypothetical data.

	After	
Before	**Yes**	**No**
Yes	50	25
No	10	15

Then,

$$\text{McNemar} = \frac{(|25-10|)^2}{25+10} = 6.43 \text{ Uncorrected}$$

$$\text{McNemar} = \frac{(|25-10|-1)^2}{25+10} = 5.6 \text{ Corrected}$$

The degree of freedom for the 2 × 2 table are $(2-1)(2-1)=1$. From the χ^2 table, we obtain $\chi^2_{0.05,1} = 3.84$. Since the calculated McNemar statistic is greater, reject H_0 and conclude otherwise. In other words, those who agreed that their governor is managing the COVID-19 pandemic well decreased significantly.

From the χ^2 table, the p-value that corresponds with the calculated McNemar statistic is between 0.01 and 0.025. Using the Excel formula CHISQ.DIST (x, degrees of freedom, cumulative), we can obtain the p-value for the uncorrected and corrected McNemar statistics: =1–CHISQ.DIST(6.43,1,TRUE) returns the p-value 0.0112. Entering =1–CHISQ.DIST(5.6,1,TRUE) returns the p-value 0.0180.

The McNemar test may also be performed using SAS. Here we present the data statement and corresponding procedure code. The ORDER=DATA option is added because otherwise SAS would have inverted the rows and columns because "N" in "NO" comes before "Y" in "Yes." The AGREE option provides McNemar's test for 2 × 2 tables.

```
DATA COVID;
  INPUT BEFORE $ AFTER $ COUNT;
DATALINES;
  Yes Yes 50
  Yes No 25
  No Yes 10
  No No 15
  ;

PROC FREQ DATA=COVID ORDER=DATA;
  TABLE BEFORE*AFTER/AGREE;
  WEIGHT COUNT;
RUN;
```

Output from this program provides the McNemar's chi-square, degrees of freedom, and the p-value, as follows:

McNemar's Test		
Chi-Square	**DF**	**Pr > ChiSq**
6.4286	1	0.0112

A statistic that is commonly used to measure the level of agreement between two observers on a binary (two level) variable is **Cohen's kappa (k)**.[17]

Equation for Cohen's Kappa

$$k = \frac{\text{Observed agreement} - \text{Expected agreement}}{1 - \text{Expected agreement}}$$

Kappa ranges from –1 (perfect disagreement) to 1 (perfect agreement). When k is zero, agreement is what might be expected by chance. If k is 1, there is perfect agreement between the raters. Expected agreement in each cell is the proportion in that cell's row multiplied by the proportion in that cell's column. Cohen's kappa measures the agreement between two raters who each classify N items into C mutually exclusive categories. The following guidelines have been suggested for interpreting k in terms of agreement:[18]

0.93–1.00	Excellent agreement
0.81–0.92	Very good agreement
0.61–0.80	Good agreement
0.41–0.60	Fair agreement
0.21–0.40	Slight agreement
0.01–0.20	Poor agreement
0.00	No agreement

Example 5.11

Suppose two voice specialists assessed 50 selected voice patients for a disorder called spasmodic dysphonia (SD).

	Specialist 2		
Specialist 1	**Yes**	**No**	**Total**
Yes	13	2	15
No	8	27	35
Total	21	29	50

Specialist 1 indicates that 15 or 30% have SD, and Specialist 2 finds that 21 or 42% have SD. On the basis of the multiplication rule, the specialists would agree by chance that 30% × 42% = 12.6% of the patients have SD. Further, by chance alone, the specialists would agree that 70% × 58% = 40.6% do not have SD. Thus, the two specialists would agree by chance 12.6% + 40.6% = 53.2% of the time. In actuality, the specialists agreed on (13 + 27)/50, or 80% of the 50 patients, such that the level of agreement beyond chance is 0.80 – 0.532= 0.268, which is the numerator of k. Kappa in this situation is therefore

$$k = \frac{0.80 - 0.532}{1 - 0.532} = \frac{0.268}{0.478} = 0.57.$$

Hence, the agreement between the two specialists in diagnosing SD among voice patients is only fair.

The kappa statistic can also be produced using SAS. The data and procedure statements are presented here, with the AGREE option producing the kappa statistic.

```
DATA Voice;
  INPUT Before $ After $ Count;
DATALINES;
  Yes Yes 13
  Yes No 2
  No Yes 8
  No No 27
;
PROC FREQ DATA=Voice ORDER=DATA;
  TABLE Before*After/AGREE;
  WEIGHT Count;
RUN;
```

Partial output from the SAS program shown here contains the kappa statistic, standard error, and corresponding confidence limits.

Simple Kappa Coefficient			
Estimate	Standard Error	95% Confidence Limits	
0.5726	0.1162	0.3448	0.8005

5.6 Hypotheses Involving Means in Two Independent Groups

In this section, we will consider hypotheses that compare parameters from two independent groups. We will begin by comparing means, then variances, and then proportions.

5.6.1 Testing the Hypothesis $\mu_1 = \mu_2$

Consider the null and alternative hypotheses about the equality of the means of two normal populations.

$$H_0: \mu_1 = \mu_2$$

$$H_a: \mu_1 \neq \mu_2$$

To evaluate these hypotheses, we rely on mean estimates from two separate samples. This situation involving two samples is characterized by three assumptions:

1. Assume the samples are independent random samples, such that knowing the values of the observations in one group do not tell us anything about the observations in the other group.
2. Assume the populations are both normally distributed—this is less a concern when the sample size is at least 30, according to the central limit theorem. For smaller sample sizes where the two separate groups are not normally distributed, a nonparametric procedure called the **Wilcoxon rank sum test** is preferred (see Chapter 9).
3. Assume that the population variances for both groups are equal. If the sample sizes are equal between the two groups, the *t* test is robust to differences in the variances.

The formula for the pooled standard deviation is

$$s_p = \sqrt{\frac{(n_1 - 1)s_1^2 + (n_2 - 1)s_2^2}{n_1 + n_2 - 2}}.$$

From the pooled standard deviation, we calculate the standard error of the difference in means as follows:

Standard Error of the Difference with Equal Variance

$$SE_{(\bar{x}_1 - \bar{x}_2)} = s_p\sqrt{\frac{1}{n_1} + \frac{1}{n_2}}$$

The standard error of the difference is used in the denominator of the *t* statistic when evaluating the difference between means from two independent groups.

Equation for the *t* Statistic for Comparing Independent Means with Equal Variances

$$t = \frac{\bar{x}_1 - \bar{x}_2}{s_p\sqrt{\frac{1}{n_1} + \frac{1}{n_2}}}$$

Degrees of freedom: $n_1 + n_2 - 2$

The *F* test is a statistical procedure that is commonly used to evaluate the equality of two variances. To calculate the *F*, the larger variance is divided by the smaller variance, and the resulting ratio is compared with the critical value from the *F* distribution (see Appendix B, Table 6). Equal variances will result in a ratio of 1. If the ratio is significantly greater than 1, we conclude that the variances are not equal. If the variances are not equal, then the pooled standard error will be underestimated.

Equality of Population Variances

As a general rule, we can say the population variances are equal if the larger standard deviation divided by the smaller standard deviation is less than 2.

The *F* distribution is an asymmetric probability distribution that ranges from 0 to infinity. It has two degrees of freedom, v_1 for the numerator, v_2 for the denominator. For each combination of these degrees of freedom, the *F* distribution differs. The distribution has the greatest spread when the degrees of freedom are small.

Hypotheses of Equality of Variances

$$H_0\colon \sigma_1^2 = \sigma_2^2 \quad H_a\colon \sigma_1^2 \neq \sigma_2^2$$

If $F > F_{\alpha/2, v_1, v_2}$, then reject H_0, where $F = s_1^2 / s_2^2$ and the degrees of freedom are $v_1 = n_1 - 1$ and $v_2 = n_2 - 1$. The largest sample variance is always placed in the numerator of the ratio.

Standard Error of the Difference with Unequal Variance

$$SE_{(\bar{x}_1 - \bar{x}_2)} = \sqrt{\left(\frac{s_1^2}{n_1} + \frac{s_2^2}{n_2}\right)}$$

Equation for the *t* Statistic for Comparing Independent Means with Unequal Variances

$$t_v = \frac{(\bar{x}_1 - \bar{x}_2) - 0}{\sqrt{\left(\frac{s_1^2}{n_1} + \frac{s_2^2}{n_2}\right)}}$$

Degrees of freedom: $n_1 + n_2 - 2$

To calculate the approximate degrees of freedom when the variances are not equal

$$v = \frac{\left[\left(\frac{s_1^2}{n_1}\right) + \left(\frac{s_2^2}{n_2}\right)\right]^2}{\frac{(s_1^2/n_1)^2}{(n_1 - 1)} + \frac{(s_2^2/n_2)^2}{(n_2 - 1)}}$$

If *v* involves a decimal place, round down to the nearest integer value. Using the Satterthwaite approximation, t_v can be approximated by a *t* distribution with *v* degrees of freedom, and we can use Appendix B, Table 4. Note that SAS computes the *t* test for both the pooled and nonpooled Satterthwaite approaches, and consultation of the *F* test for equality of variances will direct you to what *t*-statistic should be considered.

There are three possible formulations of the hypotheses:

Null Hypothesis	Alternative Hypothesis	Rejection Region
$H_0: \mu_1 \le \mu_2$	$H_a: \mu_1 > \mu_2$	$t > t_{1-\alpha,\, n_1+n_2-2}$
$H_0: \mu_1 \ge \mu_2$	$H_a: \mu_1 < \mu_2$	$t < -t_{1-\alpha,\, n_1+n_2-2}$
$H_0: \mu_1 = \mu_2$	$H_a: \mu_1 \ne \mu_2$	$\lvert t \rvert > t_{1-\alpha/2,\, n_1+n_2-2}$

Finally, the confidence interval for the difference between the two means has a similar structure as other confidence intervals, namely the statistic, plus and minus a critical value multiplied by the standard error of the statistic.

The 100(1 – α)% confidence interval for the difference between two means is given by the interval with the confidence limits

$$L = (\bar{x}_1 - \bar{x}_2) - t_{1-\alpha/2, n_1+n_2-2}\, SE_{(\bar{x}_1-\bar{x}_2)} \text{ and}$$
$$R = (\bar{x}_1 - \bar{x}_2) + t_{1-\alpha/2, n_1+n_2-2}\, SE_{(\bar{x}_1-\bar{x}_2)}.$$

The value of t is obtained from Appendix B, Table 4, using $n_1 + n_2 - 2$ degrees of freedom.

Example 5.12

Clinical studies involving random assignment of participants to an intervention or control group may be evaluated to see how well the randomization worked. Effective randomization of participants should produce groups that look similar in terms of demographics, health behaviors, and health conditions. The Coronary Health Improvement Project (CHIP) had 337 volunteers, aged 43 to 81.[19] In this example we will apply the steps to hypothesis testing to evaluate whether mean age significantly differs between participants in the intervention and control arms of the study.

1. $H_0: \mu_I = \mu_C$
2. $H_a: \mu_I \ne \mu_C$
3. $\alpha = 0.05$, $n = 337$
4. t statistic, with $(167 + 170 - 2) = 335$ degrees of freedom. On the basis of the alternative hypothesis, we see that the rejection region is in the lower and upper tails of the t distribution. Referring to Appendix B, Table 4, the critical values are –1.96 and 1.96.
5. From our sample

$$n_I = 167,\ \bar{x}_I = 50.39, \text{ and } s_I^2 = 10.97$$

$$n_C = 170,\ \bar{x}_C = 50.83, \text{ and } s_C^2 = 11.13$$

To test for equality of variances, $F = 11.13/10.97 = 1.015$. We now compare this value with $F_{0.05/2,167,170} = 1.354$. Note: the critical F was obtained in Excel, with the formula =F.INV.RT(0.025,167,170). It can also be obtained using an online calculator.[20]

Since the calculated value is smaller than the critical value, we fail to reject the null hypothesis of equality of variances. Hence, it is appropriate to use a pooled standard deviation in the t statistic.

$$t_{n_1+n_2-2} = \frac{(50.39 - 50.83)}{3.32\sqrt{\left(\frac{1}{167} + \frac{1}{170}\right)}} = -1.22$$

6. Because −1.22 is not in the rejection region, we fail to reject the null hypothesis and conclude that the mean ages are similar between the intervention and control groups.

The 95% confidence interval is calculated as follows:

$$L = (50.39 - 50.83) - 1.96 \times 0.362 = -1.15$$

$$R = (50.39 - 50.83) - 1.96 \times 0.362 = 0.270$$

Because the interval (−1.15, 0.270) overlaps 0, we conclude that there is no difference in the mean ages between the intervention and control groups.

Example 5.13

In a study involving quality of life indicators among 94 patients with obstructive sleep apnea, researchers assessed the burden of possible upper airway related symptoms (i.e., voice, cough, and diurnal dyspnea) on Short Form (SF)-36 quality of life measures.[21] Some of the data from this study are presented in **Table 5.2**. Component measures of mental and physical quality of life are shown. In this example, we will apply the steps to hypothesis testing to evaluate whether mean component physical quality of life significantly differs between patients who use continuous positive airway pressure (CPAP) and those who do not. We will also use SAS to evaluate the data.

1. H_0: $\mu_{\text{CPAP}} = \mu_{\text{NOCPAP}}$
2. H_a: $\mu_{\text{CPAP}} \neq \mu_{\text{NOCPAP}}$
3. $\alpha = 0.05$, $n = 94$
4. t statistic, with $(74 + 20 - 2) = 92$ degrees of freedom. On the basis of the alternative hypothesis, we see that the rejection region is in the lower and upper tails of the t distribution. Referring to Appendix B, Table 4, the critical value is between 1.984 and 1.99. The Excel formula =T.INV.2T(0.05,92) = 1.986.
5. The SAS program containing the data and procedure code for this data are as follows:

```
DATA T5_2;
   INPUT Subject Mental Physical VP $ CPAP $ Sex $ Sum;
   DATALINES;
   ...
   ;
PROC TTEST DATA=T5_2;
   CLASS CPAP;
   VAR Physical;
RUN;
```

SAS output in the first two boxes shows descriptive information on the outcome variable according to CPAP use. The third box shows the results for the t test of equality of means. The fourth box shows the results from the F test of equality of variances. The null hypothesis being evaluated with the F test is that the variances are equal. Given the small F value and large p-value, we fail to reject the null hypothesis of equal variances. Also, the simple rule regarding equality of population variances holds (i.e., $23.73/22.18 = 1.07 < 2$). This tells us that it is appropriate to use a pooled standard deviation in the t statistic. In the third box, the t statistic is computed based on a pooled standard deviation and also for the case where the

Table 5.2 Data on SF-36 Quality of Life, CPAP Use, and Sex for Patients with Obstructive Sleep Apnea

Subj	Mental	Physical	VP	CPAP	Sex	Sum	Subj	Mental	Physical	VP	CPAP	Sex	Sum
1	94.29	83.18	No	Yes	M	0	48	38.21	39.09	Yes	No	F	3
2	22.14	80.00	Yes	Yes	F	2	49	85.71	70.00	No	Yes	F	0
3	44.64	66.14	Yes	Yes	M	3	50	77.14	76.59	No	No	F	2
4	50.71	81.14	Yes	Yes	M	1	51	85.71	84.32	No	Yes	M	1
5	90.00	65.68	No	No	F	0	52	90.00	59.32	No	Yes	F	0
6	72.86	80.00	No	Yes	M	0	53	55.00	84.55	No	Yes	F	0
7	82.86	92.05	No	Yes	M	1	54	79.64	55.23	No	Yes	F	0
8	72.50	60.00	Yes	Yes	M	2	55	18.57	37.27	Yes	No	F	3
9	24.29	17.73	Yes	Yes	F	3	56	92.86	88.18	No	Yes	F	0
10	83.93	47.95	No	Yes	M	1	57	18.57	25.00	Yes	Yes	F	2
11	36.43	37.50	Yes	No	F	2	58	55.00	68.86	No	Yes	M	1
12	25.36	48.18	Yes	Yes	M	1	59	66.07	75.45	No	Yes	M	0
13	26.79	36.14	No	No	F	0	60	75.36	70.91	No	Yes	M	0
14	81.43	84.09	No	Yes	M	0	61	58.57	4.55	No	Yes	M	0
15	82.14	48.41	No	Yes	M	2	62	30.00	74.09	No	Yes	M	0
16	92.86	91.36	No	Yes	M	0	63	85.71	63.86	No	Yes	M	0
17	90.00	73.86	No	Yes	M	0	64	28.57	38.18	No	Yes	M	0
18	63.93	84.55	No	Yes	F	0	65	85.71	85.68	No	No	M	0
19	73.93	86.82	No	Yes	M	0	66	74.29	22.50	No	No	F	0
20	60.00	20.23	Yes	Yes	F	3	67	74.29	75.00	No	Yes	M	0
21	70.00	90.00	No	Yes	M	0	68	82.50	84.32	No	Yes	M	0
22	61.43	29.55	Yes	Yes	F	2	69	78.21	84.09	No	Yes	F	2
23	85.71	79.55	No	Yes	M	0	70	70.36	40.00	Yes	Yes	M	1
24	95.36	92.50	No	Yes	M	0	71	90.00	89.77	No	Yes	M	0

(Continues)

Table 5.2 Data on SF-36 Quality of Life, CPAP Use, and Sex for Patients with Obstructive Sleep Apnea *(Continued)*

Subj	Mental	Physical	VP	CPAP	Sex	Sum	Subj	Mental	Physical	VP	CPAP	Sex	Sum
25	61.43	74.32	No	No	M	0	72	51.07	59.77	Yes	No	F	3
26	92.86	74.32	No	Yes	F	0	73	78.57	75.68	Yes	Yes	M	2
27	92.86	90.91	Yes	Yes	F	1	74	50.71	52.73	No	Yes	M	0
28	56.43	58.64	Yes	Yes	F	3	75	87.14	84.32	No	Yes	M	0
29	72.86	71.36	No	Yes	F	0	76	74.29	57.73	No	Yes	M	0
30	55.36	26.82	No	No	F	0	77	61.07	63.18	Yes	Yes	M	3
31	81.07	18.86	Yes	No	F	3	78	33.21	16.59	Yes	Yes	F	3
32	42.86	72.73	No	Yes	M	0	79	81.43	31.36	Yes	Yes	F	2
33	65.71	53.18	No	Yes	M	0	80	78.57	74.32	Yes	No	F	3
34	75.71	70.91	Yes	No	F	1	81	53.21	11.36	Yes	Yes	M	3
35	91.43	89.77	No	Yes	M	0	82	30.00	50.68	No	Yes	M	1
36	88.57	78.86	Yes	Yes	F	1	83	58.57	16.82	Yes	Yes	F	3
37	33.93	53.86	No	Yes	M	0	84	46.43	15.45	Yes	Yes	F	1
38	78.57	63.18	Yes	Yes	F	2	85	55.71	62.73	No	No	M	0
39	94.29	75.45	No	Yes	M	0	86	60.71	70.45	Yes	Yes	M	1
40	90.00	95.45	No	Yes	M	0	87	37.14	72.95	No	Yes	M	1
41	80.00	80.91	Yes	Yes	M	2	88	80.00	93.18	No	Yes	F	0
42	64.29	73.18	No	Yes	M	0	89	69.64	57.27	Yes	No	F	2
43	62.86	80.68	Yes	Yes	M	1	90	56.43	64.09	Yes	Yes	F	3
44	62.50	49.55	No	Yes	M	1	91	62.14	55.45	Yes	Yes	M	1
45	24.29	82.50	No	No	M	0	92	46.79	13.18	Yes	Yes	F	3
46	26.07	25.00	No	No	F	0	93	71.07	50.23	Yes	Yes	M	1
47	43.57	24.55	Yes	No	F	3	94	70.00	54.77	No	No	F	0

VP: Voice problem. Sum: Total number of voice, cough, and breathing problems.

variances are not equal, based on the Satterthwaite method. Because the F test did not reject the null hypothesis of equal variances, we will refer to the t statistic based on the pooled method. This gives a t value of –2.09 and a corresponding p-value of 0.0398.

CPAP	Method	N	Mean	Std Dev	Std Err	Minimum	Maximum
No		20	51.6135	22.1820	4.9600	18.8600	85.6800
Yes		74	63.9247	23.7303	2.7586	4.5500	95.4500
Diff (1-2)	Pooled		-12.3112	23.4189	5.9020		
Diff (1-2)	Satterthwaite		-12.3112		5.6756		

CPAP	Method	Mean	95% CL Mean		Std Dev	95% CL Std Dev	
No		51.6135	41.2320	61.9950	22.1820	16.8692	32.3984
Yes		63.9247	58.4269	69.4226	23.7303	20.4273	28.3175
Diff (1-2)	Pooled	-12.3112	-24.0331	-0.5893	23.4189	20.4691	27.3700
Diff (1-2)	Satterthwaite	-12.3112	-23.8751	-0.7474			

Method	Variances	DF	t Value	Pr > |t|
Pooled	Equal	92	-2.09	0.0398
Satterthwaite	Unequal	31.78	-2.17	0.0377

Equality of Variances				
Method	Num DF	Den DF	F Value	Pr > F
Folded F	73	19	1.14	0.7706

6. Because $|-2.09| > 1.986$, we reject the null hypothesis and conclude that the mean component physical quality of life measure is significantly different between CPAP and non-CPAP users, being higher (better) in the former group.

We also see that the 95% confidence interval does not overlap 0, which is expected because the p-value is less than 0.05. Both the confidence interval and p-value indicate statistical significance.

5.6.2 Testing the Hypothesis $p_1 = p_2$

For two binomial populations, we may be interested in testing the hypothesis that the proportions are equal between both populations. In a sample from the first population, the proportion of "success" is $f_1 = x_1/n_1$. In a sample from the second population, the proportion of "success" is $f_2 = x_2/n_2$. The fraction of success for the pooled samples is

$$f_{\text{pooled}} = \frac{x_1 + x_2}{n_1 + n_2}.$$

The estimate of the standard error under the assumption that the proportions are the same is

$$SE_{f_1-f_2} = \sqrt{\frac{f_1(1-f_1)}{n_1} + \frac{f_2(1-f_2)}{n_2}}.$$

If $p_1 = p_2$, the variance can be reduced to

$$SE_{f_1-f_2} = \sqrt{f_{\text{pooled}}(1-f_{\text{pooled}})\left[\frac{1}{n_1} + \frac{1}{n_2}\right]}.$$

Under the null hypothesis, the following quantity has an approximately standard normal distribution if n_1 and n_2 are large, with

$$n_1 f_{\text{pooled}} > 5,\ n_1(1-f_{\text{pooled}}) > 5 \text{ and}$$

$$n_2 f_{\text{pooled}} > 5,\ n_2(1-f_{\text{pooled}}) > 5.$$

$$z = \frac{f_1 - f_2}{\sqrt{f_{\text{pooled}}(1-f_{\text{pooled}})\left[\frac{1}{n_1} + \frac{1}{n_2}\right]}}$$

There are three possible forms of hypotheses:

Null Hypothesis	Alternative Hypothesis	Rejection Region
$H_0: p_1 \le p_2$	$H_a: p_1 > p_2$	$z > z_{1-\alpha}$
$H_0: p_1 \ge p_2$	$H_a: p_1 < p_2$	$z < -z_{1-\alpha}$
$H_0: p_1 = p_2$	$H_a: p_1 \ne p_2$	$\lvert z \rvert > z_{1-\alpha/2}$

EXAMPLE 5.14

In the previous example, mean age was similar between those randomly assigned to the intervention and control groups. We may also ask whether the distribution of males to females was similar in both groups. We will compare the proportion of males between both groups. Applying the steps to hypothesis testing gives the following:

1. $H_0: p_I = p_C$
2. $H_a: p_I \ne p_C$
3. $\alpha = 0.05$, $n = 337$
4. z test. Referring to Appendix B, Table 3, the critical values are –1.96 and 1.96.
5. From our sample
   $n_I = 167,\ f_I = 0.2695$
   $n_C = 170,\ f_C = 0.2882$

$$f_{\text{pooled}} = \frac{45+49}{167+170} = 0.2789$$

$$z = \frac{0.2695 - 0.2882}{\sqrt{0.2789(1 - 0.2789)\left[\frac{1}{167} + \frac{1}{170}\right]}} = -0.3827$$

6. Because –0.38 is not in the rejection region, we fail to reject the null hypothesis of equal proportions of males to females between intervention and control groups.

Now we will consider the confidence interval for the difference in proportions.

Confidence Interval for $p_1 - p_2$

The 100(1 – α)% confidence interval for the population difference in proportions from two distinct groups is the interval with the following confidence limits:

$$L = (f_1 - f_2) - Z_{1-\alpha/2}\sqrt{\frac{f_1(1-f_1)}{n_1} + \frac{f_2(1-f_2)}{n_2}}$$

$$R = (f_1 - f_2) + Z_{1-\alpha/2}\sqrt{\frac{f_1(1-f_1)}{n_1} + \frac{f_2(1-f_2)}{n_2}}$$

Sample size requirement:

$$n_1 f_1 > 5,\ n_1(1 - f_1) > 5$$

$$n_2 f_2 > 5,\ n_2(1 - f_2) > 5$$

$$L = (0.2695 - 0.2882) - 1.96\sqrt{\frac{0.2695 \times (1 - 0.2695)}{167} + \frac{0.2882 \times (1 - 0.2882)}{170}}$$

$$= -0.114$$

$$R = (0.2695 - 0.2882) + 1.96\sqrt{\frac{0.2695 \times (1 - 0.2695)}{167} + \frac{0.2882 \times (1 - 0.2882)}{170}}$$

$$= 0.077$$

Because the 95% confidence interval (–0.114, 0.077) overlaps 0, we conclude that there is no difference in the proportion of males to females between the intervention and control groups.

Example 5.15

Referring to the data in Table 5.2, suppose we want to know whether having a voice disorder is associated with sex. We will apply the steps of hypothesis testing and use SAS programming to address this problem.

1. H_0: $p_M = p_F$
2. H_a: $p_M \neq p_F$
3. $\alpha = 0.05$, $n = 94$
4. The z test could be used, but the χ^2 test, which we will discuss at length in the next section, will be used. Referring to Appendix B, Table 5, the critical value is 3.84. The Excel formula =CHISQ.INV.RT(0.05,1) gives 3.84.

5. The SAS procedure we will use for this example is FREQ. The asterisk combining the variables tells SAS to create a 2 × 2 table for the two binary variables.

```
PROC FREQ DATA=T5_2;
  TABLE Sex*VP/CHISQ;
RUN;
```

Partial output from this program is shown next. The first box summarizes the number of patients according to sex and voice problem. It contains percent values in each cell and by row and by column. The second box includes several statistics. For now, we will just focus on the chi-square statistic. The chi-square value is large, and the *p*-value is small.

Frequency Percent Row Pct Col Pct	Table of Sex by VP			
		VP		
	Sex	No	Yes	Total
	F	17 18.09 41.46 29.82	24 25.53 58.54 64.86	41 43.62
	M	40 42.55 75.47 70.18	13 13.83 24.53 35.14	53 56.38
	Total	57 60.64	37 39.36	94 100.00

Statistic	DF	Value	Prob
Chi-Square	1	11.2016	0.0008
Likelihood Ratio Chi-Square	1	11.3347	0.0008
Continuity Adj. Chi-Square	1	9.8221	0.0017
Mantel-Haenszel Chi-Square	1	11.0824	0.0009
Phi Coefficient		-0.3452	
Contingency Coefficient		0.3263	
Cramer's V		-0.3452	

6. Because $\chi^2 = 11.20 > 3.84$ (or the *p*-value $= 0.0008 < 0.05 = \alpha$), we reject the null hypothesis and conclude that men and women have a different probability of having a voice problem. In the first box, we see that 58.54% of women have a voice disorder as opposed to 24.53% of men.

5.7 Chi-Square Distribution

The χ^2 test is a statistical hypothesis test that is appropriate to perform when the test statistic is distributed as a χ^2 distribution under the null hypothesis. The χ^2 test has different purposes. Three important uses of the χ^2 test are to evaluate goodness of fit, evaluate independence between categorical variables, and to determine if the variance of a population is equal to a specified value.

5.7.1 Chi-Square for Test of Goodness of Fit

The χ^2 test for assessing goodness of fit is used to determine whether sample data are consistent with a hypothesized distribution. That is, this test shows how different your data are from the expected values. The test is appropriate for a categorical variable taken from a single population.

Example 5.16

Suppose during the COVID-19 pandemic that adherence to mask wearing while in public is believed to be 75% for ages 18–29, 80% for ages 30–44, 85% for ages 45–65, and 90% for ages 65+. A random sample of 100 people is taken regarding mask wearing in public according to age. A χ^2 goodness of fit test is applied to determine whether the sample distribution differs significantly from the expected distribution. Applying the steps of hypothesis testing gives the following:

1. H_0: $p_1 = 0.75, p_2 = 0.80, p_3 = 0.85, p_4 = 0.90$
2. H_a: At least one of the proportions in the null hypothesis is false.
3. $\alpha = 0.05$, $n = 100$
4. χ^2 goodness of fit to assess difference between the observed and expected values. Degrees of freedom = levels of the categorical variable (k) minus 1; $k - 1 = 4 - 1 = 3$. Referring to Appendix B, Table 5, the critical value is 7.81. The Excel formula =CHISQ.INV.RT(0.05,3) gives 7.81.
5. From a random sample of 100 people, observed adherence to mask wearing while in public is 60% for ages 18–29, 64% for ages 30–44, 76% for ages 45–64, and 82% for ages 65+. Applying these data to the χ^2 gives the following:

$$\chi^2 = \sum_{i=1}^{4} \frac{(O_i - E_i)^2}{E_i} = \frac{(60-75)^2}{75} + \frac{(64-80)^2}{80} + \frac{(76-85)^2}{85} + \frac{(82-90)^2}{90}$$
$$= 7.86$$

   Note that $E_i = np_i$ is the expected count for the ith level of the categorical variable. The sample size is n, and the hypothesized proportion of observations in the ith level is p_i.

6. Because $\chi^2 = 7.86 > 7.81$, we reject H_0 and conclude that the sample data are not consistent with a hypothesized distribution.

5.7.2 Chi-Square for Test of Independence

A second important use of the χ^2 test is for assessing whether two categorical variables are related. No relationship means independence. In other words, this test is used to determine if the values of one categorical variable depend on the values of the other categorical variable. The null hypothesis is that the two variables are independent. The alternative hypothesis is that the two variables are not independent.

Example 5.17

Consider the example given earlier in this chapter in which we wanted to know whether men and women wear masks in public at the same level. Applying the steps of hypothesis test gives the following:

1. H_0: $p_M = p_F$
2. H_a: $p_M \neq p_F$

3. $\alpha = 0.05$, $n = 600$
4. The χ^2 distribution is used to assess counts in the contingency table. A general two-way contingency table has (Rows – 1)(Columns – 1) degrees of freedom. In the current example the degrees of freedom are 1. Referring to Appendix B, Table 5, the critical value is 3.84. The Excel formula =CHISQ.INV.RT(0.05,1) gives 3.84.
5. In this example we are interested in comparing whether sex is related to mask wearing in public, with sex represented by the rows in a contingency table and mask wearing by the columns. A cell of the table represents the intersection of a row and column.

	Mask	No Mask	Total
Men	225	75	300
Women	250	50	300
Total	475	125	600

The equation for the χ^2 for a contingency table is as follows:

$$\chi^2 = \sum_{i,j} \frac{(O_{ij} - E_{ij})^2}{E_{ij}}$$

O_{ij} = number observed to belong to the ith row and jth column
R_i = total observed number in the ith row
C_j = total observed number in the jth column
$E_{ij} = \frac{R_i C_j}{n}$
Degrees of freedom: (Rows – 1)(Columns – 1)

The expected number in each cell is obtained by multiplying the row total by the column total and dividing by the overall total. This gives the following:

	Mask	No Mask	Total
Men	237.5	62.5	300
Women	237.5	62.5	300
Total	475	125	600

The next step is, within each cell, to subtract the expected value from the observed value, square it, and then divide by the expected value.

	Mask	No Mask
Men	0.658	2.5
Women	0.658	2.5

Now, sum these values to get the calculated χ^2 value:

$$\chi^2 = 0.658 + 0.658 + 2.5 + 2.5 = 6.32$$

6. Because $\chi^2 = 6.32 > 3.84$, we reject the null hypothesis and conclude that sex and mask wearing are not independent. To obtain the p-value once we have calculated the χ^2, use the Excel formula =CHISQ.DIST.RT(6.32,1), which gives the exact p-value of 0.0119. Because p-value = $0.0119 < 0.05 = \alpha$, we come to the same conclusion about statistical significance.

Note that it is often informative to identify which cells contributed most to the χ^2 test statistic. If an individual χ^2 component is at least 4, the corresponding cell is a major contributor to the test statistic. This example has no major contributors. Further, by converting the row counts to row percentages, we can compare conditional probabilities. In this example, 75% of men wore masks and 83% of women wore masks.

5.7.3 Chi-Square for Test of Independence with Small Numbers

The χ^2 procedure, like the test for evaluating differences in proportions based on the z approximation, is an approximation method. The χ^2 test should not be used for evaluating independence if the expected frequency in any given cell is less than 5. Sometimes a less conservative approach is taken that if any expected frequency is less than 2 or if more than 20% of the expected frequencies are less than 5, then the χ^2 test should not be used. To determine whether two categorical variables have nonrandom associations when the expected frequencies in the contingency table are small, the Fisher's exact test is preferred to the χ^2 test. The Fisher's exact test was designed for a 2 × 2 contingency table with small expected frequencies or large discrepancies between cell numbers. The null hypothesis tested by both the Fisher's exact test and the χ^2 test is that two categorical variables have no correlation with each other. Most statistical programs provide the Fisher's exact test, along with the χ^2 test when analyzing 2 × 2 contingency tables.

Fisher's exact test is a statistical test used to assess contingency tables. It gives the exact probability of the occurrence of the observed frequencies, according to the assumption of independence and size of the row and column totals (marginal frequencies). The probability of obtaining the observed frequencies in the 2 × 2 contingency table is

$$P = \frac{(a+b)!(c+d)!(a+c)!(b+d)!}{a!b!c!d!n!}.$$

Example 5.18

Suppose the rate of low birth weight was greater than expected in a region. Researchers asked whether living near a high-hazard dump site compared with a low-hazard dump site increased the risk of having a low-birth-weight child. A contingency table representing randomly selected data from a study investigation appears as follows:

Low Birth Weight and Residence During Pregnancy

Residence During Pregnancy	Low Birth Weight	Normal Weight	Total
Near High-Hazard Dump Site	8	30	38
Near Low-Hazard Dump Site	3	50	53
Total	11	80	91

Applying the steps to hypothesis testing gives the following:

1. H_0: Hazardous dump site residence status is independent of low-birth-weight status
2. H_a: Hazardous dump site residence status is NOT independent of low-birth-weight status
3. $\alpha = 0.05$, $n = 91$
4. Fisher's exact test.
5. In this example we will use the following SAS program to evaluate the data.

```
DATA Hazard;
   INPUT Location $ Birth_Weight $ COUNT;
DATALINES;
   H L 8
   H N 30
   L L 3
   L N 50
   ;
PROC FREQ DATA = Hazard ORDER=DATA;
   TABLE Location* Birth_Weight/EXPECTED CHISQ;
   WEIGHT COUNT;
RUN;
```

   Including the EXPECTED option with the TABLE statement shows that one of the expected frequencies is less than 5. Hence, Fisher's exact test will be used to evaluate these data. A portion of the SAS output appears as follows:

Fisher's Exact Test	
Cell (1,1) Frequency (F)	8
Left-sided Pr <= F	0.9947
Right-sided Pr >= F	0.0295
Table Probability (P)	0.0242
Two-sided Pr <= P	0.0468

6. Because the p-value $= 0.0468 < 0.05 = \alpha$, we reject the null hypothesis and conclude that living near a hazardous dump site during pregnancy increases the risk of having a child with low birth weight (21.0% versus 5.7%).

5.7.4 Chi-Square for Test of a Single Variance

A third important use of the χ^2 test is to determine if the variance of a population is equal to a specified value. The problem should indicate whether a one-sided or a two-sided test is involved. For example, if we are interested in whether the variability inj time to process a new type of screening test is less than the variability of the current screening test, it is a one-sided test. If we want to know whether the new screening test has different variability in processing time to a standard screening test, it is a two-sided test. The hypotheses are formulated as follows:

Null Hypothesis	Alternative Hypothesis	Rejection Region
$H_0: \sigma^2 \le \sigma_0^2$	$H_a: \sigma^2 > \sigma_0^2$	$\chi^2 > \chi^2_{\alpha,n-1}$
$H_0: \sigma^2 \ge \sigma_0^2$	$H_a: \sigma^2 < \sigma_0^2$	$\chi^2 < \chi^2_{1-\alpha,n-1}$
$H_0: \sigma^2 = \sigma_0^2$	$H_a: \sigma^2 \ne \sigma_0^2$	$\chi^2 > \chi^2_{\alpha/2,n-1}$ or $\chi^2 < \chi^2_{1-\alpha/2,n-1}$

The test statistic for the χ^2 test of variance compares the sample variance to the target variance in the population. The likelihood of rejecting the null hypothesis increases the more this ratio deviates from 1.

Test Statistic for Assessing If the Variance Is a Specified Value σ_0^2

$$\chi^2 = \frac{(n-1)s^2}{\sigma_0^2}$$

A confidence interval for the standard deviation is derived as the square root of the upper and lower limits of the confidence interval for the variance.

Confidence Interval for σ

The $100(1-\alpha)\%$ confidence interval for the population standard deviation σ is the interval bounded by the confidence limits

$$L = \sqrt{\frac{(n-1)s^2}{\chi^2_{\alpha/2,n-1}}} \text{ and } R = \sqrt{\frac{(n-1)s^2}{\chi^2_{1-\alpha/2,n-1}}}.$$

Example 5.19

One study estimated the median incubation period of COVID-19 as 5.4 days with a standard deviation of 4.08 days.[22] Suppose that in another area, a random sample of 25 cases is taken and finds the incubation period has a standard deviation of 3.5 days. Let us test the null hypothesis that the true variance is 16.65.

1. $H_0: \sigma^2 = 16.65$
2. $H_a: \sigma^2 \ne 16.65$
3. $\alpha = 0.05$, $n = 25$
4. χ^2 with $25-1=24$ degree of freedom. The critical values are $\chi^2_{1-0.05/2,25-1} = 12.401$ and $\chi^2_{0.05/2,25-1} = 39.364$. These critical values were obtained from Appendix B, Table 5.

5. $\chi^2 = \dfrac{(n-1)s^2}{\sigma_0^2} = \dfrac{(25-1)12.25}{16.65} = 17.66$
6. Because the calculated value does not lie in the rejection region, we fail to reject the null hypothesis that the standard deviation is different than 4.08 days.

   The 95% confidence interval for the standard deviation is 2.73 – 4.87, which overlaps 4.08.

EXAMPLE 5.20

Researchers are often not only interested in subject responses on average, but how the response scores vary. It may be that the variance (or standard deviation) is just as or more important than the average. Referring to the data in Table 5.2 for a population of 94 patients with obstructive sleep apnea, the standard deviation for the component physical quality of life measure is 23.84. In a random sample of 50 adults from the general population without obstructive sleep apnea, their standard deviation in the component physical quality of life measure is 18.7. Suppose you are interested in whether this statistic is significantly lower than 23.84. Apply the steps of hypothesis testing for this problem.

1. $H_0: \sigma^2 = 568.35$
2. $H_a: \sigma^2 < 568.35$
3. $\alpha = 0.05$, $n = 50$
4. χ^2 with $50 - 1 = 49$ degrees of freedom.

   The critical values are $\chi^2_{1-0.05/2,50-1} = 31.55$ and $\chi^2_{0.05/2,50-1} = 70.22$. These critical values were calculated in Excel using CHISQ.INV.RT(probability, degree of freedom).
5. $\chi^2 = \dfrac{(n-1)s^2}{\sigma_0^2} = \dfrac{(50-1)349.69}{568.35} = 30.15$
6. Because the calculated value lies outside the range of the critical values, we reject the null hypothesis and conclude that the component physical quality of life scores in the general population vary less than 23.84.

   The 95% confidence interval for the standard deviation is 15.62 – 23.30, which does not overlap 23.84.

5.8 Evaluating Differences Using Error Bar Graphs

With sample data, an error bar graph shows the mean values of a variable for different groups of individuals. Error bars are connected to the estimated means to show the accuracy of the measurement. If the error bars around the mean values are 95% confidence intervals, then three general outcomes may occur (**Figure 5.1**). In the left panel of the chart, the error bars for both graphs do not overlap, so we conclude that the group means are significantly different at the 0.05 level. In the middle panel of the chart, the mean value for one group is contained within the error bars of the second group. In this situation we conclude that the means are not significantly different. In the right panel of the chart, the error bars overlap, but not enough to contain either of the other group's means, so we do not know if the means are significantly different. A statistical test is required here to assess whether the means significantly differ between the two groups.

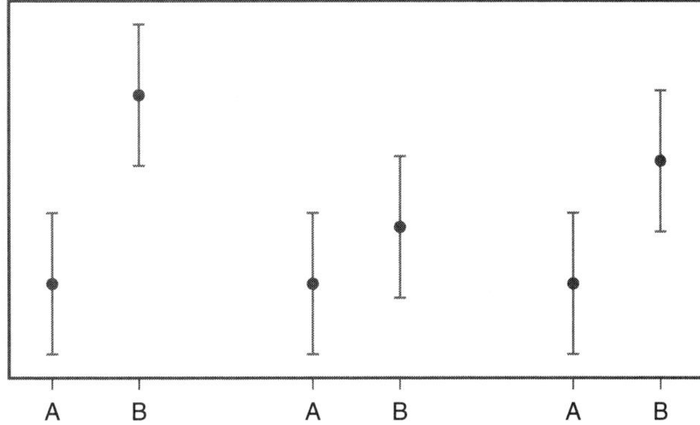

Figure 5.1 Three Visual Comparisons Between Independent Group Means and Their 95% Confidence Intervals

Example 5.21

The death-to-case ratio (%) for COVID-19 in 15 counties in the United States[23] is shown in **Figure 5.2**. As of August 3, 2020, these counties represented the highest number of cases in the country. The percentage of COVID-19 cases dying from the illness varies from 10.8% in Essex County in New Jersey to 1.4% in Miami-Dade County in Florida. Miami-Dade County has a significantly lower death-to-case ratio than the other counties. There is no significant difference between Queens and New York counties in New York. We cannot determine from the graph whether the death-to-case ratio in Essex and Wayne counties are significantly different.

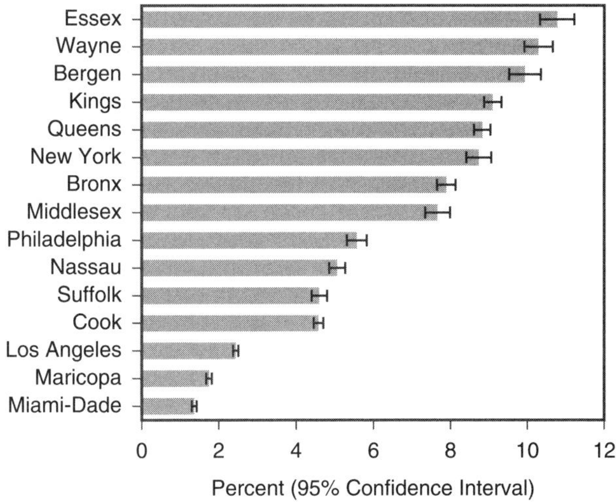

Figure 5.2 Death-to-Case (%) in 15 Counties in the United States with Leading Number of Deaths, August 3, 2020

5.9 Summary

This chapter covered methods of estimation, interval estimation, and how to establish and test hypotheses. Estimation is a process wherein we make inferences about a population using information from a sample. An estimator is a sample statistic. A point estimate is the actual numerical value of an estimator.

A single point estimate of a population characteristic is unlikely to be exactly equal to the truth. Hence, a confidence interval is often included with a point estimate to represent the range of values in which the population parameter is likely to fall. All confidence intervals have the same general form: the point estimate ± margin of error.

This chapter also presented six steps of hypothesis testing and applied them to several types of hypothesis tests. We first discussed hypotheses involving a single population and compared the sample evidence from a single sample to the hypothesized value of the population characteristic. For a single population involving a continuous variable, the sample mean was compared with the hypothesized mean. For a single binomial population, the sample relative frequency of the proportion of success was compared with the hypothesized value of the proportion of success. Hypotheses were also discussed that involved the mean of paired data and the change in proportions. The t test was shown as a way to evaluate the mean of paired data, and the McNemar test was presented as a way to evaluate change in paired proportions. Cohen's kappa k was presented as a measure of the level of agreement between two raters.

Hypotheses were then considered for evaluating means or proportions in two independent populations. First, two independent populations with the same continuous measure were evaluated by taking a sample from each population, estimating means in each group, and comparing them using an appropriate test. When two binomial populations are involved, a sample is taken from each of the populations and the same relative frequencies of successes are obtained and compared.

Hypotheses were formulated to evaluate the assumption of equal variances between two independent groups. To test this assumption, sample variances are compared between the two populations. The hypothesis of equal variance is evaluated using the F test.

Finally, three important uses of the χ^2 test were presented for evaluating goodness of fit, independence between categorical variables, and if the variance of a population is equal to a specified value.

A summary of the confidence intervals and hypothesis tests presented in this chapter is in **Table 5.3**.

Table 5.3 Summary of Confidence Intervals and Hypothesis Tests

Description	Equation
$100(1-\alpha)\%$ confidence interval for the population mean μ when the population is normally distributed and the variance σ^2 is known.	$\bar{x} \pm z_{1-\alpha/2}\frac{\sigma}{\sqrt{n}}$
$100(1-\alpha)\%$ confidence interval for the population mean μ when the population is normally distributed and the variance σ^2 is not known.	$\bar{x} \pm t_{1-\alpha/2,n-1}\frac{s}{\sqrt{n}}$
$100(1-\alpha)\%$ confidence interval for the binomial proportion of success p.	$f \pm z_{1-\alpha/2}\sqrt{\frac{f(1-f)}{n}}$ $nf > 10$ $n(1-f) > 10$

Table 5.3 Summary of Confidence Intervals and Hypothesis Tests *(Continued)*

Description	Equation
The t test statistic for one population and a continuous scaled variable. The null hypothesis is $H_0: \mu = \mu_0$.	$t = \dfrac{\bar{x} - \mu_0}{s/\sqrt{n}}$
The t test statistic for a paired design involving a continuous scaled variable. The null hypothesis is $H_0: \mu_d = 0$.	$t = \dfrac{\bar{d} - 0}{s_d/\sqrt{n}}$
The z test statistic for one binomial population. The null hypothesis is $H_0: p = p_0$.	$z = \dfrac{f - p_0}{\sqrt{p_0(1-p_0)/n}}$ $np_0 > 10$ $n(1-p_0) > 10$
The McNemar chi-square test for paired proportions. The null hypothesis is $H_0: p_1 = p_2$.	$\text{McNemar} = \dfrac{(\lvert b - c\rvert)^2}{b + c}$
The t test statistic for comparing means between two independent populations with continuous scaled measures X_1 and X_2. The null hypothesis is $H_0: \mu_1 = \mu_2$.	$t = \dfrac{\bar{x}_1 - \bar{x}_2}{SE_{(\bar{x}_1 - \bar{x}_2)}}$
The F test statistic for comparing means between two independent populations with continuous scaled measures X_1 and X_2. The null hypothesis is $H_0: \sigma_1^2 = \sigma_2^2$.	$F = \dfrac{s_1^2}{s_2^2}$
100(1 – α)% confidence interval for the difference between two means.	$(\bar{x}_1 - \bar{x}_2) \pm t_{1-\alpha/2, n_1+n_2-2} SE_{(\bar{x}_1 - \bar{x}_2)}$
The z test statistic with two binomial populations. The null hypothesis is $H_0: p_1 = p_2$. Pooled sample proportion: $f_{\text{pooled}} = \dfrac{x_1 + x_2}{n_1 + n_2}$	$z = \dfrac{f_1 - f_2}{\sqrt{f_{\text{pooled}}(1 - f_{\text{pooled}})\left[\dfrac{1}{n_1} + \dfrac{1}{n_2}\right]}}$ $n_1 f_{\text{pooled}}$; $n_1(1 - f_{\text{pooled}})$ $n_2 f_{\text{pooled}} > 5$; $n_2(1 - f_{\text{pooled}}) > 5$
100(1 – α)% confidence interval for the population difference in proportions from two distinct groups.	$(f_1 - f_2) \pm z_{1-\alpha/2}\sqrt{\dfrac{f_1(1-f_1)}{n_1} + \dfrac{f_2(1-f_2)}{n_2}}$ $n_1 f_{\text{pooled}} > 5$; $n_1(1 - f_{\text{pooled}}) > 5$ $n_2 f_{\text{pooled}} > 5$; $n_2(1 - f_{\text{pooled}}) > 5$
Independence. Equation for the χ^2 for a contingency table for testing the null hypothesis H_0: Classification of rows and columns are independent. O_{ij} = number observed to belong to the ith row and jth column. $E_{ij} = \dfrac{R_i C_j}{n}$, where R_i = total observed number in the ith row. C_j = total observed number in the jth column. Degrees of freedom = (Rows – 1)(Columns – 1)	$\chi^2 = \sum_{i,j} \dfrac{(O_{ij} - E_{ij})^2}{E_{ij}}$

(Continues)

Table 5-3 Summary of Confidence Intervals and Hypothesis Tests *(Continued)*

Description	Equation
Goodness of fit. Equation for the χ^2 for a contingency table for testing the null hypothesis H_0: Distribution is as hypothesized. Degrees of freedom = $k - 1$	$\chi^2 = \sum_i \frac{(O_i - E_i)^2}{E_i}$
Test statistic for assessing if the variance is a specified value σ_0^2; $H_0: \sigma^2 = \sigma_0^2$.	$\chi^2 = \frac{(n-1)s^2}{\sigma_0^2}$
100(1 – α)% confidence interval for the population standard deviation σ is the interval bounded by the confidence limits.	$L = \sqrt{\frac{(n-1)s^2}{\chi^2_{\alpha/2,n-1}}}$ $R = \sqrt{\frac{(n-1)s^2}{\chi^2_{1-\alpha/2,n-1}}}$

Exercises

1. For the following sample results, estimate the mean, variance, standard deviation, and standard error. Express your answer to the nearest tenth.

   a. $n = 10, \sum_i^n x_i = 40, \sum_i^n (x_i - \overline{x})^2 = 280$

   b. $n = 20, \sum_i^n x_i = 35, \sum_i^n (x_i - \overline{x})^2 = 200$

   c. $n = 5, \sum_i^n Xx_i = 50, \sum_i^n (x_i - \overline{x})^2 = 250$

2. Find the point estimates of μ, σ^2, and σ for the following data: 65, 20, 85, 45, 25, 40, 80, 40, 90, 5, 70, 5, 80, 60, 55. Note that these data represent SF-36 quality of life measures for physical functioning among a sample of morbidly obese obstructive sleep apnea patients.
3. Under what conditions is $\overline{X}$ an unbiased estimator of μ?
4. What is the difference between point and interval estimation?
5. Assuming you have random samples from normal populations with known variance, find confidence intervals for the means that have the following specifications. Express your answers to the nearest tenth.

   a. $n = 17, \overline{x} = 20, \sigma^2 = 8$, confidence level = 90%

   b. $n = 14, \overline{x} = 21, \sigma^2 = 5$, confidence level = 95%

   c. $n = 24, \overline{x} = 100, \sigma^2 = 100$, confidence level = 99%

6. What factors influence the width of a confidence interval for μ?

7. Assuming unknown variance and normal distributions, find 95% confidence intervals for the means. Note that this data was assessed in Exercise 1. Express your answer to the nearest hundredth.

   a. $n = 10, \sum_{i}^{n} X_i = 40, \sum_{i}^{n} (X_i - \bar{X})^2 = 280$

   b. $n = 20, \sum_{i}^{n} X_i = 35, \sum_{i}^{n} (X_i - \bar{X})^2 = 200$

   c. $n = 5, \sum_{i}^{n} X_i = 50, \sum_{i}^{n} (X_i - \bar{X})^2 = 250$

8. Assuming an unknown population variance and a normal distribution, and using the data from Exercise 2, find

   a. 90% confidence interval for the mean.

   b. 95% confidence interval for the mean.

   c. 99% confidence interval for the mean.

9. A dietary program was administered to a simple random sample of individuals with high cholesterol. Their cholesterol was measured before and after the intervention. The changes are as follows: 2, 4, −8, −3, −20, 5, −12, 1, −4, 10, 3, −5, −11, 7, 0, −5, −18, 14, 2, −1, 5. Find a 95% confidence interval for the mean change in cholesterol. Assume a normal distribution. Express your answer to the nearest hundredth.

10. On the basis of the interval estimate in Exercise 9, can we conclude that the intervention significantly changed cholesterol?

11. Refer to the following results from simple random samples from binomial populations. Find the best estimates for p and the standard deviation of the proportion of successes. Express your answers to the nearest thousandth.

    a. $n = 24$ and number of successes = 8

    b. $n = 65$ and number of successes = 30

    c. $n = 500$ and number of successes = 200

12. Find 95% confidence intervals for p when

    a. $n = 24$ and number of successes = 8

    b. $n = 65$ and number of successes = 30

    c. $n = 500$ and number of successes = 200

13. In a given city, a sample of 1000 individuals were interviewed. In the sample, 648 indicated that they regularly wore protective masks while in public during the COVID-19 pandemic. Give the 95% confidence interval for the proportion of people in the city who regularly wore protective masks.

14. What is a statistical hypothesis?

15. What is a statistical hypothesis test?

16. What is a p-value and its purpose?

17. What relationship does the *p*-value have with the sample size?
18. It has been reported that concern with the human spirit or soul compared with material or physical things is greater (*p*-value < 0.05) among people who attend church compared with those who do not attend church. What is a correct interpretation of this *p*-value?
19. A researcher tests the hypotheses $H_0: p = 0.10$ and $H_a: p \neq 0.10$ with $\alpha = 0.05$. The sample proportion from a random sample of 500 is 0.11. Is there sufficient evidence to reject the null hypothesis?
20. What role does hypothesis testing play in descriptive versus analytic studies?
21. A company suspects that its product may be contaminated with salmonella. The company decides to examine several randomly selected cases of the product. Its null hypothesis is that the product is contaminated.
    a. What are the Type I and Type II errors?
    b. Would the company want a small α or a small β if it had to choose for one to be smaller?
22. Define power and relate it to the probability of committing a Type II error.
23. A random sample of 17 pigs was put on a new diet for 8 weeks. Their mean weight gain over this period of time was 0.80 lb/day, with a standard deviation of 0.20 lb/day. When is it appropriate to use the formula $\overline{x} \pm t_{1-\alpha/2,n-1}\, s/\sqrt{n}$ to estimate the mean weight gain of all pigs with this new diet?
24. Assuming the conditions are met for Exercise 23, provide a 98% confidence interval for the mean weight change of the pigs. Interpret your result.

In the following exercises, assume $\alpha = 0.05$, unless otherwise indicated.

25. Suppose that the current belief is that the mean percentage of the U.S. adult population who visited the dentist in the past year is 65%. On the other hand, from your experience and observation, you believe this percentage is higher. Assume that based on a random sample of 200 adults in your community, you find $\overline{x} = 69.7\%$ and $s = 32.5\%$. Assuming a normal distribution of mean percent scores, apply the six steps to hypothesis testing.
26. Continuing with Exercise 25 but assuming a two-sided test, calculate and interpret the 95% confidence interval.

For Exercises 27–28, we will refer to a study evaluating whether a six-week coronary heart disease prevention program can lower depression and stress. This study sampled 348 individuals, ages 24 to 81.[24]

27. Mean change in the Beck Depression Inventory from baseline through follow-up was –1.53, with standard deviation of 3.38. Apply the steps of hypothesis testing to these data.
28. Continuing with Exercise 27 but assuming a two-sided test, calculate and interpret the 95% confidence interval for the mean change score in Beck Depression Inventory. Interpret your result.
29. A study wants to know whether a dietary intervention can significantly lower triglyceride scores in six weeks. A group of 10 individuals with high triglyceride scores were randomly obtained. They all participated in a dietary program. Their baseline and six week follow-up scores are as follows:

Baseline	Six Weeks
225	218
278	245
201	212
240	238
243	222
329	330
401	345
310	293
380	375
412	400

Evaluate whether the dietary intervention significantly changed triglyceride scores. Apply the six steps of hypothesis testing.

30. A change score in a measure of depression was calculated for a six-month period in both intervention and control participants. Of interest is whether the change score in different between those in the intervention group compared with those in the control group. We believe a decrease will only occur among those in the intervention group. We found the following in the intervention group: $n = 174$, $\bar{X} = -2.62$, $s = 3.02$; and for the control group: $n = 174$, $\bar{X} = -0.44$, $s = 2.73$. Test the hypothesis of equality of variance.

31. Continuing with Exercise 30, apply the steps of hypothesis testing to assess whether the mean in the intervention group is lower than the mean in the control group.

32. Calculate a 95% confidence interval for the difference in means.

33. We found that at baseline there was no difference in the level of restless sleep patterns between 100 adult participants in an intervention group and 100 adult participants in a control group. Of interest was whether an intervention could lower the percentage experiencing restless sleep. After a six-week intervention, 18% of those in the intervention group and 30% of those in the control group experienced restless sleep problems. Apply the steps of hypothesis testing using the z test.

34. Calculate the 95% confidence interval for the difference in proportions. Interpret your result.

35. It is assumed that the proportion of women in the United States ages 40 years and older that received a mammogram within the past two years is 0.80. You believe the actual proportion is less than this. Taking a random sample of 100 counties in the United States you get a proportion of 0.75. Evaluate your result using the steps of hypothesis testing. Because of the large sample size, use the z test.

36. In a random survey of 104 adults in a given community, citizens were asked in March and then again in July 2020 whether they approved of the media coverage of COVID-19. Consider the following hypothetical paired data and evaluate whether the proportion of approval significantly changed over this time. If so, comment on the direction of change.

	Follow-up Measure	
Baseline Measure	**Yes**	**No**
Yes	26	31
No	16	31

37. Suppose two students independently assessed whether several peer-reviewed articles in a given medical journal obtain a high-quality rating in terms of study design and application of appropriate statistical methods. You are interested in the level of agreement in ratings between these two students. Evaluate this observed count data for agreement.

	Student 2		
Student 1	**High Quality**	**Not High Quality**	**Total**
High Quality	22	3	25
Not High Quality	8	27	35
Total	30	30	60

38. Suppose you are interested in applying the χ^2 goodness of fit to assess whether the proportion who adhere to a dietary intervention in a clinical study in young, medium, and old age groups is $H_0: p_1 = 0.65, p_2 = 0.70, p_3 = 0.75$. Each of the age groups is equally represented. From a random sample of 100 participants, you observe for the young, medium, and old age groups that adherence is 0.64, 0.68, and 0.70. At the 0.05 level of significance, is there sufficient evidence to reject the null hypothesis?

39. Among 100 men and 100 women, the number who remained in a clinical trial through its duration was 82 and 95, respectively. Was the level of attrition similar between males and females? Show that the z test, a confidence interval for the difference in proportions, and the χ^2 test each leads to the same conclusion.

40. One COVID-19 testing site says that the average time for individuals to get their test results is 20 hours, with a standard deviation of 5 hours. To test these claims, a random sample of 10 tests was identified, with the wait times 27, 20, 29, 18, 33, 22, 42, 21, 35, and 27 hours. Apply the six steps of hypothesis testing to evaluate whether or not the mean time to get test results is 20 hours.

41. Continuing with Exercise 40, apply the six steps of hypothesis testing to assess whether the true standard deviation is 5 hours.

42. Continuing with Exercise 40, calculate the 95% confidence interval for the standard deviation and indicate what it says about statistical significance.

43. Suppose it is believed that the proportion of adults in the general population with a voice problem is 25%. However, you believe that for patients with obstructive sleep apnea the percentage having a voice problem is greater. Refer to the data in Table 5.2 and test your hypothesis, using the six steps of hypothesis testing.

44. Assess whether the mean component physical quality of life score significantly differs between those with a voice disorder versus those without a voice disorder using the data in Table 5.2. Apply the six steps of hypothesis testing.

45. Continuing with Exercise 44, calculate the 95% confidence interval for the difference in means, interpret it, and say what it tells us about statistical significance.

46. Using the data in Table 5.2, assess whether the proportion of CPAP use is similar between males and females. Apply the six steps of hypothesis testing.

47. In the obstructive sleep apnea study, information was also collected about tobacco and marijuana use. Of the 94 patients, 29 had used any tobacco products for a year or longer, of which 5 used marijuana for a year or longer. Of the 65 who had not used tobacco products for a year or longer, 2 used marijuana for a year or longer. Construct a 2×2 table and evaluate whether the expected value in any given cell is less than 5. Is use of tobacco products and marijuana use independent? Apply the six steps of hypothesis testing. Use the Fisher's Exact test if it is appropriate to do so.

48. As of August 12, 2020, death rates (per 100,000) from COVID-19 in the United States, the District of Columbia, and Puerto Rico appear in the following table.[25] An indicator variable shows if the area is in the North-East Region of the country (1 = yes, 0 = no). Test whether the mean death rate is different between areas in the North-East Region versus the other areas. Apply the six steps of hypothesis testing.

State	Rate	North East Region	State	Rate	North East Region
New Jersey	179	1	Iowa	30	0
New York	169	1	Virginia	27	0
Massachusetts	127	1	California	27	0
Connecticut	125	1	Washington	23	0
Rhode Island	96	1	Missouri	22	0
Louisiana	93	0	North Carolina	21	0
District of Columbia	84	1	Arkansas	19	0
Mississippi	65	0	Tennessee	19	0
Michigan	65	0	Kentucky	18	0
Illinois	62	0	Nebraska	18	0
Delaware	61	1	Wisconsin	17	0
Maryland	60	1	South Dakota	17	0
Arizona	58	0	Oklahoma	16	0
Pennsylvania	57	1	North Dakota	15	0
Indiana	46	0	Idaho	14	0

State	Rate	North East Region	State	Rate	North East Region
Georgia	41	0	Kansas	13	0
South Carolina	41	0	Utah	11	0
Florida	40	0	Oregon	9	0
Alabama	38	0	Puerto Rico	9	0
New Mexico	33	0	Vermont	9	1
Colorado	33	0	Maine	9	1
Texas	32	0	West Virginia	8	0
Ohio	32	0	Montana	7	0
Nevada	32	0	Wyoming	5	0
New Hampshire	31	1	Alaska	4	0
Minnesota	30	0	Hawaii	2	0

49. Continuing with Exercise 48, calculate the 95% confidence interval for the difference in means, interpret it, and say what it tells us about statistical significance.

50. Based on the confidence intervals for the death rates in the following graph, comment on whether the rates are significantly different.

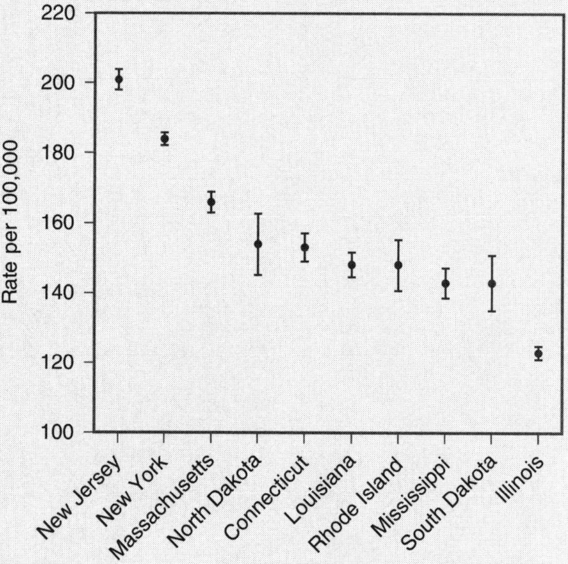

References

1. Klein, J. Francis Bacon. Stanford Encyclopedia of Philosophy; 2012. https://plato.stanford.edu/entries/francis-bacon/. First published December 29, 2003; substantive revision December 7, 2012. Accessed August 8, 2020.
2. Dweck MR, Bularga A, Hahn RT, et al. Global evaluation of echocardiography in patients with COVIC-19. *Eur Heart J Cardiovasc Imaging.* 2020;*21*(9):949–958.
3. De Bernardo G, Giordano M, Zollo, G. et al. The clinical course of SARS-CoV-2 positive neonates. *J Perinatol.* 2020;*40*(10):1462–1469.
4. Latz CA, DeCarlo C, Boitano L, et al. Blood type and outcomes in patients with COVID-19. *Ann Hematol* 2020;*99*(9):2113–2118.

5. Mizumoto K, Kagaya K, Zarebski A, Chowell G. Estimating the asymptomatic proportion of coronavirus disease 2019 (COVID-19) cases on board the Diamond Princess cruise ship, Yokohama, Japan, 2020. *Euro Surveill.* 2020;*25*(10):pii=2000180.
6. Zhang R, Wang X, Ni L, et al. COVID-19: Melatonin as a potential adjuvant treatment. *Life Sci.* 2020;*250*:117583.
7. Wang Y, Dong C, Hu Y, et al. Temporal changes of CT findings in 90 Patients with COVID-19 pneumonia: a longitudinal study. *Radiology.* 2020;*296*:E55–E64.
8. Mao L, Jin H, Wang M. Neurologic manifestations of hospitalized patients with coronavirus disease 2019 in Wuhan, China. *JAMA Neurol.* 2020;*77*(6):683–690.
9. Oxley TJ, Mocco J, Majidi S. Large-vessel stroke as a presenting feature of COVID-19 in the young. *N Engl J Med.* 2020;*382*:e60.
10. Beyrouti R, Adams ME, Benjamin L. Characteristics of ischaemic stroke associated with COVID-19. *J Neurol Neurosurg Psychiatry.* 2020;*91*(8):889–891.
11. Hassanein M, Radhakrishnan Y, Sedor J, et al. COVID-19 and the kidney. *Cleve Clin J Med.* 2020;*87*(10):619–631.
12. Ellul MA, Benjamin L, Singh B, et al. Neurological associations of COVID-19. *Lancet Neurol.* 2020;*19*(9):767–783.
13. Varatharaj A, Thomas N, Ellul MA, et al. Neurological and neuropsychiatric complications of COVID-19 in 153 patients: a UK-wide surveillance study. *Lancet Psychiatry.* 2020;*7*(10):875–882.
14. Lu Y, Li X, Geng D, et al. Cerebral micro-structural changes in COVID-19 patients — an MRI-based 3-month follow-up study. *E Clinical Medicine.* 2020;*25*:100484.
15. Abdel-Mannan O, Eyre M, Löbel U, et al. Neurologic and radiographic findings associated with COVID-19 infection in children. *JAMA Neurol.* 2020;*77*(11):1–6.
16. Merrill RM, Aldana SG. Improving overall health status through the CHIP intervention. *Am J Health Behav.* 2009;*33*(2):135–146.
17. Cohen J. A coefficient of agreement for nominal scales. *Educ Psychol Meas.* 1960; *20*(1):37–46.
18. Byrt T. How good is that agreement? *Epidemiology.* 1996;7:561.
19. Aldana SG, Greenlaw RL, Diehl HA, et al. Effects of an intensive diet and physical activity modification program on the health risks of adults. *J Am Diet Assoc.* 2005; *105*(3):371–381.
20. Social Science Statistics. Critical values calculator. https://www.socscistatistics.com/tests/criticalvalues/default.aspx. Accessed August 10, 2020.
21. Merrill RM, Roy N, Pierce J, Sundar KM. Impact of voice, cough, and diurnal breathing problems on quality of life in obstructive sleep apnea. Do they matter? *AOHNS.* 2020;*4*(2):3.
22. Yang L, Dai J, Zhao J, Wang Y, Deng P, Wang J. Estimation of incubation period and serial interval of COVID-19: analysis of 178 cases and 131 transmission chains in Hubei province, China. *Epidemiol Infect.* 2020;*148*:e117.
23. Johns Hopkins University & Medicine. COVID-19 Dashboard. https://coronavirus.jhu.edu/map.html. Accessed August 5, 2020.
24. Merrill RM, Aldana SG, Greenlaw RL, Diehl HA. The coronary health improvement project's impact on lowering eating, sleep, stress, and depressive disorders. *Am J Health Educ.* 2008;*39*(6):337–344.
25. Statista. Death rates from coronavirus (COVID-19) in the United States as of August 3, 2020, by state. https://www.statista.com/statistics/1109011/coronavirus-covid19-death-rates-us-by-state/. Accessed August 3, 2020.

CHAPTER 6

Analysis of Variance

KEY CONCEPTS

- Analysis of variance (ANOVA) is a statistical technique used to compare the means of independent groups in order to determine if there is evidence that the corresponding population means are significantly different. ANOVA is best applied when three or more population means are to be compared.
- ANOVA is a procedure that uses the computation of the variation between groups and the variation within groups (also called error variance) to test the hypothesis that *J* populations have the same mean.
- ANOVA assumes samples are randomly selected and independent of each other and that the populations are normally distributed and have equal variance.
- One-way ANOVA is appropriate when the groups are studied on one categorical variable.
- Two-way ANOVA is appropriate when the groups are studied on two categorical variables. It allows for assessing interaction between two factors.
- The *F* test is used to compare the variance between groups to the variance within groups.
- As the number of mean comparisons made increases, the chance of a Type 1 error increases.
- If comparisons are planned, they can be performed prior to completing ANOVA.
- A modified *t* statistic can be used for planned comparisons.
- When several planned comparisons are made, the α-level needs to be adjusted downward. An approach to doing this is called the Bonferroni correction.
- If the *F* test indicates overall significance in an ANOVA, then a multiple comparison method called a post hoc test can be used. Several post hoc tests are available.
- ANOVA may be used for assessing data from a complete randomized design.
- A complete randomized design involves random assignment of the same number of subjects to each treatment. When the outcome is continuous and three or more treatments are compared, ANOVA is an appropriate method to use.
- Analysis of covariance (ANCOVA) is an extension of the one-way ANOVA to include a continuous independent variable (covariate). ANCOVA is a useful approach to control for potential confounders.
- ANOVA randomized block design is another way to control for confounding and may be particularly effective when the sample size is small.
- A repeated measures ANOVA is a one-way ANOVA that involves dependent, not independent, groups. It is analogous to the paired *t* test, but with more than two groups. It is also called the within-subjects ANOVA or ANOVA for correlated samples.
- The chi-square test of independence can be used to assess hypotheses involving two categorical variables that have more than two levels.
- The Cochran-Armitage trend test will assess the trend for an ordinal variable by a categorical variable with two levels.
- The Cochran-Mantel-Haenszel test will assess the trend for an ordinal variable by a categorical variable with three or more levels.

In the current chapter, we extend the two-sample test of hypothesis to j independent, normally distributed populations. The statistical technique that allows us to evaluate whether three or more populations have the same mean is called analysis of variance (ANOVA). The hypotheses are extended as H_0: $\mu_1 = \mu_2 = \cdots = \mu_j$, H_a: At least one μ_j differs from the others. These hypotheses are evaluated using the ***F* test**, based on data from j samples. In this chapter, we will present two types of ANOVA (one way and two way), tests for multiple comparisons, ANOVA for completely randomized design, analysis of covariance (ANCOVA), ANOVA for randomized complete block design, and repeated measures ANOVA. Finally, we will cover methods for assessing categorical variables where one has two levels and the other has more than two levels, or where both have more than two levels.

6.1 Analysis of Variance Concepts and Computations

ANOVA involves partitioning the total variance of a variable into components explained by different sources of variation.

Analysis of variance (ANOVA) is a procedure that uses the computation of the variation between groups and the variation within groups to test the hypothesis that j populations have the same means.

ANOVA is a parametric procedure that has some assumptions involving independence, normality, and equality of variance. The underlying populations from which samples are taken will never exactly satisfy these assumptions. Therefore, the question is whether violations of the assumptions have serious effects on the power and significance of the F test. Studies have shown that the F test is robust against violation of the normality assumption, especially with larger sample size. Violations of constant variance is also not as critical. Violation of the independence assumption is the most serious assumption to fail. Random sampling and assignment helps ensure independence. In addition, a large sample size helps offset the effect of violations of the normality assumption.[1]

Assumptions in ANOVA

1. All the samples are randomly selected and are **independent** of one another.
2. The populations from which the samples are drawn are **normally distributed**.
3. All the populations have **equal variance**.

These assumptions can be checked by calculating descriptive statistics for each variable. For example, normality is established if the mean and median scores are similar. Equality of population variances among j groups is established if the largest standard deviation s divided by the smallest standard deviation s is less than 2.

We will discuss two types of ANOVA: one way and two way. A one-way ANOVA has one independent variable in the model. A two-way ANOVA has two independent variables in the model. For example, if you were interested in assessing whether self-reported weight differs from actual weight, on average, according to age group (young, middle, old), the single independent variable age makes this a one-way ANOVA. If you wanted to know whether self-reported weight differs from actual weight, on average, according to age group and sex, the two independent variables make it a two-way ANOVA. A two-way ANOVA is a factorial design. Factorial designs allow us to consider how multiple factors affect the outcome variable, independently as well as together.

One-way ANOVA involves data about one numerical dependent variable and one categorical independent variable. The independent variable has three or more levels. ANOVA is used to tell us whether there are significant differences among the means across the levels of the independent variable.

Two-way ANOVA involves assessment of how the means of a numerical dependent variable change across the levels of two categorical independent variables.

We will begin with one-way ANOVA. To conduct a one-way ANOVA and test the null hypothesis that three or more means are equal, we take independent samples from each of the populations of interest and obtain certain measures that allow us to compute sums of squared deviations. In the context of ANOVA, the sum of squares (SS_T) refers to the deviations of all of the observations from the mean; it is the total variance of the observations. The total variability of observed data measured as SS_T can be written as the portion of the variability explained by the model (SS_B) and the portion unexplained by the model (SS_E), as

$$SS_T = SS_B + SS_E.$$

We define these expressions as follows:

$$SS_T = \sum_{i=1}^{N}\sum_{j=1}^{J}\left(X_{ij} - \bar{\bar{X}}\right)^2$$

$$SS_B = \sum_{j=1}^{J}\left(\bar{X}_j - \bar{\bar{X}}\right)^2$$

$$SS_E = \sum_{i=1}^{N}\sum_{j=1}^{J}\left(X_{ij} - \bar{X}_j\right)^2$$

In addition, X_{ij} is the ith observation in the jth group; $\bar{X}_j$ is the mean of all observations in the jth group; and $\bar{\bar{X}}$ is the grand mean of the observations.

In the following formulas we see that the sums of squares are divided by the degrees of freedom to obtain the mean squares. The degrees of freedom for the total group are $N-1$, where N is total number of observations; between groups are $J-1$; and within groups are $N-J$.

Computational Formulas

$$SS_T = \sum_{i=1}^{N}\sum_{j=1}^{J}\left(X_{ij} - \overline{\overline{X}}\right)^2 = \sum_{i=1}^{N}\sum_{j=1}^{J}X_{ij}^2 - \frac{\left(\sum_{i=1}^{N}\sum_{j=1}^{J}X_{ij}\right)^2}{N}$$

$$SS_B = \sum_{j=1}^{N}\left(\overline{X}_j - \overline{\overline{X}}\right)^2 = \sum_{j=1}^{J}n_j\overline{X}_j^2 - \frac{\left(\sum_{i=1}^{N}\sum_{j=1}^{J}X_{ij}\right)^2}{N}$$

$$SS_E = SS_T - SS_B$$

$$MS_B = \frac{SS_B}{J-1}$$

$$MS_E = \frac{SS_E}{N-J}$$

The final step in ANOVA is to obtain the F ratio of MS_B divided by MS_E.

Hypotheses on Equality of Several Population Means and Rejection Region for ANOVA

$H_0: \mu_1 = \mu_2 = \cdots = \mu_J$

H_a: At least one μ_j differs from the others

If $F > F_{\alpha,v_1,v_2}$, then reject H_0, where $F = \frac{MS_B}{MS_E}$ and the degrees of freedom are $v_1 = J - 1$ and $v_2 = N - J$.

The ANOVA table shows the statistics involved in testing the hypotheses about the population means (**Table 6.1**). If the null hypothesis of equal means is true, then MS_B will be close to MS_E, and the **F statistic**, which is the ratio of these two values, will be close to 1. If the null hypothesis is not true, the F statistic will be greater than 1. In order to reject the null

Table 6.1 ANOVA Table

Source	DF	Sum of Squares	Mean Square	*F* Value	Pr > *F*
Between	$J-1$	$SS_B = \sum_{j=1}^{N}\left(\overline{X}_j - \overline{\overline{X}}\right)^2$	$MS_B = \frac{SS_B}{J-1}$	$F = \frac{MS_B}{MS_E}$	
Error	$N-J$	$SS_E = \sum_{i=1}^{N}\sum_{j=1}^{J}\left(X_{ij} - \overline{X}_j\right)^2$	$MS_E = \frac{SS_E}{N-J}$		
Corrected Total	$N-1$	$SS_T = \sum_{i=1}^{N}\sum_{j=1}^{J}\left(X_{ij} - \overline{\overline{X}}\right)^2$			

hypothesis, the F statistic must be greater than a critical F value, which we obtain from the F distribution table.

EXAMPLE 6.1

In this example, we will again refer to the study involving quality of life indicators in patients with obstructive sleep apnea, in which the burden of possible upper-airway–related symptoms (i.e., voice, cough, and diurnal dyspnea) on SF-36 quality-of-life measures was assessed.[2] Of interest was whether the mean SF-36 subscales and component scales for mental and physical quality of life (with the score ranging from 0 to 100, with a higher score reflecting better quality of life) related to the presence of voice, cough, and diurnal dyspnea. In this example, we will treat the physical functioning quality-of-life subscale as the dependent variable and the number of upper-airway–related symptoms as the **independent variable**. Among 94 patients, 47 (50%) had no symptoms, 18 (19%) had one, 13 (14%) had two, and 16 (17%) had three.

We are interested in whether the mean component physical score differs among the four groups.

To check the assumptions of normality and equal population variances, the following statistics were computed:

Sum	Mean	Median	s
0	69.42	74.32	20.93
1	63.81	69.66	20.29
2	57.66	60.00	21.40
3	37.61	30.91	22.85

The data are slightly skewed left for groups with zero to two upper-airway symptoms, and right for those with three upper-airway symptoms. The population variances appear to be similar in that 22.85/20.29 = 1.13 < 2.

Applying the steps to hypothesis testing results in the following:

1. $H_0: \mu_1 = \mu_2 = \mu_3 = \mu_4$
2. H_a: At least one μ_j differs from the others.
3. $\alpha = 0.05, n = 94$
4. F, $v_1 = J - 1 = 4 - 1 = 3$, $v_2 = N - J = 94 - 4 = 90$. Referring to Appendix B, Table 6, the critical value is 2.71 (also obtained using the Excel formula =F.INV.RT(0.05,3,90)).
5. Because of the computational effort required in ANOVA, statistical software is often used to obtain ANOVA tables. We used the following SAS code for this problem, applied to the data in Table 5.2. The word CLASS is used in the code to identify that Sum is a categorical variable.

```
PROC ANOVA DATA= T5_2;
   CLASS Sum;
   MODEL Physical=Sum;
   MEANS Sum;
RUN;
```

The following ANOVA table is output from SAS, where the ANOVA procedure is applied to the data.

Source	DF	Sum of Squares	Mean Square	F Value	Pr > F
Model	3	12361.34319	4120.44773	9.16	<.0001
Error	90	40482.06635	449.80074		
Corrected Total	93	52843.40954			

6. Because the calculated F value of 9.16 is greater than the critical value, we reject the null hypothesis and conclude otherwise. The p-value in the SAS output also indicates statistical significance.

6.2 Two-Sample *t* Test Following Significant *F* Test

When the F test is significant, we can conclude that the population means are not all equal but cannot conclude which specific means are not equal. We do not know whether all the means are different from one another or only some of them are different. If we reject the null hypothesis based on a significant F test, we now need to do further testing to find out which means differ.

The number of two-sample t tests that can be performed for J groups is

$$k = J \times (J - 1)/2.$$

For example, for the four groups we were considering in the previous example, there are six two-sample t tests that can be performed.

$$k = 4 \times (4 - 1)/2 = 6$$

If comparisons are planned, they can be performed without first completing ANOVA. However, performing multiple tests increases the probability of committing a Type I error. Consider that $P(\geq 1 \text{ significant result}) = 1 - P(\text{no significant results}) = 1 - (1 - \alpha)^k$. For example, if four independent comparisons are made, each at $\alpha = 0.05$, the probability of one or more significant results is $1 - (1 - 0.05)^4 = 0.185$. We can compensate for multiple comparisons by decreasing the α level. This may be completed by applying the formula $\alpha' = 1 - (1 - \alpha)^{1/k}$, where α' is the correction, α is the level of significance, and k is the number of hypotheses being tested. This is called the **Dunn-Šidàk** correction.[3] In the case of four pair-wise comparisons, $\alpha' = 1 - (1 - 0.05)^{1/4} = 0.01274$. The Italian mathematician Bonferroni also developed a correction for multiple comparisons, where $\alpha' = \alpha/k$.[3,4] For our example, $\alpha' = 0.05/4 = 0.0125$, which means that we maintain the overall probability of a Type I error at 0.05 when each of the four comparisons is evaluated for significance at the 0.0125 level. The Bonferroni correction is simpler to apply and, therefore, more commonly used.

However, the Bonferroni correction is very extreme, controlling for Type I error under the worst-case scenario. Hence, researchers sometimes use a less conservative method for controlling Type I error. Two more powerful alternatives to the Bonferroni correction are the Šidàk correction and the Holm-Bonferroni method.

If the F statistic in ANOVA is significant, then post hoc (the Latin term meaning "after this") comparisons may be performed. Post hoc tests allow us to determine where statistical significance exists in paired comparisons. Several procedures are available for making post hoc comparisons once the null hypothesis is rejected in ANOVA. These tests tend to be named after those who developed them: Tukey, Bonferroni, Fisher's LSD, Scheffe, Dunnet, Dunn-Šidàk, Holm-Bonferroni, Holm-Šidàk, and **Student-Newman-Keuls** (SNK). The examples in this book will use the SNK post hoc test. The SNK option is obtained by extending the SAS code as follows:

```
PROC ANOVA DATA=T5_2;
   CLASS Sum;
   MODEL Physical=Sum;
   MEANS Sum/SNK;
RUN;
```

The following graph is a partial output from SAS in which the ANOVA procedure is applied to the data and we requested the SNK post hoc test.

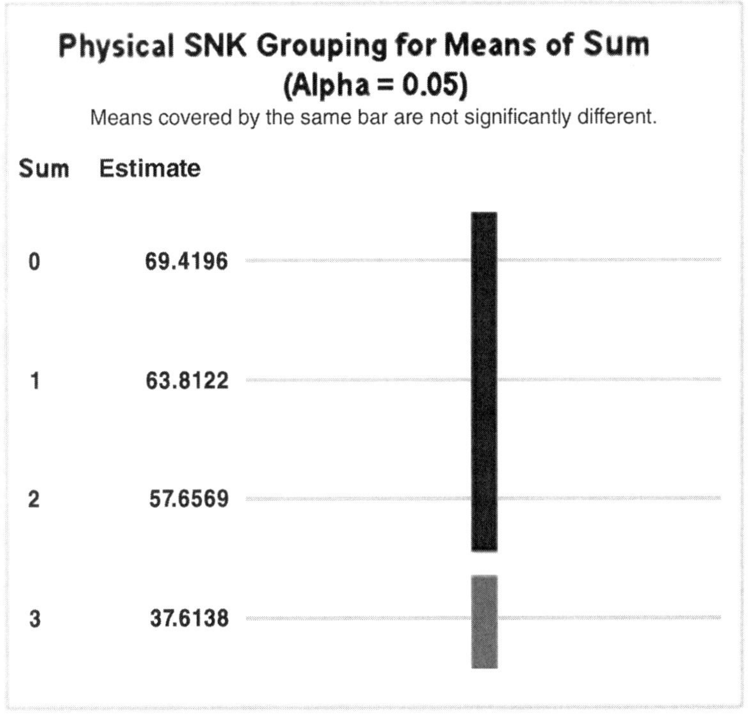

This graph tells us that although the component physical quality of life measure decreased with the increasing number of upper-airway symptoms, only those patients with all three disorders had significantly lower quality of life compared with zero, one, or two disorders.

Because only one independent variable was considered in this model (i.e., number of upper-airway symptoms), it is a one-way ANOVA. We will now provide an example of a two-way ANOVA, wherein two independent variables are considered.

Example 6.2

Suppose we are interested in whether the mean component physical quality-of-life score significantly differed according to the number of upper-airway symptoms and Sex. In this two-way ANOVA, we can ask whether differences exist in physical functioning according to number of symptoms, Sex, and whether differences exist in physical functioning quality of life owing to the combination of these variables. In this latter case, we say an interaction effect exists between the two variables. The SAS code is modified as follows in order to assess an interaction effect between the number of upper-airway symptoms and Sex. The vertical line between SUM and Sex in the MODEL and MEANS statements indicates that we have a factorial design. By including the vertical line, the main effects and interaction effects for Sum and Sex will be estimated. The GLM procedure will be used instead of the ANOVA procedure because it can perform simple or complicated ANOVA for balanced or unbalanced data.

```
PROC GLM DATA=T5_2;
  CLASS Sum Sex;
  MODEL Physical=Sum|Sex;
  MEANS Sum|Sex/SNK;
RUN;
```

The GLM output from SAS indicates that the interaction effect is not significant. In other words, the relationship between physical functioning and number of symptoms does not depend on Sex. The following table is a partial output from SAS, where the GLM procedure was applied to the data.

Source	DF	Type III SS	Mean Square	F Value	Pr > F
Sum	3	5383.295585	1794.431862	4.05	0.0096
Sex	1	1103.544501	1103.544501	2.49	0.1181
Sum*Sex	3	422.659623	140.886541	0.32	0.8123

Dropping the insignificant interaction term from the model and rerunning the GLM procedure provided greater power to estimate the effects of the independent variables.

Source	DF	Type III SS	Mean Square	F Value	Pr > F
Sum	3	7405.469858	2468.489953	5.70	0.0013
Sex	1	1969.174577	1969.174577	4.55	0.0357

Adjusted mean physical functioning scores according to the number of upper-airway symptoms and Sex are obtained using the following SAS code:

```
PROC GLM DATA=T5_2;
  CLASS Sum Sex;
  MODEL Physical= Sum Sex;
  LSMEANS Sum Sex;
RUN;
```

The LSMEANS command generates adjusted means. Mean physical functioning scores for zero, one, two, or three symptoms, adjusted for Sex, are 67.6,

60.9, 59.6, and 40.8, respectively. Mean physical functioning scores for Sex, adjusted for symptoms, are 52.1 for women and 62.4 for men.

Example 6.3

This example will provide SAS code for assessing a two-way ANOVA. Although the data are hypothetical, this example is along the lines of a study involving National Health and Nutrition Examination Survey data that showed that men and women significantly overreport their height, more so in older ages, and men tend to overreport their weight in young ages, but women underreport their weight.[5] Consequently, body mass index (BMI) is underestimated, more so for women than men at each age, and increasingly so with older age for both sexes.

Assume a group of 15 males and 15 females were asked their weight. They were then weighed to determine their actual weight. Self-reported minus actual weight is reported in the following table. The respondents in the table are also divided into age categories, young, middle, and old. Because the same number of subjects are in each cell, the design is said to be "balanced."

Sex	Young	Middle	Old
Male	5.2	1.6	0.3
Male	2.1	-0.8	0.1
Male	1.9	2.0	-0.4
Male	5.9	0.1	-1.3
Male	2.0	2.4	-2.0
Female	-2.1	-3.6	-0.3
Female	-4.3	-0.8	0.1
Female	-3.1	-2.0	0.4
Female	-5.8	0.1	1.2
Female	-2.0	-2.3	-1.8

The SAS code is as follows:

```
DATA EX_6_3;
   INPUT Sex $ Age $ Score @@;
   IF SEX='M' AND AGE='Y' THEN INTER=1; ELSE IF SEX='M' AND
   AGE='M' THEN INTER=2; ELSE IF SEX='M' AND AGE='O' THEN
   INTER=3; ELSE IF SEX='F' AND AGE='Y' THEN INTER=4; ELSE IF
   SEX='F' AND AGE='M' THEN INTER=5; ELSE IF SEX='F' AND AGE='O'
   THEN INTER=6;
DATALINES;
   M Y 5.2 M M 1.6 ...
;

PROC ANOVA DATA= EX_6_3;
   CLASS Sex Age;
   MODEL Score=Sex|Age;
   MEANS Sex|Age;
RUN;
```

Recall that the $ sign following the variables in the DATA step indicates that the variables are categorical, not numerical. The @@ symbols added at the end of this line allows us to repeat the data for each variable across the row. If these symbols were not included, we would need to enter the data in three columns.

The ANOVA table from the SAS output is as follows:

Source	DF	Sum of Squares	Mean Square	F Value	Pr > F
Model	5	139.2320000	27.8464000	13.41	<.0001
Error	24	49.8200000	2.0758333		
Corrected Total	29	189.0520000			

The ANOVA procedure table shows the sum of squares and mean square for the entire model and the error. The $F = 13.41$ and the p-value < 0.0001 show us how well the model explains the variation about the grand mean. This is important in studies where we are interested in creating a general, predictive model. However, in this situation, we are more interested in the detailed sources of variation (Sex, Age, and Sex × Age). In the two-way analysis of variance, we see that mean scores are not the same across age groups for males and females because the interaction term is statistically significant.

Source	DF	Anova SS	Mean Square	F Value	Pr > F
sex	1	68.70533333	68.70533333	33.10	<.0001
age	2	0.73400000	0.36700000	0.18	0.8390
sex*age	2	69.79266667	34.89633333	16.81	<.0001

Following are the mean difference weight values (and standard deviations) for each combination of Sex and Age. These are the mean values of the six cells in our experimental design. The results in this table indicate that young and middle-aged males tend to overestimate their weight, whereas females of all ages tend to underestimate their weight.

Level of sex	Level of age	N	score	
			Mean	Std Dev
Female	Middle	5	-1.72000000	1.42372750
Female	Old	5	-0.08000000	1.10770032
Female	Young	5	-3.46000000	1.60405736
Male	Middle	5	1.06000000	1.35572859
Male	Old	5	-0.66000000	0.97108187
Male	Young	5	3.42000000	1.96137707

Now let us modify our SAS procedure code as follows:

```
PROC ANOVA DATA= EX_6_3;
  CLASS INTER;
  MODEL Score=INTER
  MEANS INTER/SNK;
RUN;
```

This produced the following SAS graph:

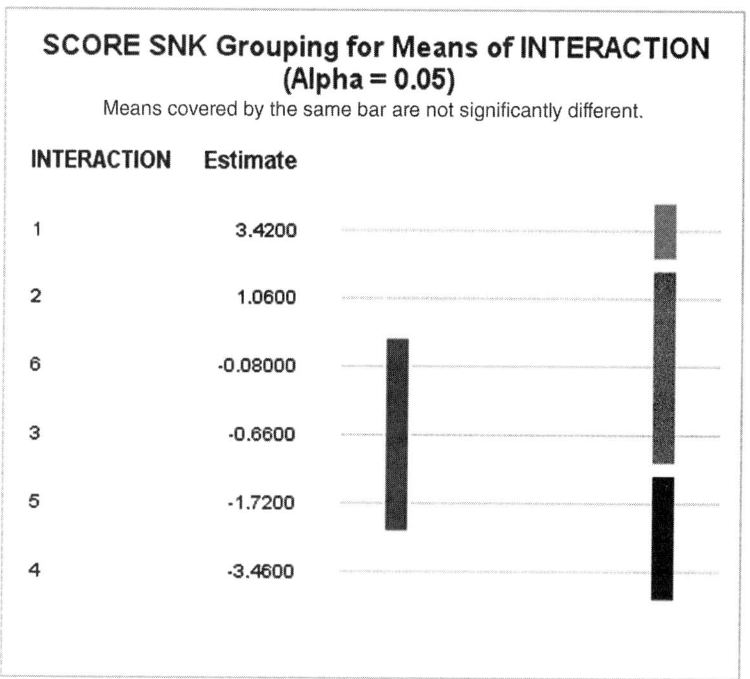

SCORE SNK Grouping for Means of INTERACTION
(Alpha = 0.05)
Means covered by the same bar are not significantly different.
INTERACTION Estimate
1 3.4200
2 1.0600
6 -0.08000
3 -0.6600
5 -1.7200
4 -3.4600

This post-hoc assessment indicates where significant differences exist in the reported weight minus the actual weight variable among the combinations of sex and age. For example, young males were significantly more likely to over-report their weight than middle or older aged males or females in any age group; young and middle aged females were significantly more likely to under-report their weight than older females or males in any age group.

News File

People usually recover from a cold in 7 to 10 days. They recover from the flu in about 3 to 7 days, but a lingering cough may last a few weeks or longer. Now, in the wake of the coronavirus pandemic, we are particularly interested in the recovery time for COVID-19. A study out of China reported a median recovery time of 11 days.[6] In a study involving mild-to-moderate COVID-19 patients in Europe, mean recover time was 11.5 days.[7] In another Chinese study, the recovery time was 10.63±1.93 days for mild to moderate patients and 18.7±2.5 for severe patients.[8] Although these and other studies have assessed mean and median survival times for COVID-19, they have not considered recovery times according to age or sex.

In response, a study out of Israel refined the assessment of recovery time for COVID-19 patients by reporting mean recovery time in days according to age and sex.[9] The study used two-way ANOVA to assess whether recovery times were significantly different among age-sex classifications. Data from this study are presented in **Figure 6.1**. Males and females ages > 30 had significantly longer recovery time versus younger patients. Hence, younger individuals are not only less likely to have severe COVID-19, but they tend to recover from SARS-COV-2 infection more quickly. In addition, in the age groups 50–59 and ≥ 60, females had significantly shorter recovery times. This is consistent with female patients tending to have less severe acute respiratory distress or fatal outcomes compared to men.[10,11]

Therefore, as we consider the time it will take to feel better and to get back to work after COVID-19, realize it will take longer for older patients and for males than females.

News File (Continued)

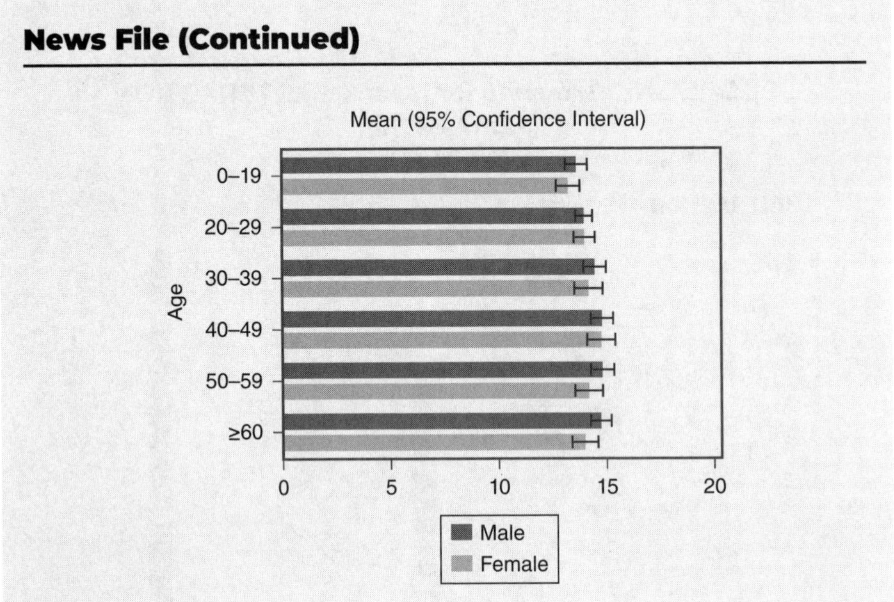

Figure 6.1 Mean Days for Recovery from COVID-19 in Israel According to Age and Sex

6.3 ANOVA for Completely Randomized Design

Recall that random sampling refers to how subjects are selected from the population to be in a study. On the other hand, random assignment refers to how subjects are placed into groups. With random assignment, chance is the only factor that determines treatment assignment, thereby allowing the application of inferential statistical tests of probability and determination of the level of significance. Randomization is often used in clinical trials where the efficacy of various levels of a treatment or combinations of treatments is investigated. The independent variable is the treatment, and the dependent variable is some characteristic the treatment is intended to modify.

A **completely randomized design** involves subjects being randomly assigned to treatments. The same number of subjects are assigned each treatment.

An important feature of randomization is that it helps balance out the effect of possible confounding (nuisance) variables, both anticipated and unanticipated confounding variables. Assuming that smoking is a potential confounder, randomization of a sufficiently large number of participants will produce a similar distribution of smokers (in terms of age started, duration, and intensity of smoking) between the intervention and control groups.

A **confounder** is a variable that affects both the independent variable and dependent variable, resulting in a spurious association; a confounder is a third variable that distorts the association between the independent and dependent variable.

With three or more treatment groups, we can use ANOVA to determine if there are any differences between the groups.

Example 6.4

Suppose that in a sample of patients with high total cholesterol (>200), three statin drugs are to be compared for their ability to lower cholesterol. High cholesterol is possibly dangerous because the body stores extra cholesterol in the arteries, potentially blocking the artery to the heart, which can cause a heart attack, or blocking the artery to the brain, which can cause a stroke. The follow-up period of the clinical trial is six weeks. The independent variable is type of treatment, and the dependent variable is cholesterol score. The null hypothesis is

$$H_0: \mu_1 = \mu_2 = \mu_3.$$

Therefore, we are interested in determining whether the mean cholesterol score significantly differs after six weeks among the treatment groups. ANOVA can be applied to evaluate whether any of the mean cholesterol scores differ, and if the F test is significant, post hoc tests can identify significant pair-wise comparisons.

Applying the steps to hypothesis testing results in the following:

1. $H_0: \mu_1 = \mu_2 = \mu_3$
2. H_a: At least one μ_j differs from the others.
3. $\alpha = 0.05, n_1 = 9, n_2 = 9, n_3 = 9.$

To randomly assign the 27 people with high cholesterol to the three treatments, assign a random number to each subject. Excel has two functions that generate random numbers, RAND and RANDBETWEEN. We introduced the latter function in an earlier chapter. Here, try typing =RAND() into a cell to obtain a random number. Copy and paste this function down the column to obtain a random number for each of the 27 subjects; sort the subjects from low to high according to their corresponding random number. Then assign the first nine subjects treatment A, and so on.

Subject	Baseline Cholesterol Score	Six-Week Cholesterol Score	Random Number	Treatment
15	226	219	0.019	A
25	233	211	0.023	A
17	226	222	0.085	A
23	239	210	0.165	A
4	245	235	0.186	A
19	202	205	0.197	A
21	216	214	0.231	A
6	230	231	0.286	A

(Continues)

Subject	Baseline Cholesterol Score	Six-Week Cholesterol Score	Random Number	Treatment
12	237	221	0.408	A
14	212	210	0.429	B
11	219	210	0.454	B
24	253	250	0.546	B
1	227	230	0.569	B
13	213	215	0.613	B
18	209	201	0.614	B
2	254	245	0.658	B
20	240	237	0.658	B
22	224	225	0.728	B
26	219	220	0.753	C
5	218	217	0.771	C
9	246	245	0.775	C
10	227	230	0.786	C
8	243	240	0.835	C
16	218	215	0.836	C
27	242	240	0.838	C
3	219	221	0.852	C
7	262	258	0.940	C

4. F, $v_1 = J - 1 = 3 - 1 = 2$, $v_2 = N - J = 27 - 3 = 24$. Referring to Appendix B, Table 6, the critical value is 3.403 (also obtained using the Excel formula =F.INV.RT(0.05,2,24)).
5. The SAS procedure code and resulting ANOVA table is as follows:

```
PROC ANOVA DATA=EX_6_4;
   CLASS Treatment;
   MODEL Chol_6wk=Treatment;
   MEANS Treatment/SNK;
RUN;
```

Source	DF	Sum of Squares	Mean Square	F Value	Pr > F
Model	2	774.740741	387.370370	1.92	0.1691
Error	24	4853.111111	202.212963		
Corrected Total	26	5627.851852			

6. Since the calculated value is less than the critical value, we fail to reject the null hypothesis. The p-value is greater than 0.05, which also tells us that these data are consistent with the null hypothesis.

If you are thinking that this analysis did not take into account the baseline cholesterol level, you are right. A better analysis would have considered the subjects baseline cholesterol. One possible solution is to calculate change scores in cholesterol from baseline through six weeks and then perform an ANOVA on this modified dependent variable. The SAS code to generate a new variable of change scores is as follows:

```
DATA EX_6_4;
   INPUT Subject Chol_0wk Chol_6wk Random Treatment $;
   Change=Chol_6wk-Chol_0wk;
DATALINES;
...

;
```

The SAS code to enact the ANOVA procedure is

```
PROC ANOVA DATA= EX_6_4;
   CLASS Treatment;
   MODEL Change=Treatment;
   MEANS Treatment/SNK;
RUN;
```

The ANOVA table from SAS is as follows:

Source	DF	Sum of Squares	Mean Square	F Value	Pr > F
Model	2	364.740741	182.370370	3.77	0.0376
Error	24	1160.000000	48.333333		
Corrected Total	26	1524.740741			

Because the p-value associated with the F statistic is < 0.05, we conclude that change scores among the groups differ significantly. The actual critical F value from the F distribution table is 3.4028.

To determine where the group differences exist, the SNK post hoc procedure was run. The following graph indicates that the decrease from baseline through six weeks was significantly greater in individuals receiving drug A compared with drug C. Mean change scores are not significantly different between drugs A and B or between drugs B and C.

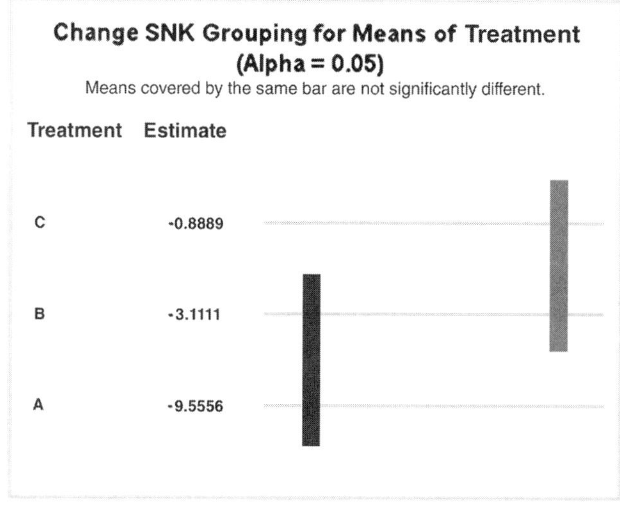

6.4 Analysis of Covariance (ANCOVA)

Analysis of covariance (ANCOVA) is a generalized linear model that combines ANOVA and regression. The idea is to combine the ANOVA model containing an independent variable to represent the group effect with one or more additional categorical or continuous variables that are related to the dependent variable. In randomized experimental studies, ANCOVA is used to increase precision when comparing treatment groups by using the relationship between the response variable and the covariates to reduce the error variability. ANCOVA often produces more powerful tests, shorter confidence intervals, and smaller required sample sizes for evaluating differences among treatment groups. ANCOVA is also used to compare the mean of a continuous variable among three or more groups while taking into account (correcting for) the variability of other variables that are not of primary interest (i.e., covariates).[12]

Analysis of covariance is an extension of the one-way ANOVA to include a continuous independent variable (covariate). The aim is to control for the potential confounding effect of the covariate.

Example 6.5

In this example, we extend the previous example by adjusting for baseline cholesterol using ANCOVA. The SAS code was modified as follows:

```
PROC GLM DATA=EX_6_4;
   CLASS Treatment;
   MODEL Chol_6wk=Treatment Chol_0wk;
   LSMEANS Treatment;
RUN;
```

LSMEANS is an option in SAS that produces adjusted means. In this example, mean cholesterol scores for the levels of treatment are adjusted for the baseline cholesterol scores. A table generated using the GLM procedure in SAS indicates that treatment is significantly different among the treatment groups after adjusting for baseline cholesterol.

Source	DF	Type III SS	Mean Square	F Value	Pr > F
Treatment	2	415.630176	207.815088	4.93	0.0165
Chol_0wk	1	3884.512555	3884.512555	92.24	<.0001

The adjusted mean cholesterol scores are as follows:

Treatment	Chol_6wk LSMEAN
A	219.788105
B	226.171999
C	229.262118

6.5 ANOVA for Randomized Block Design

While ANCOVA is one approach that can be taken to account for confounding, ANOVA applied to a randomized block design is another option to deal with confounding. This approach may be particularly useful when the sample size is small.

It is possible to isolate the effects of a confounding variable by means of a blocking procedure in which subjects who are homogeneous with respect to the confounding variable are assigned to the same block. The variability within each block is less than the variability among the blocks. The subjects within each block are then randomly assigned to the levels of treatment. The advantage of this design is that it reduces variability within levels of treatment and possible confounding. Hence, better estimates of the treatment effect result.

Example 6.6

Suppose you are interested in whether compliance to wearing face protection against COVID-19 is influenced by whether the face protection is a plain white cloth mask, a solid color mask, or a color and pattern mask. The dependent variable is the percentage of time wearing a mask while in public during a given week. The hypothesis to be tested is

$$H_0: \mu_1 = \mu_2 = \mu_3.$$

The μ_j's denote the mean percentage of time a mask is worn while in public.

Now consider that a previous study has shown that mask wearing significantly varies by age group, increasing with older age. To account for this, let's create four blocks representing the age groups 18–29, 30–44, 45–64, and ≥ 65. If we have 24 participants, six in each age group, we would randomly assign those in each block to the types of masks.

For the following hypothetical data set, subjects consisted of six individuals each in the four age groups. A random number was assigned to each subject, and the subjects with their corresponding random number were ordered from low to high. Assignment of the type of mask was given sequentially.

Subject	Percent	Age	Random Number	Face Mask
6	55	18–29	0.135	A
2	60	18–29	0.191	B
3	67	18–29	0.215	C
4	60	18–29	0.523	A
5	62	18–29	0.619	B
1	68	18–29	0.995	C
11	62	30–44	0.074	A

(Continues)

Subject	Percent	Age	Random Number	Face Mask
9	65	30–44	0.137	B
7	70	30–44	0.449	C
10	60	30–44	0.755	A
12	64	30–44	0.768	B
8	72	30–44	0.827	C
16	74	45–64	0.168	A
13	75	45–64	0.345	B
15	80	45–64	0.476	C
14	73	45–64	0.491	A
18	80	45–64	0.861	B
17	85	45–64	0.926	C
24	80	65+	0.016	A
23	82	65+	0.137	B
21	84	65+	0.552	C
22	82	65+	0.567	A
20	85	65+	0.651	B
19	90	65+	0.832	C

The data statement in SAS is as follows:

```
DATA EX_6_6;
   INPUT Subject Percent Age $ RN Mask $;
   DATALINES;
...
;
```

SAS ANOVA procedure code to evaluate these data follows

```
PROC ANOVA DATA= EX_6_6;
   CLASS Mask Age;
   MODEL Percent=Mask|Age;
   MEANS Mask Age/SNK;
RUN;
```

A table produced by this code showed that the independent variables Mask and Age both significantly influence the percentage of time masks are worn in public, but the interaction effect was not significant. The interaction term was dropped by removing the vertical line from the code and the program rerun to obtain the following table:

Source	DF	Anova SS	Mean Square	F Value	Pr > F
Mask	2	311.583333	155.791667	34.37	<.0001
Age	3	1895.791667	631.930556	139.42	<.0001

Adding the SNK option to the code resulted in the following two graphs. The first graph shows that mean percentage of time subjects wore a face mask significantly increased when a solid color mask was worn rather than a plain white cloth and when a color and pattern mask was worn rather than just a solid color mask. In addition, the mean percentage of time wearing a face mask significantly increased with age.

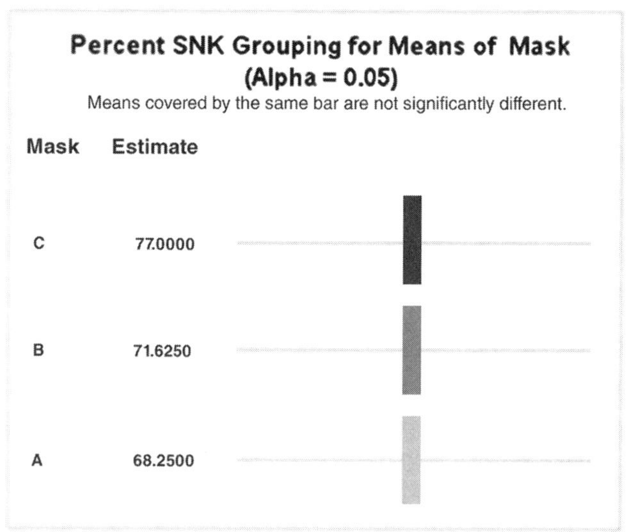

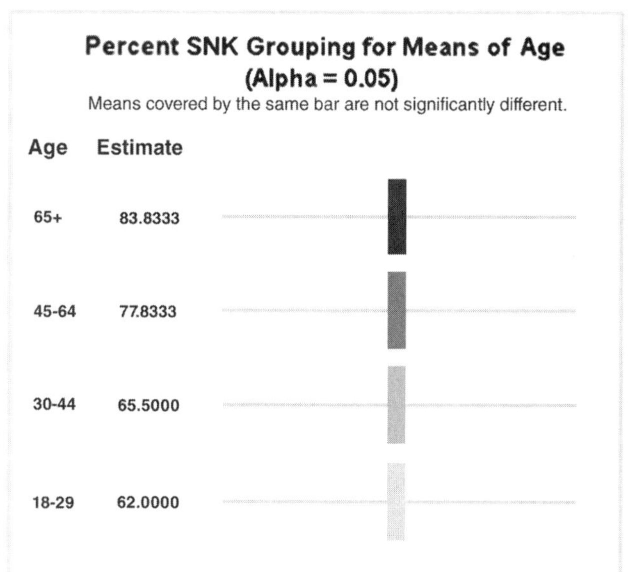

6.6 Repeated Measures ANOVA

A repeated measures ANOVA is an extension of the paired *t* test, wherein we are interested in identifying any overall differences between related means. When several measurements are taken on the same subject, the measurements tend to be correlated. If the measurements are thought of as responses to levels of time, treatment, dose, and so on, the correlation can be taken into account by performing a repeated measures ANOVA. The normal variation from subject to subject is removed from the sum of squares. An example of a repeated measures ANOVA involving time is an intervention intended to lower cholesterol over a 3-month period, measured for its effect at 1 month, 2 months, and 3 months.

An example of a repeated measures ANOVA involving different treatments is where the same subjects try a plain white mask, a solid color mask, and mixed color and pattern mask and rate each one for preference (say on a scale from 1 to 10). In these designs, the same subjects are measured multiple times at either different time points or different levels of treatment.

A **repeated measures ANOVA** is a one-way ANOVA that involves dependent, not independent, groups. It is also called a within-subjects ANOVA or ANOVA for correlated samples.

Repeated measures ANOVA are useful in three situations. First, a group of subjects is measured more than twice over time, such as BMI measured on a group at 3 months, 6 months, and 9 months. Second, a group of subjects is measured on multiple dosages of a given treatment, such as patients who are given three different dosages of an antiviral drug for COVID-19. Third, at least two groups of subjects are measured at least two times, such as a biometric measurement taken on subjects in different weight classifications before and after a dietary intervention.

The only assumption required for valid tests is that the response variables have a multivariate normal distribution with a common covariance matrix across the between-subject effects.[13]

The procedure code used in SAS for computing a repeated measures ANOVA involves specifying the class variables (e.g., group and sex), the model, the number of repeated measures, and whether an orthogonal polynomial transformation is desired of the repeated measures. The output yields information about the repeated measures effect and gives multivariate analysis results related to whether there is a time effect, whether the time effect differs by the independent variables in the model, and whether interaction effects are present. Multivariate test methods are provided in the SAS output. These tests include Pillai's trace, **Wilks' lambda**, Hotelling's trace, and Roy's largest root. Wilks' lambda is a standard test generally used for evaluating the significance of these effects. The output also indicates whether the main effects in the model are significant, along with ANOVA and contrast variables.

Example 6.7

Consider the following hypothetical data where the dependent variable is BMI, measured at three months, six months, and nine months. The independent variables consist of two interventions: diet (1 = low fat, 2 = normal) and exercise (1 = cardio exercise > 150 minutes per week, 2 = weight lifting three times per week for > 30 minutes each time, and 3 = normal exercise).

Diet	Exercise	BMI1	BMI2	BMI3
1	1	35	34	32
1	1	35	33	28
1	1	37	34	33
2	1	37	36	35
2	1	30	30	28

(Continues)

Diet	Exercise	BMI1	BMI2	BMI3
2	1	42	40	39
1	2	35	33	32
1	2	36	35	33
1	2	35	35	34
2	2	34	34	33
2	2	38	39	39
2	2	38	37	37
1	3	35	33	32
1	3	36	35	34
1	3	37	35	34
2	3	33	34	35
2	3	40	42	43
2	3	36	36	37

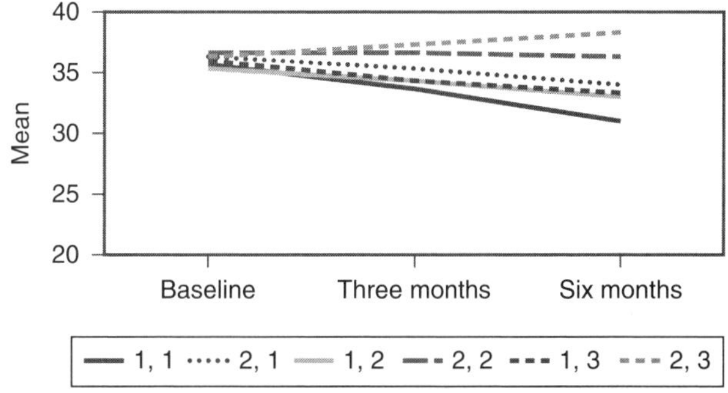

The code for the SAS data set and the repeated measures ANOVA procedure is as follows:

```
DATA EX_6_7;
  INPUT Diet $ Exercise $ BMI1 BMI2 BMI3;
  DATALINES;
...
;

PROC GLM DATA= EX_6_7;
  CLASS Diet Exercise;
  MODEL BMI1 BMI2 BMI3 = Diet|Exercise/NOUNI;
  REPEATED Time 3 (0 3 6);
RUN;
```

From the SAS output (not included here), Wilks' lambda indicates that the change in mean BMI is significant for diet (WL p-value = 0.0013) and exercise (WL p-value = 0.0146). There is not a significant time by diet by exercise effect (WL p-value = 0.4269). In other words, evidence is sufficient to reject the null hypothesis that the change in BMI is similar between types of diet and between types of exercise. The effect of diet on BMI does not depend on type of exercise. Similarly, the effect of type of exercise on BMI does not depend on diet.

As seen, an advantage of the REPEATED option of PROC ANOVA over the paired *t* test is that more than two outcome measures can be assessed and compared among groups. The model also allows us to control for potential confounders, such as age, sex, and smoking status.

6.7 Equality of Proportions and Trends

In this final section, we will consider hypotheses involving proportions of a categorical variable with three or more levels. Tests for trend provide another option for assessing whether an increasing or decreasing difference in the distribution of the dependent variable exists across independent ordinal categories. Three tests will be presented: the χ^2 test of independence, the Cochran-Armitage trend test, and the Cochran-Mantel-Haenszel test. The χ^2 test of independence will be used to assess the association between two categorical variables, one with two levels and one with three or more levels. The Cochran-Armitage trend test will assess for trend for an ordinal variable by a categorical variable with two levels. The Cochran-Mantel-Haenszel test will assess for trend for an ordinal variable by a categorical variable with three or more levels.

6.7.1 χ^2 Test of Independence for Assessing Three or More Proportions

In the previous chapter, the χ^2 test of independence between two categorical variables was presented. In the situation where one of the categorical variables has three or more levels and the other categorical variable has two levels, we can evaluate the following hypotheses using the χ^2 test of independence:

$$H_0\colon p_1 = p_2 = \cdots = p_J$$

H_a: Not all population proportions are equal.

Example 6.8

In the data for 94 patients with obstructive sleep apnea, referred to earlier in this chapter, suppose we wanted to know whether having a current voice disorder (yes versus no) was associated with postnasal drip (1 = never, 2 = occasionally with colds, 3 = seasonally, and 4 = chronically).

The steps of hypothesis testing are as follows:

1. $H_0\colon p_1 = p_2 = p_3 = p_4$
2. H_a: At least one p_i differs from the others.
3. $\alpha = 0.05, n = 94$
4. χ^2 test of independence. Degrees of freedom = (Row – 1)(Columns – 1). = (2 – 1)(4 – 1) = 3. The critical value is $\chi^2_{0.05,3} = 7.81$.

5.

	Postnasal Drip			
Voice Disorder	**Never**	**Occasionally with Colds**	**Seasonally**	**Chronically**
Yes	6	11	5	15
No	20	22	10	5

In SAS, we can apply the χ^2 test to these data. SAS code for the data statement and the frequency procedure with the χ^2 test option is as follows:

```
DATA EX_6_8;
   LABEL VD = 'Voice Disorder';
   LABEL PND = 'Postnasal Drip';
   INPUT VD $ PND $ COUNT;
DATALINES;
   Yes Never 6
   Yes Occasional 11
   Yes Seasonal 5
   Yes Chronic 15
   No Never 20
   No Occasional 22
   No Seasonal 10
   No Chronic 5
   ;

PROC FREQ DATA= EX_6_8 ORDER=DATA;
   TABLE VD*PND/CHISQ;
   WEIGHT COUNT;
RUN;
```

Resulting output follows:

Frequency Percent Row Pct Col Pct	Table of VD by PND					
		PND(Post Nasal Drip)				
	VD(Voice Disorder)	Never	Occasion	Seasonal	Chronic	Total
	Yes	6 6.38 16.22 23.08	11 11.70 29.73 33.33	5 5.32 13.51 33.33	15 15.96 40.54 75.00	37 39.36
	No	20 21.28 35.09 76.92	22 23.40 38.60 66.67	10 10.64 17.54 66.67	5 5.32 8.77 25.00	57 60.64
	Total	26 27.66	33 35.11	15 15.96	20 21.28	94 100.00

The column percentage shows a positive trend in the proportion with a voice disorder across the ordered levels of postnasal drip. The CHISQ option gives the following output, with our primary interest in this example being the chi-square statistic, which indicates statistical significance.

Statistics for Table of VD by PND

Statistic	DF	Value	Prob
Chi-Square	3	14.2621	0.0026
Likelihood Ratio Chi-Square	3	14.3343	0.0025
Mantel-Haenszel Chi-Square	1	11.4393	0.0007
Phi Coefficient		0.3895	
Contingency Coefficient		0.3630	
Cramer's V		0.3895	

Because $\chi^2 = 14.26 > \chi^2_{0.05,3} = 7.81$ (obtained using the Excel formula =CHISQ .INV.RT(0.05,3)), we fail to reject the null hypothesis of equal proportions. This conclusion is also gotten by the fact that p-value $= 0.0026 < 0.05 = \alpha$.

6.7.2 Cochran-Armitage Trend Test

The Cochran-Armitage test assesses for trends in binomial proportions across levels of a single factor. It is appropriate for a contingency table where one variable is ordinal and the other variable has two levels (binary). The binary variable is the dependent variable, and the ordinal variable has three or more ordered categories. It tests the null hypothesis that no ordered differences exist in the proportions of the dependent variable across the levels of the ordinal independent variable.[14,15]

Example 6.9

For the data in the previous example, the independent variable, presence of postnasal drip, represent four ordered categories. Of interest is whether the trend in the proportion with a voice disorder across the levels of the postnasal drip variable differs from those without a voice disorder.

To perform the Cochran-Armitage trend test in SAS, in the TABLE statement, we need to include a cross tabulation of voice disorder and postnasal drip classifications, along with the TREND and NOPRINT options:

```
PROC FREQ DATA= EX_6_8 ORDER=DATA;
  TABLE VD*PND/TREND NOPRINT;
  WEIGHT COUNT;
RUN;
```

Partial output from this program follows:

Cochran-Armitage Trend Test	
Statistic (Z)	3.4003
One-sided Pr > Z	0.0003
Two-sided Pr > |Z|	0.0007

This trend test contains the z statistic for one-sided and two-sided p-values. Both are statistically significant. The one-sided p-value tests the hypothesis that there is a significant increasing relationship between a voice disorder and the presence and severity of postnasal drip. The two-sided p-value tests against either an increasing or decreasing alternative. This is an appropriate hypothesis if we want to determine whether presence and severity of postnasal drip has progressive effects on the probability of a voice disorder but the direction is unknown. By looking at how the proportions change across postnasal drip, we can state that the proportion of those with a voice disorder significantly increases with the presence and severity of postnasal drip.

6.7.3 Cochran-Mantel-Haenszel Trend Test

The Cochran-Mantel-Haenszel statistic is useful for assessing the overall ordered difference in proportions for a dependent categorical variable with three or more levels across the ordered categories of an independent variable. The Cochran-Mantel-Haenszel statistic tests the null hypothesis that the proportions of the dependent categorical variable are the same across the ordered levels of the independent categorical variable.

Example 6.10

Data in the next table represent the distribution of deaths involving COVID-19 by race-Hispanic origin and age in the United States, as of July 15, 2020.[16]

	< 34	35–54	55–74	≥ 75
Non-Hispanic white	171	1576	15,624	46,702
Non-Hispanic black	318	2546	12,089	12,895
Hispanic	422	3320	8857	8250
Non-Hispanic Asian	46	439	2253	3284
Non-Hispanic other	67	231	606	507

The code for the SAS dataset follows:

```
DATA EX_6_10;
   INPUT AGE $ RACE_ETH $ COUNT;
DATALINES;
...
;
```

The SAS frequency procedure code with the Cochran-Mantel-Haenszel option follows:

```
PROC FREQ ORDER=DATA DATA= EX_6_10;
   TABLE RACE_ETH*AGE/CMH;
   WEIGHT COUNT;
RUN;
```

Partial output from this program produces the following:

Cochran-Mantel-Haenszel Statistics (Based on Table Scores)				
Statistic	**Alternative Hypothesis**	**DF**	**Value**	**Prob**
1	Nonzero Correlation	1	8732.0335	<.0001
2	Row Mean Scores Differ	4	12203.6364	<.0001
3	General Association	12	12957.9045	<.0001

The output shows three alternative hypotheses.

Test	Alternative Hypothesis	Assumption
Nonzero Correlation	A linear association exists between rows and columns for at least one stratum.	Ordinal scale required for both row and column variables.
Row Mean Scores Differ	Mean scores for the R rows are not equal for at least one stratum.	The column variable has an ordinal scale.
General Association	An association exists between variables for at least one stratum.	Ordinal scale is not required for either the row or column variable.

Because we are interested in whether a trend exists between race/ethnicity (not ordinal) and age (ordinal) categories, we will refer to the *p*-value for the hypothesis about Row Mean Scores Differ. This is a two-sided *p*-value, which tells us that an overall significant relationship exists between race-Hispanic origin and age categories since the p-value < 0.05.

6.8 Summary

In this chapter, we presented a procedure for testing the equality of three or more means known as ANOVA. Similar to the *t* test, ANOVA is a parametric procedure that has important assumptions involving independence, normality, and equality of variance. When the sample size is large, the normality assumption is less important than the other assumptions. To conduct an ANOVA and test the null hypothesis that three or more means are equal, we take randomly selected independent samples from each of the populations of interest and obtain certain measures that allow us to compute sums of squared deviations. The sum of squares between groups is divided by $J - 1$ degrees of freedom to obtain an estimate of the variance among groups. The sums of squares within groups is divided by $N - J$ to obtain an estimate of the variance within groups.

The F statistic is the ratio of these two variances and is used to test the null hypotheses of equality of means among groups. A one-way ANOVA involves one categorical independent variable. A two-way ANOVA involves two categorical independent variables. Interaction effects can be assessed when two independent variables are involved.

If comparisons between groups are planned, they can be done prior to performing ANOVA, but the α-level needs to be adjusted downward. This can be done using the Bonferroni correction. If the F test rejects the null hypothesis of equality of means, multiple comparison methods called post hoc tests can be used. These adjust for the number of comparisons between group means that are made.

This chapter also discussed ANOVA for a completely randomized design, analysis of covariance (ANCOVA), ANOVA for randomized complete block design, and repeated measures ANOVA. A complete randomized design involves random assignment of the same number of subjects to each treatment being considered. When a continuous outcome variable is compared across three or more treatments, ANOVA is a useful method for assessing overall treatment differences. ANCOVA extends one-way ANOVA to include one or more continuous independent variables. These are called covariates. If the covariate is a confounder, then its nuisance effect is adjusted for by including it in the model. An ANOVA randomized block design first divides subjects into homogeneous blocks. Then subjects from each block are randomly assigned to each level of the treatment. This study design is very useful in laboratory experiments and is an effective way to control for confounding, particularly for small sample sizes. Finally, repeated measures ANOVA is a counterpart to the paired t test, but with three or more outcome measures. A strength of this design is that it controls for individual variation, which can be large in research studies involving human subjects. In this design, subjects serve as their own controls. Thus, variability because of individual differences is not part of the error term, thereby increasing the chances of finding significant differences between the levels of the treatment.

The chapter concluded by presenting the χ^2 test of independence for assessing three or more proportions, the Cochran-Armitage trend test, and the Cochran-Mantel-Haenszel trend test. The χ^2 test of independence can evaluate the following null hypotheses H_0: $p_1 = p_2 = \cdots = p_J$. The Cochran-Armitage trend test was presented to assess trend for an ordinal variable by a categorical variable with two levels. The Cochran-Mantel-Haenszel test was presented to assess trends for an ordinal variable by a categorical variable with three or more levels. Important formulas are summarized in **Table 6.2**.

Table 6.2 Summary of Key Formulas in Analysis of Variance

Description	Equation
Analysis of variance with H_0: $\mu_1 = \mu_2 = \cdots = \mu_J$. The F test statistic has two corresponding degrees of freedom, $J - 1$ and $N - J$. Each population is assumed to be normally distributed and have equal variance.	$F = \frac{MS_B}{MS_E}$ $MS_B = \frac{SS_B}{J-1}$ $MS_E = \frac{SS_E}{N-J}$
The number of two-sampled t tests possible for J groups.	$k = J \times (J-1)/2$ or $\binom{J}{2} = \frac{J!}{2!(J-2)!}$

Exercises

1. Sample size for normal weight is 67, for overweight is 101, and obese is 180. What are the degrees of freedom for the *F* test?
2. Refer to Exercise 1. $SS_B = 366.895$; $SS_T = 7469.526$. What is the *F* value?
3. Refer to the previous exercise. What is the critical value for the *F* test, and what is your conclusion?
4. If you found that the model was significant and you were interested in where the means differed, what approach would you take to discover this?
5. What type of ANOVA was just performed, one way or two way? Explain.
6. Many companies are incorporating worksite wellness programs. Three types of programs that are now popular are (1) personal fitness campaigns and challenges, (2) health-risk appraisal and health coaching, and (3) on-site fitness center. Random samples of employee satisfaction, measured on a scale from 1 (low) to 10 (high) were taken from five employees in each of the programs. The results are in the accompanying table.
   a. What is the grand mean for all the sample data and the sample means for each group?
   b. What is the between-groups sum of squares?
   c. What is the between-groups degrees of freedom?
   d. What is the mean square between groups?
   e. What is the error-groups sum of squares?
   f. What is the error-groups degrees of freedom?
   g. What is the mean square error?
   h. Test the hypothesis that the mean satisfaction values are the same for all three work schedules. Use 0.05 for the level of significance.
   i. Show the ANOVA table.
   j. If the *F* test is significant, apply the SNK post hoc test and indicate where differences lie.

Personal Fitness Campaigns and Challenges	Health-Risk Appraisal and Health Coaching	On-Site Fitness Center
8	8	6
7	7	5
10	7	6
10	7	7
8	8	5

7. Studies have shown that diet is influenced by marital status (married, never married, divorced, and widowed). The average number of fruit and vegetables consumed each day were taken from a random sample of seven individuals in each marital status group. The results are in the accompanying table.
   a. What is the grand mean for all the sample data and the sample means for each group?
   b. What is the between-groups sum of squares?
   c. What is the between-groups degrees of freedom?
   d. What is the mean square between groups?
   e. What is the within-groups sum of squares?

f. What is the within-groups degrees of freedom?
g. What is the mean square within groups?
h. Test the hypothesis that the mean satisfaction values are the same for all three work schedules. Use 0.05 for the level of significance.
i. Show the ANOVA table.
j. If the *F* test is significant, apply the SNK post hoc test and indicate where differences lie.
k. Suppose you planned to compare married and divorced, married and never married, and married and widowed prior to performing your ANOVA. If you performed these tests using the *t* test statistic, what is the appropriate alpha level for assessment based on the Bonferroni method?

Never Married	Married	Divorced	Widowed
3	8	3	5
3	5	3	6
2	7	2	7
3	4	4	4
2	5	1	5
4	3	4	6
2	3	4	7

8. An intervention was implemented, intended to increase fruit and vegetable consumption. Average fruit and vegetable consumption was measured at baseline and 6 weeks follow-up. Random samples were taken of change in average fruit and vegetable consumption according to intervention and education status and are shown in the accompanying table.
   a. Perform an ANOVA and assess the significance of the main effects and the interaction effect.
   b. Show the ANOVA table, without the interaction effect if it is not significant.
   c. Test the hypothesis that the means are the same in the three education groups. Use 0.05 for the level of significance.

Intervention	High School	College	Post-College
Yes	0.6	0.1	1.9
Yes	0.1	0.8	1.1
Yes	0.9	2.0	3.1
Yes	-0.04	0.3	2.4
Yes	1.0	2.4	1.8
No	0.1	-1.0	-0.3
No	-1.3	-0.8	0.1
No	-0.4	2.0	0.4
No	0.5	0.1	1.2
No	-0.07	-0.05	-0.8

9. Two groups of patients suffering from depression were identified, one with a genetic deficiency and the other without the deficiency (i.e., "normal").[17] They were randomly assigned a drug for treating depression or a placebo.

A standardized depression survey was administered to all the subjects, and the accompanying results were obtained.

a. Conduct a two-way ANOVA.
b. Is there an interaction effect? Interpret the findings.

	Anti-Depressant Drug	Placebo
Genetic deficiency	10	6
	10	9
	11	6
	9	7
Normal	7	11
	4	10
	5	12
	7	11

10. Thirty individuals volunteered to participate in a program intended to reduce body fat. Three programs were evaluated: physical activity, diet, and both physical activity and diet. The 30 subjects were randomly assigned to one of the three interventions. Percent body fat was measured at baseline and again at 6 months. The data are presented in the accompanying table.
    a. For the baseline data, evaluate H_0: $\mu_1 = \mu_2 = \mu_3$ using the steps of hypothesis testing.
    b. Create a variable that is the change in percent body fat from baseline to 6 month follow-up. The dependent variable is now the change score. Evaluate H_0: $\mu_1 = \mu_2 = \mu_3$ using the steps of hypothesis testing. Perform and discuss the results of a post hoc assessment.
    c. Perform an ANCOVA where the dependent variable is percent body fat at 6 months and the independent variables are the categorical intervention and percent body fat at baseline. Also, calculate the mean change in body fat for the three drugs, adjusting for baseline percent body fat.

Subject	Baseline	6 Months	Random #	Intervention
9	62	60	0.006	A
18	26	25	0.061	A
12	55	53	0.086	A
19	38	36	0.118	A
14	35	33	0.136	A
22	35	34	0.154	A
2	36	34	0.176	A
10	30	30	0.245	A
15	57	54	0.284	A
5	25	24	0.378	A
24	39	36	0.428	B
1	45	44	0.433	B
27	37	35	0.461	B

Subject	Baseline	6 Months	Random #	Intervention
8	58	55	0.473	B
28	29	27	0.474	B
13	53	50	0.556	B
26	43	40	0.572	B
11	20	19	0.620	B
20	45	44	0.629	B
16	22	20	0.673	B
21	37	30	0.679	C
25	46	29	0.744	C
17	30	24	0.745	C
3	29	27	0.815	C
4	60	50	0.821	C
29	58	52	0.827	C
23	38	32	0.832	C
6	40	35	0.840	C
7	32	27	0.905	C
30	37	32	0.932	C

11. Consider that we have four drugs designed to relieve pain. Eight subjects are given each of the four drugs. Pain tolerance is then measured on the subjects. Assume a sufficient washout time period between successive drugs so that no residual drug effect exists. The null hypothesis is H_0: $\mu_1 = \mu_2 = \mu_3 = \mu_4$.
    a. What are the sample means for each group?
    b. Perform a repeated measures ANOVA.
    c. What does Wilk's lambda say about statistical significance?
    d. If you reject the null hypothesis, which drug(s) is/are preferred?

Subject	Drug A	Drug B	Drug C	Drug D
1	5	8	6	9
2	3	12	8	8
3	7	12	10	11
4	11	9	5	14
5	5	10	7	9
6	5	7	8	10
7	6	10	10	11
8	8	8	7	8

12. Consider a two-factor experiment with repeated measures on both factors where a group of subjects is tested in the morning and afternoon on two separate dates.[17] Subjects were given a strong sleeping medication the night before the experiment on one day, but a placebo on the other. Reaction times to a stimulus measure were then obtained for each subject. Reaction times by treatment and time are in the accompanying table. When more than one factor is repeated, specify the number of

levels of each factor after the factor name; that is, the REPEATED line of the SAS code should read as follows: REPEATED TIME 2, TREAT 2 / NOM;

a. Perform the repeated measures ANOVA.
b. Is the time effect significant? Treatment effect significant? Time by treatment effect significant?
c. Calculate mean reaction times. What conclusions can be drawn?

	Control		Drug	
Subject	**A.M.**	**P.M.**	**A.M.**	**P.M.**
1	70	65	75	70
2	72	64	78	68
3	65	55	70	60
4	90	80	97	85

13. Of interest is whether CPAP use is independent of overall severity of obstructive sleep apnea. CPAP and severity variables are both categorical. Apply the steps of hypothesis testing to these data.

CPAP	Mild Problem	Moderate Problem	Severe Problem
Yes	26	30	18
No	12	7	1

14. Suppose that for our 94 patients with obstructive sleep apnea, we are interested in whether the number of upper-airway symptoms (i.e., voice, cough, and breathing problems) is associated with social anxiety.

Anxiety	0	1	2	3
Yes	7	8	9	12
No	40	10	4	4

Is there an association between anxiety and symptoms? Consider using a trend test.

15. Patients with obstructive sleep apnea were asked to rate their general health as good, fair, or poor. They also rated their daytime sleepiness on a scale from 0–3. Data results are in the following table:

	Daytime Sleepiness			
General Health	**0—no problem**	**1—mild problem**	**2—moderate problem**	**3—severe problem**
Excellent	13	12	4	3
Good	6	15	11	8
Poor	3	6	5	8

Evaluate whether a linear trend exists between general health and daytime sleepiness.

References

1. Kirk RE. *Experimental Design*, 2nd ed. Belmont, California: Brooks/Cole Publishing Company; 1982.
2. Merrill RM, Roy N, Pierce J, Sundar KM. Impact of voice, cough, and diurnal breathing problems on quality of life in obstructive sleep apnea. Do they matter? *AOHNS*. 2020;*4*(2):3.
3. Abdi H. The Bonferroni and Šidák corrections for multiple comparisons. In: Salkind N, ed. *Encyclopedia of Measurement and Statistics*. Thousand Oaks, CA: Sage; 2007.
4. Miller, RG. *Simultaneous Statistical Inference, 2nd ed.* New York, NY: Springer-Verlag; 1981.
5. Merrill RM, Richardson JS. Validity of self-reported height, weight, and body mass index: findings from the National Health and Nutrition Examination Survey, 2001–2006. *Prev Chronic Dis*. 2009;6(4):A121.
6. Chen J, Qi T, Liu L, Ling Y, Qian Z, Li T. Clinical progression of patients with COVID-19 in Shanghai, China. *J Infect*. 2020;*80*(5):e1–e6. doi: 10.1016/j.jinf.2020.03.004.
7. Lechien JR, Chiesa-Estomba CM, Place S, Van Laethem Y, Cabaraux P, Mat Q. Clinical and epidemiological characteristics of 1420 European patients with mild-to-moderate coronavirus disease 2019. *J Intern Med*. 2020;288(3):335–344.
8. Wu J, Li W, Shi X, Chen Z, Jiang B, Liu J. Early antiviral treatment contributes to alleviate the severity and improve the prognosis of patients with novel coronavirus disease (COVID-19). *J Intern Med*. 2020;288(1):128–138.
9. Voinsky I, Baristaite G, Gurwitz D. Effects of age and sex on recovery from COVID-19: analysis of 5769 Israeli patients. *J Infect*. 2020;*81*(2):e102-3103.
10. Conti P, Younes A. Coronavirus COV-19/SARS-CoV-2 affects women less than men: clinical response to viral infection. *J Biol Regul Homeost Agents*. 2020;*34*(2):339–343.
11. Gudbjartsson DF, Helgason A, Jonsson H, Magnusson OT, Stefansson K. Spread of SARS-CoV-2 in the Icelandic population. *N Engl J Med*. 2020 doi: 10.1056/NEJMoa2006100.
12. Keppel G. *Design and Analysis: A Researcher's Handbook*. 3rd ed. Englewood Cliffs, NJ: Prentice-Hall Inc.; 1991.
13. SAS Institute Inc. *SAS/Stat User's Guide. Vol* 2. 4th ed. Cary, NC: SAS Inc.; 1989;954.
14. Park C, Hsiung J, Soohoo M, Streja E. Choosing wisely: using the appropriate statistical test for trend. https://www.lexjansen.com/wuss/2019/175_Final_Paper_PDF.pdf. Accessed June 3, 2020.
15. SAS. Cochran-Armitage test for trend. https://v8doc.sas.com/sashtml/stat/chap28/sect24.htm. Published 1999. Accessed May 23, 2020.
16. Centers for Disease Control and Prevention. Weekly updates by selected demographic and geographic characteristics. https://www.cdc.gov/nchs/nvss/vsrr/covid_weekly/index.htm#Race_Hispanic. Accessed July 15, 2020.
17. Cody RP, Smith JK. *Applied Statistics and the SAS Programming Language*. 5th ed. Upper Saddle River, NJ: Pearson Prentice Hall; 2006.

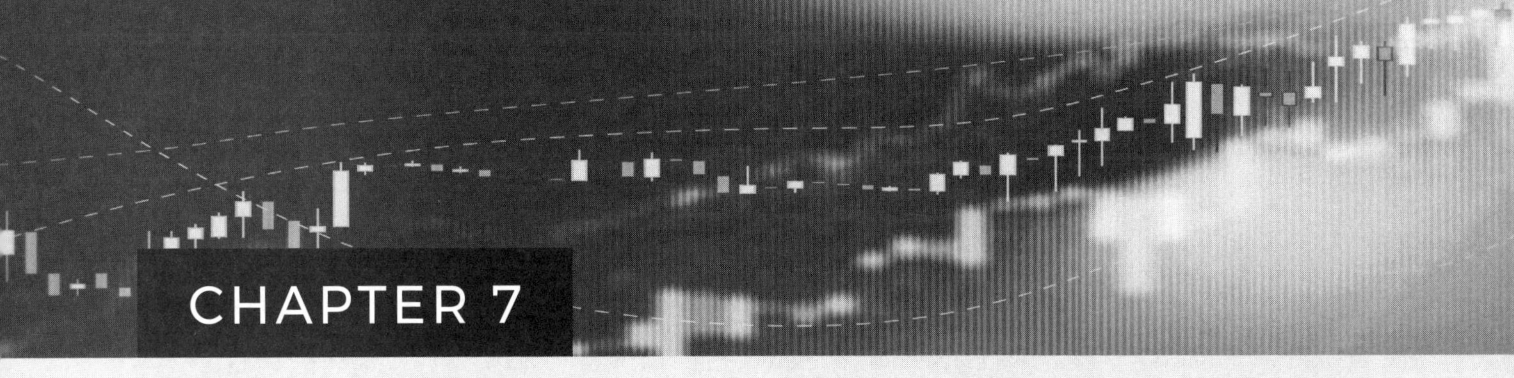

Measures of Association

KEY CONCEPTS

- A measure of association is a type of statistic that quantifies the relationship between variables.
- The statistical technique used to measure the strength of association between variables depends on the process of data collection and whether the variables are categorical or continuous.
- Categorical variables are measured on a nominal or ordinal scale, and continuous variables are measured on an interval or ratio scale.
- The categorical or continuous dependent variable depends on or responds to change in the categorical or continuous independent variable or variables. The independent variable does not depend on other variables in the study. The independent variable is sometimes called the predictor, exposure, or experimental variable.
- In experimental research, the independent variable is manipulated by the investigator in order to assess its effect on the dependent variable.
- The measurement technique for evaluating the association between two dichotomous (two-level) nominal variables is the risk ratio or rate ratio when cohort data are involved, the odds ratio when case-control or ecologic data are involved, and the prevalence ratio when cross-sectional data are involved.
- The relative risk (risk ratio) is a measure of the strength of association between dichotomous exposure and outcome variables that involves the ratio of two attack rates.
- The rate ratio is a measure of the strength of association between dichotomous exposure and outcome variables that involves the ratio of two person–time rates.
- The odds ratio is the ratio of the odds of exposure among cases divided by the odds of exposure among noncases.
- The prevalence ratio is analogous to the risk ratio but involves cross-sectional data in which the prevalence (proportion of all existing cases) is compared between exposed and unexposed subjects.
- Matching is a useful approach to control for confounding in case-control studies. It is a process that ensures that the confounding variable is similarly distributed among the groups being compared. With matched data, a modified formula for the odds ratio is used.
- The Mantel-Haenszel method is an approach for computing a weighted risk ratio, rate ratio, odds ratio, or prevalence ratio. It provides a pooled estimate across strata. It is used to adjust (control) for confounding.
- The chi-square (χ^2) test is used for evaluating hypotheses about the population risk ratio, rate ratio, odds ratio, and prevalence ratio.
- Other measures of association for dichotomous nominal data presented are risk and rate differences, the attributable fraction in the population, and the attributable fraction in the exposed group.
- The Pearson correlation coefficient (or correlation coefficient) is a measure of the linear association between two variables, ranging from −1 (perfect negative relationship) to +1 (perfect positive relationship).
- Spearman's correlation coefficient (also called Spearman's rho) is an alternative to the correlation coefficient when outlying data exist, such that one or both the distributions for the variables being correlated are skewed.
- The coefficient of determination is a measure of the proportion of the total observed variability among the dependent variable that is explained by the independent variable.
- Fisher's z-transformation is introduced because it allows us to test hypotheses and construct confidence intervals when the population correlation coefficient is assessed to be some value other than 0.

The fourth general area of biostatistics involves statistical techniques, which consist of a number of approaches that utilize statistical methods to investigate research questions. Various statistical techniques have already been presented in the context of addressing descriptive and inferential research questions. For example, the mean and standard deviation can be used to characterize a normal distribution, rates can be used to describe the risk of health outcomes, and comparisons of means, proportions, and rates can be used in statistical inference.

We are often interested in addressing research questions about the direction and magnitude of relationship between two variables. A statistic that measures the strength of relationship (effect size) between variables is a measure of association. Measures of association are different than statistical significance in that a weak association may be statistically significant or a strong association may be statistically insignificant. This is because statistical significance is based on more than just effect size; it is also based on variation in the data and sample size.

Several statistical techniques have been developed for measuring the strength of association between variables. Their use depends on the study design used for collecting, analyzing, and interpreting data. The process of data collection and the measurement scale of the variables involved indicate the type of measure of association that should be used. The purpose of this chapter is to present common measures of association according to the study design used, the measurement scale of the variables involved, and the underlying assumptions.

7.1 Questions About Statistical Associations

In scientific and scholarly investigation, the research question is matched with an appropriate study design. The study design is used to provide direction in collecting, analyzing, and interpreting data. A list of common study designs is presented in **Table 7.1**. Addressing some research questions provide descriptive information, while answering other research questions tell us something about how variables are associated. In biological research, we often address questions in which we assume the variables are logically ordered. That is, the dependent variable depends on or responds to change in the independent variable or variables. The independent variable (also called the predictor, exposure or experimental variable) does not depend on other variables in the study.

In experimental research, the independent variable is manipulated in order to assess its effect on the dependent variable. The experimental study design is a type of cohort study involving a time sequence of events in that the independent variable precedes the dependent variable. For example, in one study, three different allergy medications were randomly assigned to a group of subjects to be taken before bed (independent variable). Sleep quality was then measured (dependent variable). The experimental study design provides greater evidence about causality because the researcher is able to better control for temporality and remove effects of **bias** through blinding and confounding through random assignment.

Manipulating the independent variable is often not practical or ethical. For example, a researcher may want to know the effect of marijuana on psychosis. It would be unethical to assign some subjects to take marijuana and others not. However, a researcher could ask a sample of both marijuana users and nonusers to complete a questionnaire that indicates the extent both groups display psychotic behavior.

Table 7.1 Description and Examples of Questions Associated with Selected Study Designs

Study Design	Description	Questions
Case study	A qualitative description of a problem or situation for a subject or small group of subjects.	What effect does a new drug have on a given patient? What symptoms are manifest in a small group of individuals infected by SARS-CoV-2?
Ecological	Aggregate data involved, such as an infection rate or a proportion of people affected in the population; takes advantage of existing data.	What are COVID-19 death rates among U.S. counties? What proportion of the population is ⩾ 65 years among U.S. counties? Is there an association between COVID-19 death rates and the proportion of the population ⩾ 65 years among U.S. counties?
Cross-sectional	All of the variables are measured at a point in time; an effective way to collect prevalence data.	Have you used marijuana for a year or more? Do you have a history of psychosis? Is there an association between marijuana use and psychosis?
Case-control	Cases are compared to controls in terms of previous exposure status.	Are women with breast cancer compared with women without breast cancer more likely to have their first child after the age of 30? Do women with breast cancer compared with women without breast cancer have a shorter duration of breastfeeding?
Cohort	A group of subjects who share a defining characteristic are followed over time to describe the incidence or the natural history of a condition. The condition may be assessed according to exposure status.	In a foodborne outbreak among people who attended a community dinner, are those who ate the egg salad more likely to experience salmonellosis? In a group of nurses followed over time, is there evidence that eating nuts is protective against heart disease?
Experimental	A type of cohort study in which effects of an assigned intervention on an outcome are evaluated; if conducted in a medical setting to assess a new drug, medical device, or procedure, it is called a clinical trial; other types of trials are prophylactic, therapeutic, and community.	Does pre-exposure prophylaxis protect against HIV infection? Does remdesivir improve survival among people with severe COVID-19?

We refer to studies in which the levels of the independent variable are not determined by the researcher as **observational studies**. Several research questions are addressed using these types of studies (Table 7.1). Questions about statistical association may be addressed with each type of study design, except the case study design, which involves a qualitative description. In the following sections, statistical measures of association will be presented for the different study designs.

7.2 Measurement Scales

Recall that variables are measured on nominal, ordinal, interval, or ratio scales (see Table 1.2). A categorical variable is classified as either nominal or ordinal. A continuous variable is measured on either an interval or ratio scale. Categorical and continuous variables are described and assessed using different statistical methods. They are also evaluated for association using different methods. Further, the reference for no association differs. When continuous variables are being compared, a measure of association yielding 0 signifies no relationship. On the other hand, when the ratio of proportions or rates is being assessed, a measure of association resulting in 1 means no relationship.

Classifying a variable as categorical or continuous is also not always straightforward. For example, an ordinal scale variable may be treated as continuous. For example, a preference rating on a scale from 1 to 5 is an ordinal variable, but some may choose to evaluate it using the mean and standard deviation instead of proportions. In addition, how a variable is categorized is a matter of subjective choice. For example, the categories of race may or may not include ethnicity; a current voice disorder may require the problem to exist in the past week, month, or some other time period; and smokers may be classified into light, medium, or heavy smokers.

The specific type of measure of association used is presented according to study design and type of data employed in **Table 7.2**. Some study designs by variable types are not reflected in this table (e.g., ANOVA). The regression techniques listed are used to estimate slope coefficients, which measure the strength of the association between independent and dependent variables. These regression techniques will be covered in the next chapter.

Table 7.2 Measures of Association Used with Types of Independent and Dependent Variables

	Independent Variable/Dependent Variable			
Study Design	**Nominal 2 Levels/ Nominal 2 Levels**	**Nominal 2 Levels/ Continuous, Normally Distributed**	**Continuous, Normally Distributed/ Continuous, Normally Distributed**	**Continuous, Not Normally Distributed or Ordinal with > Two Categories/ Continuous, Not Normally Distributed or Ordinal with > Two Categories**
Ecological	Odds ratio; Logistic regression	Comparison of means	Correlation coefficient; Regression	Spearman rank correlation
Cross-sectional	Prevalence ratio; Log-binomial regression Prevalence difference	Comparison of means	Correlation coefficient; Regression	Spearman rank correlation
Case-control	Odds ratio; Logistic regression			
Cohort/ Experimental	Risk ratio; Log-binomial regression Risk difference (comparison of proportions) Rate ratio; Poisson regression Rate difference	Comparison of means	Correlation coefficient; Regression	Spearman rank correlation

7.3 Nominal Data

To begin, consider the following 2 × 2 contingency table, which is a common way to express the data relationship between two nominal (two-level) scale variables (**Table 7.3**). The frequency of data in each cell is represented by letters a, b, c, and d. The independent variable is exposure status, and the dependent variable is case status.

Table 7.3 2 × 2 Contingency Table for Cohort Data

	Cases	Noncases	Total
Exposed	a	b	$a + b$
Not Exposed	c	d	$c + d$
Total	$a + c$	$b + d$	$n = a + b + c + d$

7.3.1 Risk Ratio

To obtain a measure that compares the risk of a given health outcome between exposed and unexposed subjects, we can either take the ratio of two risks to provide a relative measure of the effect of the exposure, or we can take the difference of two risks to yield an absolute measure of the effect of the exposure. Risk ratios are measures of association that can be derived from cohort data. Risk ratios are commonly reported in the literature. For example, one study showed an inverse association between adherence to the Mediterranean diet and cancer mortality and incidence.[1] Based on a pooled analysis of several cohort studies, the paper reported a lower risk of cancer mortality (RR = 0.82, 95% CI 0.81–0.91) colorectal cancer (RR = 0.82, 95% CI 0.75–0.88), breast cancer (RR = 0.43, 95% CI 0.21–0.88), gastric cancer (RR = 0.72, 95% CI 0.60–0.86), liver cancer (RR = 0.58, 95% CI 0.46–0.73), and head and neck cancer (RR = 0.49, 95% CI 0.37, 0.67). The fact that the confidence intervals for these estimates do not overlap 1 indicates statistical significance at the 0.05 level. In addition, each estimate is less than 1, indicating that those adhering to the Mediterranean diet have lower risk of dying from these cancers than those not on the Mediterranean diet. For example, the RR = 0.43 indicates that those who adhere to the diet are 0.43 times as likely (or 57% less likely) to die from breast cancer. In a study of hospitalized patients with COVID-19 in Wuhan, China, those who were ≥ age 65 years versus younger were 3.8 (95% CI 1.15–17.39) times as likely to die.[2]

Suppose the data in Table 7.3 represent a cohort from the population of interest. The risk ratio consists of the proportion of the outcome for those exposed divided by the proportion of the outcome for those not exposed.

The **risk ratio** for a cohort study is

$$\text{Risk Ratio} = \frac{P(\text{outcome} \mid \text{exposed})}{P(\text{outcome} \mid \text{not exposed})} = \frac{R_e}{R_o}.$$

R_e = risk of being a case in the exposed group:
$P(\text{outcome} \mid \text{exposed}) = a/(a+b)$

R_o = risk of being a case in the unexposed group:
$P(\text{outcome} \mid \text{not exposed}) = c/(c+d)$

R = risk of being a case in the whole group: $P(\text{outcome}) = \dfrac{a+c}{a+b+c+d}$

We evaluate the risk ratio for statistical significance using the chi-square test statistic.

The **chi-square test statistic for evaluating the risk ratio** is

$$\chi^2 = \frac{(|ad-bc| - n/2)^2 \times n}{(a+b)(c+d)(a+c)(b+d)}$$

The 95% confidence interval is also useful for saying something about the precision of our estimate and whether the risk ratio is significantly different than 1.

The **95% confidence interval for a risk ratio** is

$$CI(RR) = e^{\ln(\text{Risk Ratio}) \pm \left(z_{1-\alpha/2} \times \sqrt{\frac{b/a}{a+b} + \frac{d/c}{c+d}}\right)}.$$

The risk difference tells us the excess risk of the outcome among the exposed group compared with the unexposed group, typically expressed per 100, 1000, or 100,000.

The **risk difference** for the difference in risk exposed minus the risk not exposed:

$$RD = P(\text{outcome} \mid \text{exposed}) - P(\text{outcome} \mid \text{not exposed}) = R_e - R_o$$

Example 7.1

A group of 348 adults in the United States were randomly assigned a dietary and physical activity intervention versus continuing with their normal dietary and physical activity.[3] Resulting data are shown in the following table. Apply the six steps of hypothesis testing to evaluate whether the intervention was effective at lowering percent body fat.

	Lowered Percent Body Fat	
Intervention	**Yes**	**No**
Yes	142	32
No	101	73

1. H_0: Risk Ratio $= 1$
2. H_a: Risk Ratio $\neq 1$
3. $\alpha = 0.05$, $n = 348$
4. χ^2, the critical value is $\chi^2_{0.05,1} = 3.841$.
5. $RR = \dfrac{142/174}{101/174} = 1.41$

$$\chi^2 = \frac{(|142 \times 73 - 32 \times 101| - 348/2)^2 \times 348}{(142 + 32)(101 + 73)(142 + 101)(32 + 73)} = 21.82$$

6. Referring to Appendix B, Table 5, the calculated χ^2 value is in the rejection region and corresponds with p-value < 0.005. Hence, we reject H_0 and conclude that those receiving the intervention are 1.41 times (41%) more likely to lower body fat over the six-week study period.

The 95% confidence interval does not overlap 1, which also indicates statistical significance.

$$95\%\ CI(1.41) = e^{\ln(1.41) \pm 1.96\sqrt{\frac{32/142}{142+32} + \frac{73/101}{101+73}}} \rightarrow 1.22 - 1.62$$

The risk difference is as follows:

$$\text{Risk Difference} = 0.8161 - 0.5805 = 0.2356.$$

Hence, body fat reduction in the intervention group is 23.56% higher.

7.3.2 Rate Ratio

In some cases, we are interested in measuring a rate, where the numerator in the calculation represents new cases during a given time period and the denominator is the time each person is observed, totaled for all persons. The ratio of two rates is called a **rate ratio**. A comparison of rates can be very informative. For example, the incidence rate ratio of COVID-19 in Italy compared with the United States, as of August 18, 2020, is 0.25.[4] The mortality rate ratio of COVID-19 in Italy compared with the United States on this same date is 1.11. Thus, Italy's incidence rate is 75% lower and its mortality rate is 11% higher than the United States. In another example, COVID-19 hospitalization rates are reported by race and Hispanic origin in the United States as of August 8, 2020.[5] From these data, the rate ratio of non-Hispanic American Indian or Alaska Native, non-Hispanic black, Hispanic, and non-Hispanic Asian or Pacific Islander compared with non-Hispanic white is 5.00 4.74, 4.71, and 1.31, respectively.

Table 7.4 provides the information we need to calculate a rate ratio from a cohort involving **person–time** data.

Table 7.4 2 × 2 Contingency Table for Cohort Person–Time Data

	Cases	Noncases	Person–Time
Exposed	a	b	PT_e
Not Exposed	c	d	PT_0
Total	$a + c$	$b + d$	PT

The **rate ratio** for a cohort study is

$$\text{Rate Ratio} = \frac{R_e}{R_o} = \frac{a/PT_e}{c/PT_o}.$$

R_e = rate of cases in the exposed group: $= a/PT_e$

R_o = rate of cases in the unexposed group: $= c/PT_o$

R = rate of cases in the whole group: $= (a+c)/PT$

We can evaluate the rate ratio for statistical significance using the chi-square test statistic.

The **chi-square test statistic for evaluating the rate ratio** is

$$\chi^2 = \frac{\{a - [PT_e(a+c)]/PT\}^2}{PT_e[PT_o(a+c)]/PT^2}.$$

The confidence interval allows us to see the precision in our estimate and determine statistical significance.

The **95% confidence interval for a rate ratio** is

$$CI(\text{Rate Ratio}) = e^{\ln(\text{Rate Ratio}) \pm z_{1-\alpha/2} \times \sqrt{\frac{1}{a} + \frac{1}{c}}}.$$

The rate difference tells us the excess rate of the outcome among the exposed group attributed to the exposure, typically expressed per 100, 1000, or 100,000.

The **rate difference** for the difference in the rate exposed and the rate not exposed is

$$RD = R_e - R_o.$$

Example 7.2

A cohort study was conducted among males, ages 40–79, in Japan.[6] Researchers investigated whether smoking was related to increased risk of cardiovascular disease. The data appear as follows:

Current Smoker	Cardiovascular Disease	Person-Years
Yes	882	220,965
No	673	189,254

1. H_0: Rate Ratio = 1
2. H_a: Rate Ratio ≠ 1

3. $\alpha = 0.05$, $n = 94{,}683$
4. χ^2, the critical value is $\chi^2_{0.05,1} = 3.841$
5. $RR = \dfrac{882/220{,}965}{673/189{,}254} = 1.12$

$$\chi^2 = \frac{\{882 - [220{,}965(882+673)]/410219\}^2}{220{,}965[189{,}254(882+673)]/410219^2} = 5.10$$

6. Referring to Appendix B, Table 5, the calculated χ^2 value is in the rejection region and corresponds with p-value = 0.0240. Hence, we reject H_0 and conclude that smokers are 1.12 times (or 12%) more likely than nonsmokers to die from cardiovascular disease. The confidence interval also supports the conclusion about statistical significance.

$$95\%\ CI(1.12) = e^{\ln(1.12) \pm 1.96\sqrt{\frac{1}{882}+\frac{1}{673}}} \rightarrow 1.02 - 1.24$$

The rate difference is calculated as follows:

$$\text{Rate Difference} = 0.003992 - 0.003556 = 0.0004355.$$

Therefore, the excess risk of cardiovascular disease attributed to smoking is 43.6 per 100,000.

7.3.3 Attributable Fraction in the Population (AF_p)

Another measure of association is the attributable fraction in the population, also called the population attributable risk percent.

$$AF_p = \frac{R - R_o}{R} \times 100$$

This measure reflects the expected proportional reduction in risk that would occur if the exposure were removed from the population. The numerator in the AF_p is the excess of disease in the population attributed to the exposure. For example, $AF_p = 25\%$ means that eliminating the exposure from the population would reduce the number of cases by 25%.

Example 7.3

Returning to Example 7.1, $R_o = 101/174 = 0.5805$ and $R = 243/348 = 0.6983$. Then

$$AF_p = \frac{0.6983 - 0.5805}{0.6983} \times 100 = 16.87\%.$$

Thus, if everyone were exposed to the intervention, we would expect a 16.87% increase in the percent who lowered their percent body fat over a 6-week period.

7.3.4 Attributable Fraction in the Exposed Cases (AF_e)

A related measure is the attributable fraction in the exposed cases, also called the attributable risk percent.

$$AF_e = \frac{R_e - R_o}{R_e} \times 100$$

This measure reflects the expected proportional reduction in cases who were exposed had the exposure not occurred. The numerator in the AF_e is the excess of disease among the exposed group attributed to the exposure. For example, $AF_e = 50\%$ means that among cases who were exposed, 50% of those cases are attributed to their exposure. Both the attributable fraction in the population and the attributable fraction in the exposed cases assumes a causal association between the independent and dependent variables.

EXAMPLE 7.4

Returning to Example 7.1, $R_e = 142/174 = 0.8161$ and $R_o = 101/174 = 0.5805$. Then

$$AF_e = \frac{0.8161 - 0.5805}{0.8161} \times 100 = 28.87\%.$$

Hence, among those who lowered their percent body fat that were also in the intervention group, 28.87% of the lower percent body fat is attributed to the intervention.

7.3.5 Prevalence Ratio

If the data in the table represent the prevalence (all existing cases) of the outcome or event at a point in time, then the prevalence for subjects exposed versus not exposed is calculated in the same way as the risk ratio. The χ^2 and confidence interval are also calculated the same way.

EXAMPLE 7.5

Among 94 obstructive sleep apnea patients, 28 had a snoring problem, and 66 did not. Of those with a snoring problem, 23 had esophageal reflux. Of those without a snoring problem, 38 had esophageal reflux.[7] Evaluate the prevalence ratio using the six steps of hypothesis testing.

1. H_0: Prevalence Ratio $= 1$
2. H_a: Prevalence Ratio $\neq 1$
3. $\alpha = 0.05$, $n = 94$
4. χ^2, the critical value is $\chi^2_{0.05,1} = 3.841$.
5. $PR = \dfrac{23/28}{38/66} = 1.43$

$$\chi^2 = \frac{(|23 \times 28 - 5 \times 38| - 94/2)^2 \times 94}{(23 + 5)(38 + 28)(23 + 38)(5 + 28)} = 4.19$$

6. Referring to Appendix B, Table 5 in the calculated χ^2 value is in the rejection region and corresponds with p-value = 0.0408. Hence, we reject H_0 and conclude that those with a snoring problem are 1.43 times (43%) more likely to have esophageal reflux than those without a snoring problem.

   The 95% confidence interval does not contain 1, which also indicates statistical significance at the 0.05 level.

$$95\%\ CI(1.43) = e^{\ln(1.43) \pm \left(1.96 \times \sqrt{\frac{5/23}{23+5} + \frac{28/38}{38+28}}\right)} \rightarrow 1.09 - 1.87$$

7.3.6 Odds Ratio

The odds ratio compares the odds of exposure among cases to the odds of exposure among non-cases. Like the other types of ratios considered thus far, when the odds ratio equals 1, there is no association between the exposure and the outcome. For example, a recent study asked about certain factors associated with hospitalization for COVID-19.[8] The study comprised six acute care hospitals and associated outpatient clinics in metropolitan Atlanta, Georgia, March 1–April 7, 2020. Researchers calculated odds ratios to evaluate associations. The odds ratio of hospitalization (yes versus no) according to sex (male versus female) was 1.86 (95% confidence interval = 1.31–2.64). In other words, the odds of being male among those who were hospitalized was 1.86 times greater than the odds of being male among those not hospitalized. The authors further used a technique called multiple logistic regression to estimate the odds ratio, adjusting for several potential confounding factors. We will address this technique of adjusting for potential confounders in the next chapter.

Now suppose the information in Table 7.3 represents **case-control** data. In this situation, an entire cohort is not represented in the table. Hence, the odds ratio is not interpreted the same way as the risk ratio or rate ratio. Instead of measuring the risk or rate of the outcome variable per exposure status, we measure the odds of exposure among cases versus the odds of exposure among noncases.

The formula for the **odds ratio** is

$$\text{Odds Ratio} = \frac{P(\text{exposed} \mid \text{outcome})/P(\text{unexposed} \mid \text{outcome})}{P(\text{exposed} \mid \text{no outcome})/P(\text{unexposed} \mid \text{no outcome})} = \frac{a/c}{b/d} = \frac{a \times d}{b \times c}.$$

The χ^2 formula for evaluating the odds ratio is the same as for the risk ratio and prevalence ratio. However, the formula is different for calculating the 95% confidence interval.

The **95% confidence interval for an odds ratio** (OR) is

$$CI(OR) = e^{\ln(OR) \pm z_{1-\alpha/2} \times \sqrt{\frac{1}{a} + \frac{1}{b} + \frac{1}{c} + \frac{1}{d}}}.$$

The attributable fraction can also be estimated in case-control studies when OR is an estimate of the RR. The OR is a good estimate of RR for rare outcomes where less than 10% of the population is affected. The proportion of exposed subjects in the population (p_e) in a case-control study is typically estimated by the exposure prevalence in the controls.

The **attributable fraction in the population for a case-control study** is

$$AF_p = \frac{p_e(OR-1)}{p_e(OR-1)+1} \times 100.$$

If the OR is a good estimate of RR, then we can also estimate the attributable fraction in exposed cases from a case-control study.

The **attributable fraction in exposed cases in a case-control study** is obtained as

$$AF_e = \frac{OR-1}{OR} \times 100.$$

Example 7.6

In a study examining the association between vitamin D intake with fracture risk in children under 6 years of age, 206 cases were recruited between May 2009 and April 2003 along with 343 controls.[9] The data are shown in the following table. Apply the six steps of hypothesis testing.

		Fracture	
		Yes	**No**
Vitamin D Supplement	No	170	229
	Yes	32	105

1. H_0: Odds Ratio $= 1$
2. H_a: Odds Ratio $\neq 1$
3. $\alpha = 0.05$, $n = 536$
4. χ^2, the critical value is $\chi^2_{0.05,1} = 3.841$
5. $\text{Odds Ratio} = \dfrac{170/32}{229/105} = 2.44$

   $$\chi^2 = \frac{(|170 \times 105 - 229 \times 32| - 536/2)^2 \times 536}{(170+229)(32+105)(170+32)(229+105)} = 15.28$$

6. Referring to Appendix B, Table 5, the calculated χ^2 value corresponds with p-value < 0.005. Hence, we reject H_0 and conclude that the odds of not using vitamin D supplements among cases is significantly greater than the odds of not using vitamin D supplements among noncases.

   The 95% confidence interval does not contain 1, which supports this conclusion.

   $$95\%\ CI(2.44) = e^{\ln(2.44) \pm 1.96 \times \sqrt{\frac{1}{170}+\frac{1}{229}+\frac{1}{32}+\frac{1}{105}}} \rightarrow 1.56 - 3.79$$

   The attributable fraction in the population for these data is

   $$AF_p = \frac{0.69(2.44-1)}{0.69(2.44-1)+1} \times 100 = 49.8\%.$$

In other words, if all children took vitamin D supplements, we would expect a decrease in fractures among children under 6 by almost 50%.

The attributable fraction in the exposed group is

$$AF_e = \frac{2.44 - 1}{2.44} \times 100 = 59.02\%.$$

This means that of those children who had a fracture who did not take vitamin D supplements, 59.02% of those cases are attributed to not taking the supplements.

7.3.7 Odds Ratio for Matched Case-Control Study

The potential for confounding is always present in observational studies. Matching is a strategy where the distribution of potential confounding factors is forced to be similar between cases and controls. In the example assessing the association between exercise and heart disease, a control of a similar age and gender could be selected for each case in order to control for the potential confounding effects of these factors.

In a **matched-paired case-control study**, the odds ratio is modified as follows:

$$\text{Odds Ratio} = \frac{P(\text{exposed} \mid \text{no outcome})}{P(\text{not exposed} \mid \text{outcome})} = \frac{b}{c}$$

The **chi-square test statistic** for a matched case-control study is

$$\chi^2 = \frac{(|b-c|-1)^2}{(b+c)}.$$

The **95% confidence interval** for a matched case-control study is

$$CI(OR) = e^{\ln(OR) \pm z_{1-\alpha/2} \times \sqrt{\frac{1}{b} + \frac{1}{c}}}.$$

Example 7.7

In a matched case-control study conducted in Morocco, investigators wanted to assess whether a relationship existed between using candles for light and lung cancer.[10] Controls were matched to cases on smoking status, age, and gender. Applying the steps to hypothesis testing for this matched case-control study gives the following:

1. H_0: Odds Ratio $= 1$
2. H_a: Odds Ratio $\neq 1$
3. $\alpha = 0.05$, $n = 160$
4. χ^2, the critical value is $\chi^2_{0.05,1} = 3.841$
5. The data appear (set up differently than previous tables) in the following contingency table:

		Controls	
		Candle Lighting	**No Candle Lighting**
Cases	Candle Lighting	25	25
	No Candle Lighting	10	100

$$OR = \frac{25}{10} = 2.5$$

$$\chi^2 = \frac{(|25-10|-1)^2}{(25+10)} = 5.6$$

6. Referring to Appendix B, Table 5, the calculated χ^2 value corresponds with $0.025 < P < 0.01$. Because the calculated value is in the rejection region, we reject H_0 and accept that there is an association between using candles for lighting and lung cancer in Morocco. This conclusion is also supported by the confidence interval.

$$95\%\, CI(2.5) = \exp\left[\ln(2.5) \pm 1.96 \times \sqrt{\frac{1}{25} + \frac{1}{10}}\right] \rightarrow 1.20 - 5.21$$

News File

Psychotic breaks from reality appears to be more common in cannabis users. A study of 901 patients with first-episode psychosis across 11 sites and 1237 controls found that daily cannabis use was associated with increased odds (odds ratio = 3.2, 95% *CI* = 2.2–4.1) of psychotic disorder compared with never users.[11] For daily users of high-potency cannabis compared with never users, that odds ratio was 4.8 (2.5–6.3). The attributable fraction in the population (*AFp*) for daily use of cannabis was 20.4% (17.6–22.0) in 11 European areas combined. In other words, 20.4% of psychotic disorder in these areas is attributed to daily cannabis use. The *AFp* in London (UK) was 21.0% (17.6–22.0), in Amsterdam (Netherlands) was 43.8% (34–69.1), and in Paris was 20.8% (13.5–36.1). The *AFp* for high-potency cannabis (THC ⩾ 10%) was 12.2% (3.0–16.1) in the 11 areas, 30.3% (15.2–40.0) in London (UK), 50.3% (27.4–66.0) in Amsterdam (Netherlands), and 18.9% (14.6–36.0) in Paris. Thus, daily use of cannabis and daily use of high-potency cannabis have a strong contribution to psychotic disorder. As the availability of cannabis and high-potency cannabis increases, society should be aware of the adverse consequences this will likely have on public health.

7.4 Mantel-Haenszel Method to Estimate an Adjusted Measure of Association

A pooled odds ratio across i homogeneous strata has been proposed by Mantel-Haenszel.[12] Stratification eliminates the association between the confounder and exposure within the strata. However, if the strata odds ratios are not homogeneous, then the odds ratio depends on the levels of the stratified variable. In this situation, it is informative to report the odds ratio for each strata.

$$\text{Odds Ratio}_{MH} = \frac{\sum_i \frac{a_i d_i}{n_i}}{\sum_i \frac{b_i c_i}{n_i}}$$

The 95% confidence interval for a stratified odds ratio in a case-control study requires the estimated chi-square value.

$$CI(OR_{MH}) = OR_{MH}^{1 \pm z_{1-\alpha/2}/\sqrt{\chi^2_{MH}}}$$

The chi-square test statistic for the summary odds ratio is complicated, best derived by the computer.

$$\chi^2_{MH} = \frac{\left\{\sum_i a_i - \sum_i [(a_i + c_i)(a_i + b_i)/n_i]\right\}^2}{\sum_i (a_i + b_i)(c_i + d_i)(a_i + c_i)(b_i + d_i)/[n_i^2(n_i - 1)]}$$

The Mantel-Haenszel method can also apply to the risk ratio or rate ratio in cohort studies. Again, we adjust for the potential confounder by stratifying across the levels of this variable. However, if the risk ratio or rate ratio is not homogeneous across strata, do not report a pooled estimate but report its value for each strata.

$$\text{Risk Ratio}_{MH} = \frac{\sum_i \frac{a_i(c_i + d_i)}{a_i + b_i + c_i + d_i}}{\sum_i \frac{c_i(a_i + b_i)}{a_i + b_i + c_i + d_i}}$$

$$\text{Rate Ratio}_{MH} = \frac{\sum_i \frac{a_i PTo_i}{PT_i}}{\sum_i \frac{c_i PTe_i}{PT_i}}$$

$$CI(RR_{MH}) = RR_{MH}^{1 \pm z_{1-\alpha/2}/\sqrt{\chi^2_{MH}}}$$

The **Breslow-Day test** for homogeneity can be used to assess whether it is appropriate to pool the stratified odds ratios or risk ratios.[13] The null hypothesis tested by this test is that the estimates across the strata are homogeneous. If the χ^2 value is larger than the critical value and, equivalently, the corresponding p-value < 0.05, then reject the null hypothesis of homogeneity and do not pool the stratified estimates but report them separately for each strata. The Breslow-Day test is available in most statistical software packages. This test is valid if the sample size is sufficiently large in each stratum, such that at least 80% of the expected cell counts are greater than 5. We can test for homogeneity among stratified rate ratios using an interaction term in a Poisson regression model.

EXAMPLE 7.8

In a case-control study involving a group of women aged 30 years and older, researchers wanted to know whether there was a relationship between coffee drinking and osteoporosis. Smoking is thought to be a confounder, so data were collected on this variable so a stratified analysis could be performed. Applying the steps to hypothesis testing for this study gives the following:

1. H_0: Odds $\text{Ratio}_{MH} = 1$
2. H_a: Odds $\text{Ratio}_{MH} \neq 1$
3. $\alpha = 0.05$, $n = 400$
4. χ^2, the critical value is $\chi^2_{0.05,1} = 3.841$
5. The hypothetical data appear in the following contingency tables:

Coffee Drinking and Osteoporosis, Crude Data

	Osteoporosis	
Coffee Drinker	Yes	No
Yes	136	119
No	62	85

$$OR_{Crude} = \frac{136 \times 85}{119 \times 62} = 1.57$$

Coffee Drinking and Osteoporosis Among Smokers

	Osteoporosis	
Coffee Drinker	Yes	No
Yes	96	62
No	24	19

$$OR_S = \frac{96 \times 19}{62 \times 24} = 1.23$$

Coffee Drinking and Osteoporosis Among Nonsmokers

	Osteoporosis	
Coffee Drinker	Yes	No
Yes	40	57
No	38	66

$$OR_{NS} = \frac{40 \times 66}{57 \times 38} = 1.22$$

Because the crude odds ratio is larger than the stratified odds ratios, it appears that smoking is a positive confounder. The stratified odds ratios are about the same, so we pool them using the Mantel-Haenszel method.

$$OR_{MH} = \frac{\frac{(96 \times 19)}{201} + \frac{(40 \times 66)}{201}}{\frac{(62 \times 24)}{201} + \frac{(57 \times 38)}{201}} = 1.22$$

The χ^2 test statistic obtained from SAS is 0.8059.

6. Referring to Appendix B, Table 5, the calculated χ^2 value corresponds with p-value > 0.100. Its exact value obtained by SAS is 0.3693. So we fail to reject the null hypothesis.

   The bounds of the 95% confidence interval contain 1, which also indicates no significant relationship between coffee drinking and osteoporosis.

$$95\%\ CI(1.22) = 1.22^{1 \pm 1.96/\sqrt{0.8059}} \rightarrow 0.79 - 1.89$$

Example 7.9

A group of adults were randomly assigned to either an intervention or control group. The intervention involved a dietary program. Each group had their body mass index (BMI) determined at baseline and 6 months. We suspect that sex may confound the results. Let's calculate a risk ratio that adjusts for the potential confounding effect of gender. Application of the steps of hypothesis gives the following:

1. H_0: Risk Ratio$_{MH} = 1$
2. H_a: Risk Ratio$_{MH} \neq 1$
3. $\alpha = 0.05$, $n = 360$
4. χ^2, the critical value is $\chi^2_{0.05,1} = 3.841$
5. The hypothetical data are presented in contingency tables for men and women:

	Lowered BMI	
Intervention	Yes	No
Yes	148	36
No	98	78

$$RR_{Crude} = \frac{\frac{148}{(148+36)}}{\frac{98}{(98+78)}} = 1.44$$

Men

	Lowered BMI	
Intervention	Yes	No
Yes	40	7
No	35	13

$$RR_M = \frac{\frac{40}{(40+7)}}{\frac{35}{(35+13)}} = 1.17$$

Women

	Lowered BMI	
Intervention	Yes	No
Yes	108	29
No	63	65

$$RR_W = \frac{\frac{108}{(108+29)}}{\frac{63}{(63+65)}} = 1.60$$

The χ^2 test statistic is 26.36 and the Breslow-Day test statistic's p-value is 0.3126 (obtained by SAS). We do not reject the null hypothesis for homogeneity of the risk ratios. Therefore, it is appropriate to obtain a pooled risk ratio, which adjusts for the confounding effect of sex.

$$RR_{MH} = \frac{40(35+13)/95+108(63+65)/265}{35(40+7)/95+63(108+29)/265} = 1.45$$

6. Referring to Appendix B, Table 5, the calculated $\chi^2 = 26.36$ corresponds with p-value < 0.0001. Hence, we reject H_0 and conclude that the intervention does significantly lower BMI through 6 months of follow-up, after controlling for sex.

The 95% confidence interval tells us something about the precision of our estimate and also indicates statistical significance.

$$95\%\ CI(1.45) = 1.45^{1\pm1.96/\sqrt{26.36}} \rightarrow 1.25 - 1.68$$

EXAMPLE 7.10

Suppose you recently read a study indicating that high levels of caffeinated soda consumption can lead to psychosis. You want to test this for yourself in a cohort study. However, you are also aware that psychosis can be associated with marijuana consumption, and you also suspect that people who drink a lot of caffeinated soda are also more likely to use marijuana. Hence, you suspect that adjusting for marijuana in the study is important.

Application of the steps of hypothesis gives the following:

1. H_0: Rate Ratio$_{MH} = 1$
2. H_a: Rate Ratio$_{MH} \neq 1$
3. $\alpha = 0.05$, $n = 4000$
4. χ^2, the critical value is $\chi^2_{0.05,1} = 3.841$
5. The hypothetical data presented in contingency tables are

	Psychosis	
Heavy Caffeinated Soda Use	Yes	Person-Years
Yes	146	2000
No	99	2000

$$RR_{Crude} = \frac{\frac{146}{2000}}{\frac{99}{2000}} = 1.47$$

Marijuana Users

	Psychosis	
Heavy Caffeinated Soda Use	Yes	Person-Years
Yes	100	1000
No	55	1000

$$RR_{MU} = \frac{\frac{100}{1000}}{\frac{55}{1000}} = 1.82$$

Marijuana Nonusers

	Psychosis	
Heavy Caffeinated Soda Use	Yes	Person-Years
Yes	46	1000
No	44	1000

$$RR_{MNU} = \frac{\frac{46}{1000}}{\frac{44}{1000}} = 1.05$$

The interaction term in a Poisson regression gives a p-value = 0.041 (obtained by SAS). We reject the null hypothesis for homogeneity of the rate ratios and do not estimate a pooled rate ratio.

6. Of interest is whether the association between heavy caffeinated soda use and psychosis depends on marijuana use. For marijuana nonusers who consume heavy amounts of caffeinated soda, their level of psychosis is 1.05 (5%) greater than those who do not consume heavy amounts of caffeinated soda. For marijuana users, on the other hand, those who consume heavy amounts of caffeinated soda are 1.82 (82%) more likely to experience psychosis than those who do not consume heavy amounts of caffeinated soda.

7.5 Continuous Data

If two continuous variables are obtained, a scatter plot is an appropriate way to display the data. The scatter plot can tell us whether the variables are normally distributed and linearly related. The correlation coefficient and the regression model are standard techniques to measure the association between continuous variables. Both assume a linear relationship between the independent and dependent variables. Here is a scatter plot showing the association between BMI and SF-36 general health quality of life among 94 patients with obstructive sleep apnea (**Figure 7.1**).[7] The data were obtained from a cross-sectional survey, with each dot representing individual level information. The distribution of BMI scores is slightly skewed to the right (mean = 35.37 and median = 33.40). The distribution of general health quality-of-life scores is slightly skewed to the left (mean = 52.93 and median = 55.00). A linear line

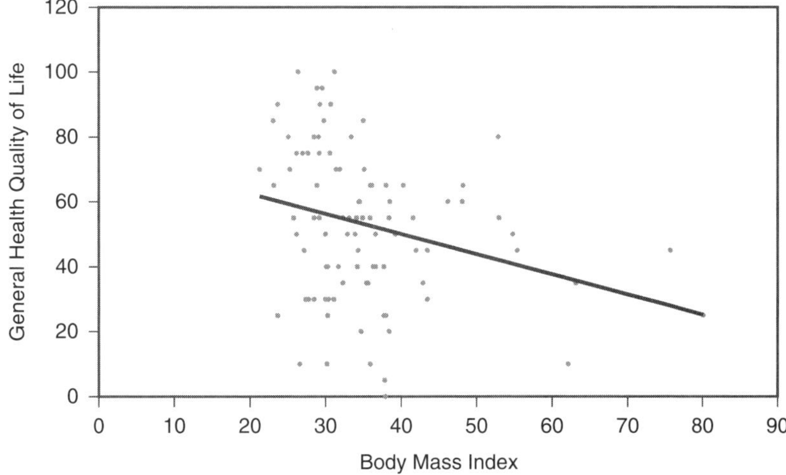

Figure 7.1 BMI by General Health Quality of Life

fit to the data indicates a negative (or inverse) association between the variables. In other words, as BMI increases, general health quality of life tends to decrease.

This next graph displays ecologic data, with each data point representing aggregated information on the population level (**Figure 7.2**). The case-fatality rate (per 100) for COVID-19 on August 18, 2020, is shown by life expectancy for 176 countries around the world.[4,14] The graph shows that the life expectancy and case-fatality rate variables are not linearly related. The lowest case-fatality rates are in countries with life expectancy about 68 years of age.

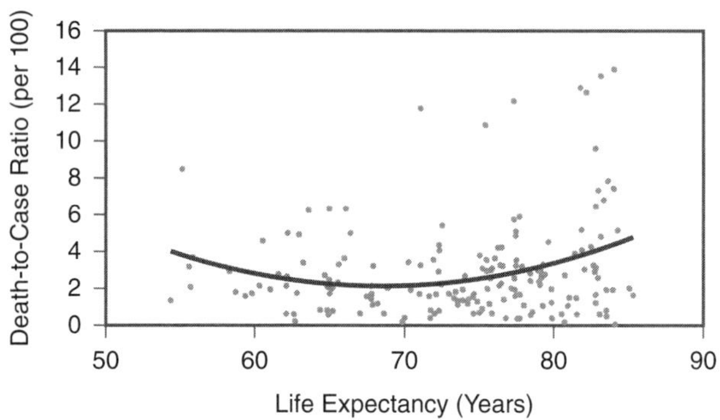

Figure 7.2 Life Expectancy by Case-Fatality Fate of COVID-19 as of August 18, 2020

7.5.1 Correlation Coefficient

A popular statistic that measures the strength of the linear association between numerical variables is the correlation coefficient. Assumptions for this statistic are bivariate normality and linearity. The correlation coefficient is a scaled range from –1 (perfect negative association) to +1 (perfect positive association). A 0 value means there is no association between the variables. The population parameter for this measure is ρ (the lowercase Greek letter rho), which is estimated by r.

Correlation Coefficient

$$r = \frac{\Sigma_i (x_i - \bar{x})(y_i - \bar{y})}{\sqrt{\Sigma_i (x_i - \bar{x})^2 \, \Sigma_i (y_i - \bar{y})^2}}$$

If the population parameter ρ is set to 0 in the null hypothesis, significance of the estimated correlation coefficient can be assessed using the t-ratio.

***t*-Ratio for Evaluating** $H_0\!: \rho = 0$

$$t = \frac{r\sqrt{n-2}}{\sqrt{1-r^2}}$$

Degrees of freedom $= n - 2$

For the data in Figure 7.1, the correlation coefficient is –0.274. It follows that

$$t = \frac{-0.274\sqrt{94-2}}{\sqrt{1-(-0.274)^2}} = -2.73.$$

Referring to Appendix B, Table 5, the calculated t corresponds with a p-value = 0.0075. Since the p-value < 0.05, we reject H_0 and conclude that as BMI increases, general health quality of life among patients with obstructive sleep apnea decreases.

For the data in Figure 7.2, the correlation coefficient is misleading because the data are not bivariate normal or linear. The distribution of life expectancy among the countries is skewed to the left (mean = 73.80 and median = 75.50). The case-fatality rate data are skewed right (mean = 2.93 and median 2.15). In addition, the association between the variables is first negative and then positive. A linear relationship may fit the data adequately for countries with life expectancy below 68 and for countries with life expectancy of 68 years and older. Stratifying the data in this manner resulted in correlation coefficients of –0.164 (p-value = 0.2811) and 0.260 (p-value = 0.0027), respectively. However, in both groups the data have outliers, such that the normality assumption does not hold.

7.5.2 Spearman Rank Correlation Coefficient

When outliers are present, an alternative to the correlation coefficient is the Spearman rank correlation coefficient (also called Spearman's rho), denoted by r_s. The Spearman rank correlation coefficient is essentially the correlation coefficient applied to ranked data for each variable.

Spearman Rank Correlation Coefficient

$$r = \frac{\Sigma_i (R(x_i) - R(\overline{x}))(R(y_i) - R(\overline{y}))}{\sqrt{\Sigma_i (R(x_i) - R(\overline{x}))^2 \, \Sigma_i (R(y_i) - (\overline{y}))^2}}$$

The Spearman rank correlation coefficients for the life expectancy and case-fatality data for those countries with life expectancy < 68 years of age is –0.100 (p-value = 0.5189) and for those countries with life expectancy ≥ 68 years of age is 0.212 (p-value = 0.0151). Thus, the Spearman rank correlation coefficient, which adjusts for outliers, also indicates that there is no association between life expectancy and the death-to-case ratio in countries with poorer life expectancy, but confirms a significant positive correlation between these variables in countries with better life expectancy.

7.5.3 Coefficient of Determination

A related statistic is the coefficient of determination, denoted as r^2. This measure represents the proportion of the total variation in the dependent variable Y that is determined by the independent variable X. For example, if $r = 1$ then all of the variation in the dependent variable is explained by the independent variable. However, typically only part of the variation in the dependent variable is explained by a single independent variable. For the data in Figure 7.1, the coefficient of determination is 0.075, which means that 7.5% of the variation in general health quality of life is explained by BMI.

EXAMPLE 7.11

COVID-19 case, death, and testing information on August 18, 2020, is shown for selected countries in **Table 7.5**.[4] Also included in the table is the percentage of the population 60 years of age and older.[15] Research has shown that older people are more susceptible to COVID-19. Hence, in our data we would expect that older people would be more likely to get tested and have a higher case rate, death rate, and death-to-case ratio. Relationships between being at least 60 years of age (%) and the selected COVID-19 variables are shown in **Figure 7.3**.

Table 7.5 COVID-19 Information and Percentage Aged 60 Years and Older by Selected Countries

	Test Rate per 1M	Case Rate per 1M	Death Rate per 1M	Death-to-case ratio %	≥ 60 %
United States	219,822	17,143	531	3.1	23.2
Brazil	64,532	16,066	518	3.2	13.6
India	22,972	2052	39	1.9	10.2
Russia	227,606	6423	110	1.7	22.6
South Africa	57,744	9968	206	2.1	9.2
Peru	85,341	16,630	807	4.9	11.8
Mexico	9269	4115	447	10.9	11.4
Colombia	45,124	9599	307	3.2	12.8
Chile	109,069	20,380	553	2.7	17.2
Spain	170,147	8298	616	7.4	24.5
Iran	34,943	4163	239	5.7	9.4
United Kingdom	220,629	4727	609	12.9	24.3
Argentina	22,386	6762	135	2.0	16.5
Saudi Arabia	125,515	8677	101	1.2	6.1
Pakistan	10,568	1312	28	2.1	6.9
Bangladesh	8450	1729	23	1.3	10.1
Italy	127,596	4223	586	13.9	28.5
Turkey	70,682	2997	72	2.4	12.5
Germany	121,658	2729	111	4.1	30.2
France	91,893	3447	466	13.5	26.5
Iraq	33,357	4681	152	3.2	5.0
Philippines	19,705	1583	25	1.6	7.6
Indonesia	6992	529	23	4.3	12.0
Canada	129,153	3264	239	7.3	25.8
Israel	233,898	10,631	85	0.8	16.0
Ukraine	30,551	2206	49	2.2	23.9
Ireland	148,756	5571	359	6.4	18.8
Australia	212,984	939	18	1.9	21.4

	Test Rate per 1M	Case Rate per 1M	Death Rate per 1M	Death-to-case ratio %	≥ 60 %
Denmark	350,230	2751	107	3.9	25.8
Luxembourg	1,099,843	11,955	198	1.7	20.9

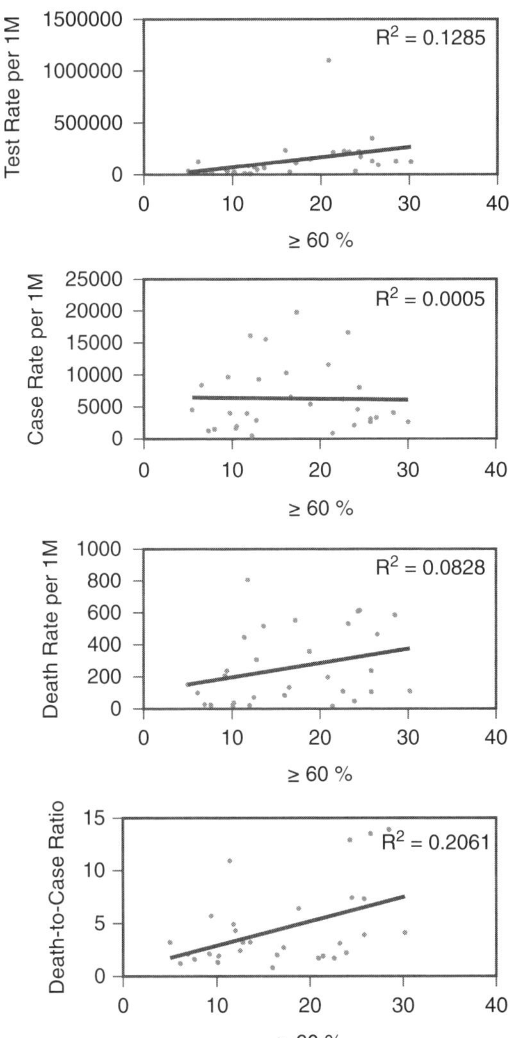

Figure 7.3 Scatter Plots Showing COVID-19 Variables by the Percentage Age 60 and Older

The correlation coefficients can be readily calculated in SAS, Excel, etc. (see Section 7.3). The t ratios were computed as 2.03, –0.11, 1.59, and 2.69. Referring to Appendix B, Table 5, the critical value of t is 2.048. Hence, the association between COVID-19 testing and ≥ 60 years of age (%) is marginally insignificant, and the association between the death-to-case ratio and ≥ 60 years of age is significant.

You may have noticed a few outliers in the data, especially for the COVID-19 test rate data. Spearman's correlation coefficient for the association between COVID-19 testing and ≥ 60 years of age (%) is 0.617, and $r_s^2 = 0.381$, resulting in a t ratio of 4.15 and a p-value of 0.0003. This statistic can be calculated in Excel by first computing the rank values for each variable, and then deriving the correlation coefficient from the ranked data.

Therefore, for the countries considered, COVID-19 testing is positively associated with a higher percentage of the population being at least 60 years of age. Approximately 38.1% of the variation in COVID-19 testing is explained by the percentage at least 60 years of age. The death-to-case ratio is also greater in countries with a higher percentage of their population being ≥ 60 years of age. Approximately 20.6% of the variation in the COVID-19 death-to-case ratio is explained by the percentage at least 60 years of age.

7.5.4 Fisher's z-Transformation for Testing the Correlation Coefficient

Although we are generally interested in testing H_0: $\rho = 0$ when the correlation coefficient is under consideration, sometimes there may be an interest in testing whether the correlation is equal to a value other than 0.[16] The Fisher's z-transformation can be used to test the null hypothesis about the correlation that equals any value in the range 0–1. In that sense, it is more flexible than the t test. It can also form confidence intervals.

Steps for Fisher's Exact Test

1. Transform the correlation coefficient

$$z(r) = \frac{1}{2}\ln\left(\frac{1+r}{1-r}\right)$$

where ln is the **natural logarithm**.

2. Apply the standard normal z

$$z = \frac{z(r) - z(\rho)}{\sqrt{1/(n-3)}}$$

Example 7.12

The correlation coefficient measuring the linear association between voice-related quality of life and SF-36 social functioning quality of life for a group of adults is 0.38. Suppose we wanted to know whether the correlation is significantly greater than 0.20. To proceed we will consider the six steps of hypothesis testing.

1. $H_0: \rho = 0.2$
2. $H_a: \rho > 0.2$
3. $\alpha = 0.05$. Referring to Appendix B, Table 3, the critical value of z = 1.645.
4. Fisher's z transformation
5. $z = \frac{z(0.38) - z(0.20)}{\sqrt{1/(94-3)}} = \frac{0.400 - 0.203}{\sqrt{1/(94-3)}} = 1.88$
6. The calculated z statistic is greater than the critical value, so we reject H_0 and conclude that the relationship between voice-related quality of life and SF-36 social functioning quality of life is greater than 0.2.

7.5.5 Confidence Interval for a Correlation Coefficient

The Fisher's z-transformation makes it possible to form confidence intervals for the correlation coefficient. The process of obtaining confidence limits is to first estimate transformed confidence limits and then transform them back to values that correspond to the correlation coefficient.

Confidence Interval for Fisher's z-Transformed r

$$z \text{ transform of } r \pm z_{1-\alpha/2}\sqrt{(1/(n-3))}$$

$$\text{Confidence Interval} = \left[\frac{e^{2L}-1}{e^{2L}+1}, \frac{e^{2U}-1}{e^{2U}+1}\right]$$

EXAMPLE 7.13

Continuing with the previous example, Fisher's z-transformation for the correlation coefficient 0.38 is 0.400. Let us use a level of significance of 0.1, such that

$$\begin{aligned} z(0.38) &\pm 1.645\sqrt{(1/(94-3))} \\ &= 0.400 \pm 0.172 \\ &= 0.228, 0.572 \end{aligned}$$

$$\text{Confidence Interval} = \left[\frac{e^{2\times0.228}-1}{e^{2\times0.228}+1}, \frac{e^{2\times0.572}-1}{e^{2\times0.572}+1}\right] = 0.224, 0.517.$$

Hence, we are 90% confident that the true value of the correlation in the population is bounded in the interval 0.224–0.517. Because 0.2 is not contained in the confidence interval, this further supports that the 0.38 is significantly greater than 0.2.

7.6 Comparing Two Correlation Coefficients

In some situations, it may be of interest to identify whether there is a difference between two correlation coefficients. In this section, we will present the situation where the correlation coefficient is compared between two independent groups. When a correlation coefficient involving two variables is constructed in two independent groups, we can use Fisher's z-transformation to test hypotheses and construct confidence intervals.

Test Statistic for Comparing Correlations in Two Independent Groups

$$z = \frac{z(r_1) - z(r_2)}{\sqrt{\frac{1}{n_1-3} + \frac{1}{n_2-3}}}$$

EXAMPLE 7.14

We are interested in whether the correlation coefficient measuring the strength of the linear association between muscle mass and age among adults differs between men and women. Suppose the correlation coefficient for men is –0.549 and for women is –0.949 and the sample size in each group is 10.

1. $H_0: \rho_1 = \rho_2$
2. $H_a: \rho_1 \neq \rho_2$
3. $\alpha = 0.05$, and n per group is 10.
4. Fisher's z transformation. Refer to Appendix B, Table 3, to obtain the two-tailed critical value of $z = 1.96$.
5. $z = \dfrac{-0.617 - (-1.826)}{\sqrt{\dfrac{1}{10-3} + \dfrac{1}{10-3}}} = 2.25$
6. Since the value of the test statistic is greater than 1.96, we reject H_0 and conclude that there is a significant difference in the correlation coefficients for muscle mass and age between men and women.

7.7 Statistical Software

Statistical software can compute many of the measures of association that will be covered in this text. In this section, SAS data and procedure statements are presented for computing the statistics for most of the examples in this chapter.

SAS Data Statement	SAS Procedure Code
DATA EX7_1; INPUT X Y Count; DATALINES; 1 1 142 1 2 32 2 1 101 2 2 73 ;	PROC FREQ DATA=EX7_1; TABLE X*Y/RELRISK RISKDIFF CHISQ; WEIGHT Count; RUN;
DATA EX7_2; INPUT Smoke $ Cases PYEARS; LPYEARS=LOG(PYEARS); DATALINES; 1 882 220965 2 673 189254 ;	PROC GENMOD DATA=EX7_2; CLASS Smoke; MODEL CASES=Smoke/ DIST=POISSON LINK=LOG OFFSET=LPYEARS; ESTIMATE 'Smoke' Smoke 1 -1/EXP; RUN;
DATA EX7_5; INPUT X Y COUNT; DATALINES; 1 1 23 1 2 5 2 1 38 2 2 28 ;	PROC FREQ DATA=EX7_5; TABLE X*Y/RELRISK CHISQ; WEIGHT COUNT; RUN;

<table>
<tr><th>SAS Data Statement</th><th>SAS Procedure Code</th></tr>
<tr><td>DATA EX7_6;
INPUT X Y COUNT;
DATALINES;
1 1 170
1 2 229
2 1 32
2 2 105
;</td><td>PROC FREQ DATA=EX7_6;
TABLE X*Y/RELRISK CHISQ;
WEIGHT COUNT;
RUN;</td></tr>
<tr><td>The following SAS data statement is another way to create a SAS data set in a 2 × 2 table.
DATA EX7_7;
  DO CASE = 'PRESENT','ABSENT';
  DO CONTROL = 'PRESENT','ABSENT';
  INPUT COUNT @@;
  OUTPUT;
  END;
END;
DATALINES;
25 25
10 100
;</td><td>The following SAS code computes the odds ratio and corresponding confidence interval for matched paired data.
DATA New;
SET EX7_7;
RETAIN ID 0;
DO ID=ID+1 TO ID+COUNT;
FACTOR=CASE;
RESPONSE='CASE';OUTPUT;
FACTOR=CONTROL;
RESPONSE='CONTROL';OUTPUT;
END;
KEEP ID FACTOR RESPONSE;
RUN;
PROC PRINT DATA=New;
ID ID;
RUN;
PROC FREQ DATA=New ORDER=DATA;
TABLE ID*FACTOR*RESPONSE/CMH NOPRINT;
RUN;</td></tr>
<tr><td>DATA EX7_8;
INPUT S X Y COUNT;
DATALINES;
1 1 1 96
1 1 2 62
1 2 1 24
1 2 2 19
2 1 1 40
2 1 2 57
2 2 1 38
2 2 2 66
;</td><td>PROC FREQ DATA=EX7_8;
TABLE S*X*Y/CMH;
WEIGHT COUNT;
RUN;</td></tr>
<tr><td>DATA EX7_9;
INPUT S X Y COUNT;
DATALINES;
1 1 1 40
1 1 2 7
1 2 1 35
1 2 2 13
2 1 1 108
2 1 2 29
2 2 1 63
2 2 2 65
;</td><td>PROC FREQ DATA=EX7_9;
TABLE S*X*Y/CMH;
WEIGHT COUNT;
RUN;</td></tr>
</table>

SAS Data Statement	SAS Procedure Code
DATA EX7_10; INPUT M $ S $ Cases PY; LPY=LOG(PY); DATALINES; 1 1 100 1000 1 2 55 1000 2 1 46 1000 2 2 44 1000 ;	PROC GENMOD DATA+EX&_10; CLASS M S; MODEL CASES=M S M*S/DIST=POISSON LINK=LOG OFFSET=LPYEARS; ESTIMATE 'Caffinated Soda' S 1 -1/EXP; RUN;
DATA EX7_11; INPUT TR CR DR DCR X60_P; DATALINES; 219822 17143 531 3.1 23.2 64532 16066 518 3.2 13.6 22972 2052 39 1.9 10.2 227606 6423 110 1.7 22.6 57744 9968 206 2.1 9.2 85341 16630 807 4.9 11.8 9269 4115 447 10.9 11.4 45124 9599 307 3.2 12.8 109069 20380 553 2.7 17.2 170147 8298 616 7.4 24.5 34943 4163 239 5.7 9.4 220629 4727 609 12.9 24.3 22386 6762 135 2.0 16.5	PROC CORR DATA=EX7_11 PEARSON SPEARMAN; VAR TR CR DR DCR; WITH X60_P; RUN;
125515 8677 101 1.2 6.1 10568 1312 28 2.1 6.9 8450 1729 23 1.3 10.1 127596 4223 586 13.9 28.5 70682 2997 72 2.4 12.5 121658 2729 111 4.1 30.2 91893 3447 466 13.5 26.5 33357 4681 152 3.2 5 19705 1583 25 1.6 7.6 6992 529 23 4.3 12 129153 3264 239 7.3 25.8 233898 10631 85 0.8 16 30551 2206 49 2.2 23.9 148756 5571 359 6.4 18.8 212984 939 18 1.9 21.4 350230 2751 107 3.9 25.8 1099843 11955 198 1.7 20.9 ;	

The correlation coefficient is also easily obtained in Excel, using the formula =CORREL(array1, array2). In Excel, to obtain the coefficient of determination, we raise the correlation coefficient to the second power using the formula $= r\text{^}2$.

To obtain ranks, the following formula in Excel is useful: =RANK(number, array, order). For order, enter 0 for descending and 1 for ascending.

The following input and formulas are used in Excel for computing Examples 7.12–7.14.

FORMULAS FOR EXAMPLE 7.12

	A	B	C	D	E	F
1	r	$z(r)$	ρ	$z(\rho)$	n	z
2	.38	=1/2*ln((1 + A2)/(1 – A2))	.2	=1/2*ln((1 + C2)/(1 – C2))	94	=(B2 – D2)/sqrt(1/(E2 – 3))

FORMULAS FOR EXAMPLE 7.13

	A	B	C	D	E	F
1	r	$z_{1-\alpha/2}$	n	$z(r)$	L	U
2	0.38	1.645	94	=1/2*ln((1 + A2)/(1 – A2))	=D2 – B2*sqrt(1/(C2 – 3))	=D2 + B2*sqrt(1/(C2 – 3))
3					Lower confidence limit	Upper confidence limit
4					=(exp(2*E2) – 1)/(exp(2*E2) + 1)	=(exp(2*F2) – 1)/(exp(2*F2) + 1)

FORMULAS FOR EXAMPLE 7.14

	A	B	C	D	E	F	G
1	r_1	n_1	r_2	n_2	$z(r_1)$	$z(r_2)$	z
2	–.549	10	–.949	10	=1/2*ln((1 + A2)/(1 – A2))	=1/2*ln((1 + C2)/(1 – C2))	=(E2 – F2)/sqrt(1/(B2 – 3)+1/(D2 – 3))

7.8 Summary

In this chapter, we have studied the strength of relationship (effect size) between two variables *X* and *Y*. A number of statistical techniques used to measure the strength of association between variables were presented, with the technique depending on the process of data collection and whether the variables involved were categorical (nominal or ordinal) or continuous (interval or ratio). Study designs tend to involve data obtained through observation: case series, ecologic, cross-sectional, case-control, and cohort. In contrast, the experimental research design involves data in which the independent variable is manipulated by the researchers in order to assess its effect on the dependent variable.

The measurement techniques presented for evaluating the association between two dichotomous nominal variables are the risk ratio or rate ratio (for cohort data), the odds ratio (for case-control or ecologic data), and the prevalence ratio (for cross-sectional data). The risk ratio is a measure of the strength of association between dichotomous exposure and outcome variables that involves the ratio of two attack rates. The rate ratio is a measure of the strength of association between dichotomous exposure and outcome variables that involves the ratio of two person–time rates. The odds ratio is the odds of exposure among cases divided by the odds of exposure among noncases. The prevalence ratio is a measure of the strength of association between dichotomous exposure and outcome variables that involves the ratio of prevalence proportions. Two methods for controlling for confounding variables were presented, matching and the **Mantel-Haenszel method** to provide a pooled estimate across strata. Other related statistics that often yield informative information are the risk difference and rate difference, the attributable fraction in the population, and the attributable fraction in the exposed group.

Correlation analysis was presented to measure the direction and strength of the relationship between two random variables. The measurement of linear association between two continuous variables was the correlation coefficient r. Spearman's correlation coefficient is related to the correlation coefficient in that the data for the independent and dependent variables are ranked and then the ranked values are derived using the correlation coefficient. This method is used when outlying data exist for one or both variables, thus causing the distribution of data to be skewed. By simply squaring the value of the correlation coefficient we get the coefficient of determination, which is the proportion of the total observed variability among the dependent variable that is explained by the independent variable.

In some instances, the research question may ask about a hypothesis that the correlation coefficient is different from some value other than 0. In this case, the Fisher's z-transformation can be used for testing the hypothesis and constructing confidence intervals. Fisher's z-transformation can also be used in comparing the correlation coefficient between two independent groups.

Important formulas have been shown in this chapter. These are summarized in **Table 7.6**.

Many research questions involve both correlation and regression analysis. Regression is a powerful statistical technique used to explore the relationship between variables. It has numerous applications and plays an important role in biological and medical research. In the next chapter, we will present simple (one independent variable) and multiple (more than one independent variables) linear regression.

Table 7.6 Summary of Selected Formulas Involving Association

Statistic	Equation
Risk ratio	$\frac{P(\text{outcome} \mid \text{exposed})}{P(\text{outcome} \mid \text{not exposed})} = \frac{R_e}{R_o} = \frac{a/(a+b)}{c/(c+d)}$
Chi-square for evaluating the risk ratio	$\chi^2 = \frac{(\lvert ad-bc \rvert - n/2)^2 \times n}{(a+b)(c+d)(a+c)(b+d)}$
Confidence interval for the risk ratio	$e^{\ln(\text{Risk Ratio}) \pm \left(z_{1-\alpha/2} \times \sqrt{\frac{b/a}{a+b} + \frac{d/c}{c+d}} \right)}$
Risk difference	$P(\text{outcome} \mid \text{exposed}) - P(\text{outcome} \mid \text{not exposed}) = R_e - R_o = a/(a+b) - c/(c+d)$
Rate ratio	$\text{Rate Ratio} = \frac{R_e}{R_o} = \frac{a/PT_e}{c/PT_o}$
Chi-square for evaluating the rate ratio	$\chi^2 = \frac{\{a - [PT_e(a+c)]/PT\}^2}{PT_e[PT_o(a+c)]/PT^2}$

Statistic	Equation
Confidence interval for the rate ratio	$e^{\ln(\text{Rate Ratio}) \pm z_{1-\alpha/2} \times \sqrt{\frac{1}{a}+\frac{1}{c}}}$
Attributable fraction in the population (AF_p)	$\frac{R - R_o}{R} \times 100$ $R_o = c/(c+d)$; $R = \frac{a+c}{a+b+c+d}$ for risk ratio $R_o = c/PT_o$; $R = (a+c)/PT$ for rate ratio
Attributable fraction in the exposed group (AF_e)	$\frac{R_e - R_o}{R_e} \times 100$ $R_e = a/(a+b)$; $R_o = c/(c=d)$ for risk ratio $R_e = a/PT_e$; $R_o = c/PT_o$ for rate ratio
Odds ratio	$\frac{P(\text{exposed} \mid \text{outcome})/P(\text{not exposed} \mid \text{outcome})}{P(\text{exposed} \mid \text{no outcome})/P(\text{not exposed} \mid \text{no outcome})} = \frac{a/c}{b/d} = \frac{a \times d}{b \times c}$
Chi-square test for the odds ratio	$\chi^2 = \frac{(\lvert ad - bc \rvert - n/2)^2 \times n}{(a+b)(c+d)(a+c)(b+d)}$
Confidence interval for the odds ratio	$e^{\ln(OR) \pm z_{1-\alpha/2} \times \sqrt{\frac{1}{a}+\frac{1}{b}+\frac{1}{c}+\frac{1}{d}}}$
Attributable fraction in the population (AF_p) for a case-control study	$\frac{p_e(OR-1)}{p_e(OR-1)+1} \times 100$ $p_e = \frac{b}{b+d}$
Attributable fraction in the exposed group (AF_e) for a case-control study	$\frac{OR-1}{OR} \times 100$
Matched-paired case-control study odds ratio	$\frac{P(\text{exposed} \mid \text{no outcome})}{P(\text{not exposed} \mid \text{outcome})} = \frac{b}{c}$
Chi-square test statistic for a matched case-control study	$\chi^2 = \frac{(\lvert b-c \rvert - 1)^2}{(b+c)}$
Confidence interval for the matched odds ratio	$e^{\ln(OR) \pm z_{1-\alpha/2} \times \sqrt{\frac{1}{b}+\frac{1}{c}}}$
Mantel-Haenszel summary odds ratio	$\frac{\sum_i \frac{a_i d_i}{n_i}}{\sum_i \frac{b_i c_i}{n_i}}$

Statistic	Equation
Confidence interval for the Mantel-Haenszel summary odds ratio	$95\%\ CI(OR_{MH}) = OR_{MH}^{1 \pm z_{1-\alpha/2}/\sqrt{\chi^2_{MH}}}$
Mantel-Haenszel summary risk ratio	$\text{Risk Ratio}_{MH} = \dfrac{\sum_i \frac{a_i(c_i + d_i)}{a_i + b_i + c_i + d_i}}{\sum_i \frac{c_i(a_i + b_i)}{a_i + b_i + c_i + d_i}}$
Confidence interval for the Mantel-Haenszel summary risk ratio	$95\%\ CI(RR_{MH}) = RR_{MH}^{1 \pm z_{1-\alpha/2}/\sqrt{\chi^2_{MH}}}$
Mantel-Haenszel summary rate ratio	$\text{Rate Ratio}_{MH} = \dfrac{\sum_i \frac{a_i PTo_i}{PT_i}}{\sum_i \frac{c_i PTe_i}{PT_i}}$
Confidence interval for the Mantel-Haenszel summary rate ratio	$95\%\ CI(RR_{MH}) = RR_{MH}^{1 \pm z_{1-\alpha/2}/\sqrt{\chi^2_{MH}}}$
Correlation coefficient	$r = \dfrac{\sum_i (x_i - \bar{x})(y_i - \bar{y})}{\sqrt{\sum_i (x_i - \bar{x})^2 \sum_i (y_i - \bar{y})^2}}$
t-ratio for evaluating $H_0: \rho = 0$, $n-2$ degrees of freedom	$\dfrac{r\sqrt{n-2}}{\sqrt{1-r^2}}$
Fisher's exact test	$z = \dfrac{z(r) - z(\rho)}{\sqrt{1/(n-3)}}$, where $z(r) = \dfrac{1}{2}\ln\left(\dfrac{1+r}{1-r}\right)$
Confidence interval for Fisher's *z*-transformed *r*	z transform of $r \pm z_{1-\alpha/2}\sqrt{(1/(n-3))}$ Confidence Interval $= \left[\dfrac{e^{2L}-1}{e^{2L}+1}, \dfrac{e^{2U}-1}{e^{2U}+1}\right]$
Test statistic for comparing correlations between two independent groups	$z = \dfrac{z(r_1) - z(r_2)}{\sqrt{\dfrac{1}{n_1 - 3} + \dfrac{1}{n_2 - 3}}}$

Exercises

1. Match the description in the left column with the measures study design in the right column.

___ Entire group of interest is followed over time without manipulation of the independent variable.	A. Case series
___ Unit of analysis is an aggregate measure.	B. Ecological study
___ It is retrospective, beginning with the outcome.	C. Case-control study
___ Entire group of interest is followed over time with manipulation of the independent variable.	D. Cohort study
___ The description is qualitative.	E. Experimental study

2. Calculate and interpret the risk ratio for $a = 17$, $b = 7$, $c = 7$, $d = 20$. Express your answer to the nearest hundredth.
3. Refer to Exercise 2, what is the 95% confidence interval for the risk ratio?
4. Refer to Exercise 2, what is the risk difference per 100 for these data?
5. Calculate and interpret the rate ratio for $a = 20$, $b = 11$, $c = 10$, $d = 18$, $PT_e = 852$, and $PT_o = 924$. Express your answer to the nearest hundredth.
6. What is the 95% confidence interval for the rate ratio?
7. What is the rate difference per 1,000 for these data?
8. Consider the following data and then complete the table. Round your answers to the nearest tenth.

Population	Lung Cancer Incidence Rate per 100,000 Person-Years	Coronary Heart Disease Incidence Rate per 100,000 Person-Years
Overall	$R = 60$	$R = 240$
Cigarette smokers	$R_e = 180$	$R_e = 420$
Nonsmokers	$R_o = 20$	$R_o = 180$

Statistic	Equation	Lung Cancer	Coronary Heart Disease	Interpretation
Rate ratio	$\frac{R_e}{R_o}$			
Rate difference	$R_e - R_o$			
AF_p	$\frac{R - R_o}{R} \times 100$			
AF_e	$\frac{R_e - R_o}{R_e} \times 100$			

9. Calculate the odds ratio for $a = 20$, $b = 10$, $c = 8$, $d = 16$. Express your answer to the nearest hundredth.
10. Calculate the 95% confidence interval for the odds ratio in the previous exercise. Express your answer to the nearest hundredth.
11. Calculate AF_e for the data in Exercise 9.
12. Calculate AF_p for the data in Exercise 9.
13. A cohort of fifth grade school children were identified as to whether they had been bullied by their peers or not. After 3 years they were classified as being happy or not. Let $a = 100$, $b = 125$, $c = 270$, $d = 200$.
    a. What is the risk ratio? Interpret.
    b. What is the 95% confidence interval? Interpret.
    c. What is the risk difference? Interpret.
14. The data in the previous exercise can be stratified by sex: $a = 13$, $b = 26$, $c = 62$, $d = 219$ for males and $a = 20$, $b = 48$, $c = 37$, $d = 190$ for females.
    a. Are the stratified rate ratios homogeneous?
    b. Calculate the Mantel-Haenszel estimator for a common rate ratio.
    c. Calculate the 95% confidence interval for the common rate ratio.
15. Under what conditions will the odds ratio approximate the risk ratio?
16. A sample was taken of students from a given school district. They were asked if they thought marijuana use was risky. The investigators wanted to determine if the prevalence of perceived riskiness varied according to school grade. The following data were collected. Evaluate these data using three prevalence ratios 8th grade versus 6th grade, 10th grade versus 6th grade, and 12th grade versus 6th grade. Report confidence intervals with each of your prevalence ratios. What conclusions can you make from your results?

School Grade	Marijuana Use Risky	Marijuana Use Not Risky
6th	150	9
8th	120	15
10th	145	20
12th	110	27

17. We are interested in whether there is an association between the value placed on religion and general health for a population of adults. The following sample data were collected from a cross-sectional survey.

	Men		**Women**	
My religious faith is very important to me.	Perceived health is excellent or very good		Perceived health is excellent or very good	
	Yes	No	Yes	No
Yes	257	94	149	113
No	50	30	17	20

a. Use prevalence ratios (and 95% confidence intervals) to evaluate the relationship between these two variables separately for men and women.
b. Is the relationship similar for males and females?
c. Is it appropriate to collapse the data over sex and present a summary prevalence ratio?
d. If so, what is the summary prevalence ratio and 95% confidence interval? Interpret your result.

18. Researchers assessed the association between self-reported type 2 diabetes and primary open-angle glaucoma (POAG) in a cohort of black women.[17]

	POAG	
Type 2 Diabetes	**Case**	**Person-Years**
Yes	57	23,488
No	308	389,470

a. Apply the steps of hypothesis testing to this cohort data.
b. Calculate the 95% confidence interval for the rate ratio. Interpret the result and say what the interval tells us about statistical significance.

19. A case-control study design was used to evaluate the association between oral contraceptive use and breast cancer risk in Chinese women.[18] Data are presented as follows:

	Breast Cancer	
Oral Contraceptive Use	**Yes**	**No**
Ever	419	426
Never	1654	1657

a. Apply the steps of hypothesis testing to this data, using an appropriate measure of association.
b. Calculate the 95% confidence interval. Interpret the result and say what the interval tells us about statistical significance.

20. In a case-control study researchers investigated whether there was an association between living near a high-hazard dump site versus a low-hazard dump site and risk of having a low birth weight child.[19] The study found that in a group of women living near a high-hazard dump site while pregnant there were 181 low birth weight children and 4268 normal birth weight children. Corresponding numbers for women living near a low-hazard dump site were 126 and 4236, respectively.
a. Formulate the null and alternative hypotheses.
b. Estimate the odds ratio and 95% confidence interval. Interpret the result and say what the interval tells us about statistical significance.

21. Match the descriptions in the left column with the measures of association in the right column.

___ Measure of association between two continuous variables that is robust to outliers	A. Correlation coefficient
___ Assumes two continuous variables are bivariate normal and linearly related	B. Coefficient of determination
___ Proportion of the total variation in the dependent variable explained by the independent variable	C. Spearman rank correlation coefficient

22. Why is it important to create a scatter plot of the data when evaluating the relationship between two continuous random variables?
23. For the following information, calculate the sample correlation coefficient and test $H_0: \rho = 0,\ H_a: \rho \neq 0$. Let $\alpha = 0.05$.
    a. $n = 12,\ \sum(X - \overline{X})(Y - \overline{Y}) = 395,\ \sum(X - \overline{X})^2 = 630,$ $\sum(Y - \overline{Y})^2 = 400$
    b. $n = 21,\ \sum(X - \overline{X})(Y - \overline{Y}) = 37,\ \sum(X - \overline{X})^2 = 38,$ $\sum(Y - \overline{Y})^2 = 101$
24. Consider the heights for a group of father and son pairs. Heights are presented in inches.

Father's Height	Son's Height	Father's Height	Son's Height
69	72	69	70
66	78	67	70
67	70	75	79
68	68	73	78
71	72	70	75
73	73	68	70
70	71	69	69

    a. Construct a two-way scatter plot for these data.
    b. Is there a linear relationship between the heights of the fathers and sons?
    c. Compute the correlation coefficient.
    d. At the 0.05 level of significance, test the null hypothesis that the population correlation is equal to 0. What do you conclude?
    e. Calculate the Spearman rank correlation coefficient.
    f. How does the value of the correlation coefficient compare with the Spearman rank correlation coefficient? Which is more appropriate for these data?
    g. Using the Spearman correlation coefficient, test the null hypothesis that the population correlation is equal to 0. What do you conclude?
25. Data were obtained on life expectancy, fruit and vegetable servings, obesity, and college graduates among adults in states across the United States.[20,21] Suppose you are interested in identifying how having a college education correlates with life expectancy, fruit and vegetable consumption, and obesity.

	Life Expectancy			Fruit 1+ Serving %	Vegetable 1+ Serving %	Obese %	College Graduate %
	Overall	Black	White				
Alabama	75.4	72.9	76.0	55.2	80.7	36.2	22.0
Alaska	78.3	79.3	79.4	63.1	81.0	29.5	25.9
Arizona	79.6	76.5	79.8	63.0	79.4	29.5	25.4
Arkansas	76.0	72.2	76.3	55.6	80.8	37.1	19.9
California	80.8	75.1	79.8	67.5	78.6	25.8	29.3
Colorado	80.0	76.7	80.2	67.0	82.6	23.0	35.8
Connecticut	80.8	77.8	81	68.8	83.2	27.4	34.7
Delaware	78.4	75.4	78.6	64.6	82.8	33.5	28.4
Florida	79.4	75.8	79.1	65.7	80.7	30.7	26.1
Georgia	77.2	74.7	77.6	61.4	81.9	32.5	26.7
Hawaii	81.3	79.7	81.2	63.0	79.0	24.9	29.4
Idaho	79.5	83.3	79.4	64.6	84.1	28.4	23.6
Illinois	79.0	73.7	79.3	66.7	78.7	31.8	30.5
Indiana	77.6	73.8	77.7	59.4	80.8	34.1	23.1
Iowa	79.7	75.3	79.8	64.4	80.7	35.3	25.4
Kansas	78.7	73.6	78.8	62.5	82.7	34.4	29.1
Kentucky	76.0	73.5	76.0	57.3	83.0	36.6	21.1
Louisiana	75.7	72.4	76.7	55.0	76.1	36.8	21.1
Maine	79.2	81.8	79.1	68.6	87.6	30.4	28.4
Maryland	78.8	75.5	79.4	65.7	81.7	30.9	35.3
Massachusetts	80.5	78.8	80.4	68.8	83.3	25.7	38.2
Michigan	78.2	73.4	79.0	63.6	81.6	33.0	25.6
Minnesota	81.1	82.5	80.4	67.8	82.0	30.1	31.6
Mississippi	75.0	72.4	76.1	53.7	78.7	39.5	19.1
Missouri	77.5	74.2	77.7	60.1	83.1	35.0	25.7
Montana	78.5	83.4	79.1	63.6	84.9	26.9	27.3
Nebraska	79.8	73.9	80.0	63.2	80.0	34.1	27.9
Nevada	78.1	75.9	76.7	62.4	77.9	29.5	21.4
New Hampshire	80.3	86.8	80.1	69.9	86.5	29.6	33.1
New Jersey	80.3	75.5	80.3	66.4	80.9	25.7	35.0
New Mexico	78.4	75.2	79.0	62.6	79.6	32.3	23.8
New York	80.5	77.4	80.5	66.5	79.7	27.6	32.5
North Carolina	77.8	74.7	78.3	62.6	84.4	33.0	26.9
North Dakota	79.5	84.2	80.2	63.2	80.2	35.1	26.2

(*Continues*)

	Life Expectancy			Fruit 1+ Serving %	Vegetable 1+ Serving %	Obese %	College Graduate %
	Overall	Black	White				
Ohio	77.8	73.9	78.1	62.3	81.3	34.0	24.8
Oklahoma	75.9	72.8	76.0	54.2	82.9	34.8	22.5
Oregon	79.5	77.2	79.2	67.1	83.6	29.9	29.2
Pennsylvania	78.5	73.4	78.9	66.0	83.7	30.9	27.5
Rhode Island	79.9	71.6	79.7	66.6	82.3	27.7	29.9
South Carolina	77.0	74.0	77.8	59.4	82.0	34.3	24.6
South Dakota	79.5	81.7	80.4	63.1	83.1	30.1	25.2
Tennessee	76.3	72.9	76.7	61.1	84.2	34.4	23.8
Texas	78.5	74.4	78.0	60.6	78.1	34.8	25.5
Utah	80.2	74.3	80.1	67.9	82.7	27.8	27.9
Vermont	80.5	84.4	80.4	70.4	87.2	27.5	33.2
Virginia	79.0	75.3	79.4	63.4	84.2	30.4	34.0
Washington	79.9	77.5	79.7	68.2	83.4	28.7	31.4
West Virginia	75.4	72.8	75.4	55.1	81.7	39.5	18.5
Wisconsin	80.0	74.0	80.3	67.6	81.0	32.0	26.5
Wyoming	78.3	83.5	78.4	62.4	84.7	29.0	24.2

a. Construct a scatter plot and evaluate whether a linear line fits the association between percent with a college education and each of the other variables.
b. Calculate the correlation coefficient for the college education variable by each of the other variables.
c. Calculate the coefficient of determination for the college education variable by each of the other variables.
d. Does the correlation coefficient indicate a stronger linear association between the college education variable and life expectancy for blacks or whites?
e. Does the correlation coefficient indicate a stronger linear association between the college education variable and the fruit variable or the vegetable variable?
f. Describe the association between the college education variable and the obesity variable.
g. Calculate the Spearman correlation coefficient for the college education variable by each of the other variables.
h. The Spearman correlation coefficient is most different than the correlation coefficient for the association between college education and life expectancy for blacks. What does this say about the normality assumption?
i. Is life expectancy most strongly correlated with the variable fruit, vegetable, obesity, or college education?
j. Are the correlation coefficients measuring the association between life expectancy and fruit, vegetable, obesity, and college education stronger for whites or blacks?

26. The correlation coefficient measuring the linear association between a college education (%) and overall life expectancy in the previous exercise is 0.77. Suppose you are interested in whether the correlation is significantly greater than 0.65, with $\alpha = 0.05$. Proceed with the six steps of hypothesis testing.
27. What is the 95% confidence interval for the correlation coefficient measuring the association between college education and overall life expectancy?
28. The correlation coefficient measuring the association between a college education and overall life expectancy is 0.351 for blacks and 0.773 for whites. Are these two correlation coefficients significantly different? Apply the steps of hypothesis testing to address this question.

References

1. Schwingshackl L, Schwedhelm C, Galbete C, Hofmann G. Adherence to Mediterranean diet and risk of cancer: an updated systematic review and meta-analysis. *Nutrients.* 2017;*9*(1):1063.
2. Du RH, Liang LR, Yang CQ, et al. Predictors of mortality for patients with COVID-19 pneumonia caused by SARS-CoV-2: A prospective cohort study. *Eur Respir J.* 2020;*55*(5):2000524.
3. Aldana SG, Greenlaw RL, Diehl HA, et al. The behavioral and clinical effects of therapeutic lifestyle change on middle-aged adults. *Prev Chronic Dis.* 2006;*3*(1):A05.
4. Worldometer. COVID-19 coronavirus pandemic. https://www.worldometers.info/coronavirus/?utm_campaign=instagramcoach1? Accessed September 24, 2020.
5. Centers for Disease Control and Prevention. Coronavirus disease 2019 (COVID-19). https://www.cdc.gov/coronavirus/2019-ncov/covid-data/covidview/index.html. Accessed October 11, 2020.
6. Iso H, Date C, Yamamoto A, et al. Smoking cessation and mortality from cardiovascular disease among Japanese men and women. The JACC study. *Am J Epidemiol.* 2005;*161*(2):170–179.
7. Merrill RM, Roy N, Pierce J, Sundar KM. Impact of voice, cough, and diurnal breathing problems on quality of life in obstructive sleep apnea. Do they matter? *Arch Otorhinol Head Neck Surg.* 2020;*4*(2):3.
8. Killerby M, Link-Gelles R, Haight SC, et al. Characteristics associated with hospitalization among patients with COVID-19—Metropolitan Atlanta, Georgia, March-April 2020. *MMWR Morb Mortal Wkly Rep.* 2020;*69*(25);790–294.
9. Anderson LN, Heong SW, Chen Y, et al. Vitamin D and fracture risk in early childhood: a case-control study. *Am J Epidemiol.* 2017;*185*(12):1255–1262.
10. Sasco AJ, Merrill RM, Dari I, Benhaïm-Luzon V, Carriot F, Cann CI, Bartal M. A case-control study of lung cancer in Casablanca, Morocco. *Cancer Causes Control.* 2002;*13*(7):609–616.
11. Forti MD, Quattrone D, Freeman TP, et al. The contribution of cannabis use to variation in the incidence of psychotic disorder across Europe (EU-GEI): A multicentre case control study. *Lancet Psychiatry.* 2019;*6*(5):427–436.
12. Mantel N, Haenszel W. Statistical aspects of the analysis of data from the retrospective analysis of disease. *J Natl Cancer Inst.* 1959;*22*(4)710–748.
13. Breslow NE, Day NE. *Statistical Methods in Cancer Research Vol. 1: The Analysis of Case-Control Studies*. Lyon, France: IARC Scientific Publications; 1980.
14. Worldometer. Life expectancy of the world population. https://www.worldometers.info/demographics/life-expectancy/. Accessed October 11, 2020.
15. United States Census Bureau. International data base. https://www.census.gov/programs-surveys/international-programs/about/idb.html. Accessed October 11, 2020.
16. Fisher RA. *Statistical Methods for Research Workers*. 14th ed. New York, NY: Hafner Publishing; 1973.
17. Wise LA, Rosenberg L, Radin RG, et al. A prospective study of diabetes, lifestyle factors, and glaucoma among African-American women. *Ann Epidemiol.* 2001;*21*(6):430–439.
18. Xu WH, Shu XO, Long J, et al. Relation of FGFR2 genetic polymorphisms to the association between oral contraceptive use and the risk of breast cancer in Chinese women. *Am J Epidemiol.* 2011;*173*(8):923–931.

19. Gillbreath S, Kass PH. Adverse birth outcomes associated with open dump sites in Alaska Native villages. *Am J Epidemiol.* 2006;*164*:518–528.
20. Life expectancy by state 2020. https://worldpopulationreview.com/state-rankings/life-expectancy-by-state. Accessed October 11, 2020.
21. Centers for Disease Control and Prevention. BRFSS Prevalence & Trends Data. https://www.cdc.gov/brfss/brfssprevalence/index.html. Accessed October 11, 2020.

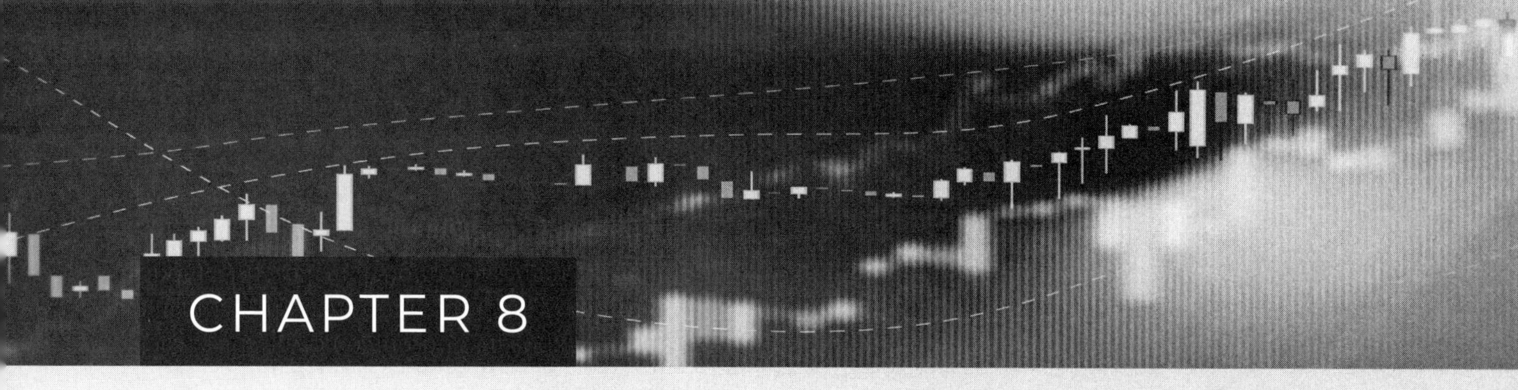

Regression

KEY CONCEPTS

- A regression function describes the relationship between the dependent variable and one or more independent variables.
- The researcher decides which variable is dependent and which is independent, based on observation and experience.
- Simple linear regression involves one dependent variable and one independent variable.
- Multiple regression involves one dependent variable and two or more independent variables.
- Multivariate regression involves more than one dependent variable with different distributions and one or more independent variables.
- Assumptions for simple linear regression are (1) the values of X are known (not random); (2) for each value of X, the distribution of Y is normally distributed; (3) the standard deviation of the Y does not change over X; (4) the Y values are independent; and (5) a linear relationship exists between X and Y.
- The standard approach used to obtain the intercept and slope of the regression line is the least squares method.
- The standard error of the estimated intercept or slope is used to test hypotheses or to construct confidence intervals.
- A regression model should include an interaction term if the association between a dependent variable and an independent variable differs according to the levels of a third variable.
- Logistic regression is used to describe the relationship between a categorical dependent variable and one or more independent variables, with different possible scales.
- Poisson regression is useful when the dependent variable Y has a Poisson distribution, and the logarithm of its expected value is modeled as a linear combination of a set of parameters. We assume the observations are independent of one another and the mean of the Poisson random variable equals its variance.
- Log-binomial regression is useful for estimating risk ratios for binary response variables, adjusting for confounders.
- The Cox proportional hazard model allows us to assess the effect of several risk factors on survival.
- Multiple regression models are important because independent variables may simultaneously affect the dependent variable or confound or modify the relationship between dependent and independent variables.
- A residual is the difference between the observed and predicted values. Residual plots are an effective way to evaluate whether a linear model is a good fit to the data. The coefficient of determination r^2, multiple R^2, and adjusted R^2 are also useful statistics for evaluating models.

Statistical models describe patterns of association and interaction among variables. Model specification is the process of choosing a model form, which best describes the relationship between variables. Model fitting is the process by which data are used to estimate the parameters in a model. Parameter estimates provide measures of the strength and statistical importance of effects. Many parametric models used in biostatistics involve fitting a linear line to observed data and testing hypotheses about the fitted model parameters.

Regression analysis plays a primary role in biostatistics research. This technique is used to estimate the association between variables that are not perfectly associated. The method is also useful when evaluating associations between variables while adjusting for one or more potential confounding variables. A regression model estimates the association between a dependent variable and an independent variable or variables, but unlike the correlation coefficient, it produces an estimate that represents the original scale of the data.

Regression is a method used to estimate the functional relationship between a dependent variable and an independent variable or variables. Multivariate regression is used to estimate the functional relationship between more than one correlated dependent variable and an independent variable or variables. In this text, we will focus on regression involving just one dependent variable. Each type of regression model considered in this chapter has a linear function. The only difference among these models is the nature of the dependent variable. Such models are collectively referred to as generalized linear models. Five of the most common generalized linear models are (1) linear regression, which has a continuous dependent variable; (2) logistic regression, which has a categorical dependent variable; (3) Poisson regression, which has a count or person–time rate as the dependent variable; (4) log-binomial regression, which has an attack rate as the dependent variable; and (5) Cox proportional hazards regression, which has hazard rate (risk of failure) as the dependent variable. The purpose of this chapter is to introduce these important generalized linear models.

8.1 Questions

Regression analysis is a commonly used method for identifying whether certain variables predict a primary variable of interest. In other words, regression analysis allows us to answer questions about which variables matter most, which are irrelevant, and how the variables affect each other (confound, interact). Researchers are often interested in answering questions about whether selected demographic variables (e.g., age, sex, race/ethnicity) and risk factors variables (e.g., environmental exposure, poor nutrition, tobacco smoking) impact a dependent variable like a disease (e.g., COVID-19, influenza, cancer), event (e.g., injury, drug abuse, suicide), or condition (e.g., obesity, asthma, arthritis).

As an example of the widespread use of regression analysis in health research, in the September 2020 issue of the *American Journal of Epidemiology*, regression models were used to study the association between predisaster social capital and changes in social capital following a disaster with subsequent mental disorders;[1] association between women's work and family histories and cognitive performance in later life;[2] associations between gastric atrophy and poor oral health and the risk of esophageal squamous cell carcinoma;[3] associations between two key kidney diseases (estimated glomerular filtration rate and urinary albumin-to-creatinine ratio) and cancer incidence;[4] association between categories of peripheral artery disease and mortality, cardiovascular events, and cardiovascular mortality;[5] and association between menopausal hormone therapy and chronic disease.[6]

8.2 Regression Function

A regression function describes the association between the dependent variable and one or more independent variables. The frequentist view of regression, which will be considered in this chapter (versus the Bayesian interpretation), describes how the dependent variable Y changes according to the independent variable X. The regression function can be expressed as $E(Y \mid X = x)$, which is the expected average (population mean) of the dependent variable Y when the independent variable X takes on a specific value x.

The investigator chooses the relevant independent variable or variables and decides on the functional form of the model. The specific form of the relationship between Y and X is based on judgment and experience. Further, the relationship is stochastic in that an error term is included in the model.

$$E(Y \mid X = x) = f(x)$$

Note that $f(x)$ is a function that indicates the relationship between variables. An error term is added to capture the influence of variables that were not considered in the model. A statistical relation is not a perfect one, unlike an algebraic functional relation.

The slope (gradient) of a straight line in mathematics is the rise over the run. In the following graph (**Figure 8.1**), the slope is 3/1 = 3. In this example, the equation is $E(Y \mid X = x) = f(x) = 1 + 3x$. The functional relationship is a perfect relationship. In contrast, a statistical relationship is generally not a perfect one in which each observation falls on the line, but there is a scattering of points about the line. A linear line fits the data in Figure 7.1, but a curvilinear line fits the data in Figure 7.2. In statistics, we use a technique called regression to provide the best fitting line to the data.

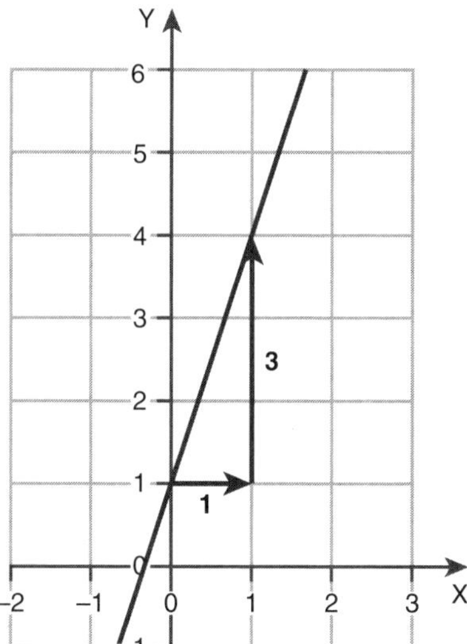

Figure 8.1 Slope of a Straight Line

8.3 Simple Linear Regression

Simple linear regression is a statistical technique that is used to identify the relationship between a continuous dependent variable and a continuous or categorical independent variable. Regression analysis allows us to identify how a dependent variable changes given a unit increase in an independent variable. Of primary interest is to estimate the value of the dependent variable that relates to a fixed independent variable. The researcher decides on which variable is dependent and which is independent.

Simple Linear Regression Model

$$Y_i = \beta_0 + \beta_1 X_i + \epsilon_i$$

Y_i = value of the dependent variable for observation i
X_i = value of the independent variable for observation i
ϵ_i = value of random fluctuation or error for observation i
β_0 = a parameter that represents the population regression line intercept; mean of Y when $X = 0$
β_1 = a parameter that represents the slope of the population regression line; mean change in Y for a unit increase in X

EXAMPLE 8.1

Given that COVID-19 patients who are older are more likely to die from the illness, we are interested in whether countries with longer life expectancy (in years) have greater COVID-19 death rates. The model $Y_i = \beta_0 + \beta_1 X_i + \epsilon_i$ says that a COVID-19 death rate is some base value β_0 plus an average of β_1 increase in death rate for every year increase in life expectancy.

In order to make inferences about the population from a simple linear regression model, certain assumptions must be met. The first assumption is that the values of the independent variable X are known. The second assumption is that for each value of X, the Y values will be normally distributed around the population regression line. The third assumption is that the variability around the regression line is constant across the values of X. If the variability about the regression line is the same as we increase over X, the data are referred to as homoscedastic. Otherwise, the data are heteroscedastic. The fourth assumption is that the Y values are not related to one another over the levels of X. The fifth assumption is that the independent and dependent variables are linearly related.

Assumptions for Simple Linear Regression

1. The values of X are known (not random).
2. For each value of X, the distribution of Y is normal.
3. The standard deviation of the dependent variable Y does not change over x.
4. The dependent variables Y are independent.
5. A linear relationship exists between X and Y.

We assume $\epsilon_i \sim N(0,\sigma^2)$ and independent. This expression means the errors are normally distributed with mean 0 and variance σ^2. The relationship between X and Y is linear in the parameter β_1. If X is fixed, then $Y_i \sim N(\mu_i,\sigma^2)$. The mean of the expected value of Y is

$$E(Y_i) = E(\beta_0 + \beta_1 X_i + \epsilon_i) = \beta_0 + \beta_1 X_i + E(\epsilon_i) = \beta_0 + \beta_1 X_i$$

If y_i is the observed outcome of Y_i for a particular value x_i, and $\hat{y}_i$ is the corresponding predicted value, then

$$e_i = y_i - \hat{y}_i$$

The distance e_i is known as the residual, which estimates the random population error. When the regression equation is used to describe the relationship in the sample, it is often written as

$$\hat{y}_i = b_0 + b_1 x_i.$$

The statistic b_0 represents the estimated y-intercept of the linear fitted line, and the statistic b_1 represents the estimated slope. The slope is a measure of association that reflects how y changes when x changes by one unit.

8.3.1 Least Squares Method

The standard method used to obtain the intercept and slope of the regression line that passes through data points on a scatter plot is the least squares method. To understand this method, refer to the fitted regression line and residuals in **Figure 8.2**. The least squares method minimizes the distance from each of the observations to the regression line. The components of the regression model are shown in **Figure 8.3**.

Corresponding to each observed y_i is a predicted value $\hat{y}_i$, which equals $b_0 + b_1 x_i$. The sample deviation is $e_i = y_i - \hat{y}_i$. The sum of squares is then

$$\sum_i e_i^2 = \sum_i (y_i - \hat{y}_i)^2 = \sum_i (y_i - b_0 - b_1 x_i)^2.$$

The estimators b_0 and b_1 are estimated to minimize the sum of squares. On the basis of calculus, equations are obtained to derive estimates of the slope and intercept.

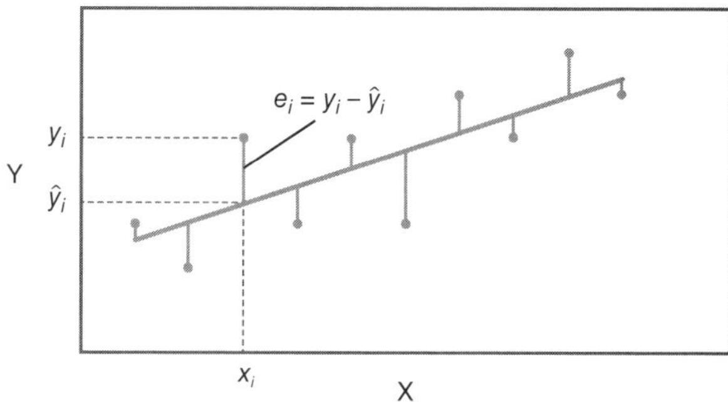

Figure 8.2 Estimated Regression Line for Selected Sample Points

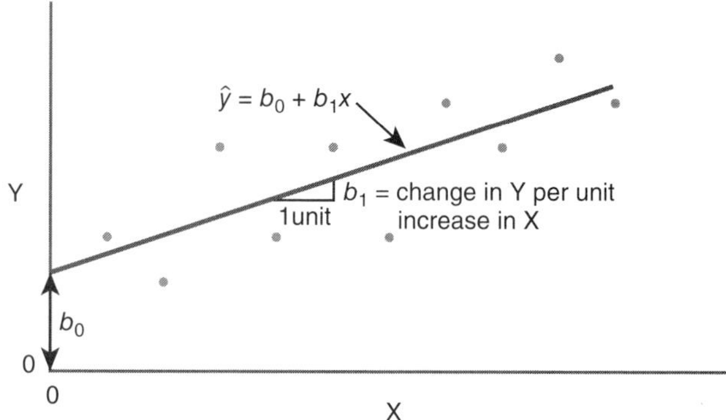

Figure 8.3 Intercept and Slope of the Regression Line

Equation for estimating the slope coefficient

$$b_1 = \frac{\sum(x_i - \bar{x})(y_i - \bar{y})}{\sum(x_i - \bar{x})^2}$$

Equation for estimating the intercept coefficient

$$b_0 = \bar{y} - b_1\bar{x}$$

In the previous chapter, the correlation coefficient was estimated for the association between the death-to-case ratio per 100 and the percent ≥ 60 years of age. The estimated regression line for these data is

$$\text{Death-to-case ratio} = 0.598 + 0.229 \times \%\ \text{Ages} \geq 60.$$

The slope is interpreted as for each unit increase in percent ≥ 60 years of age, the death-to-case ratio increased by 0.229, on average. The regression model can predict the death-to-case ratio for a given percent ≥ 60 years of age. It is generally a good idea to avoid extrapolating beyond the range of the data. In addition, interpretation of the slope requires that the dependent variable be a function of the independent variable and not the other way around.

It is also interesting to show the relationship between the correlation coefficient and the slope coefficient:

$$b_1 = r\frac{\sqrt{\sum(y_i - \bar{y})^2}}{\sqrt{\sum(x_i - \bar{x})^2}}$$

$$r = b_1\frac{\sqrt{\sum(x_i - \bar{x})^2}}{\sqrt{\sum(y_i - \bar{y})^2}}$$

If the correlation coefficient is statistically significant, the corresponding slope coefficient in our regression model will also be statistically significant.

8.3.2 Statistical Inference About the Slope

The sample slope coefficient is the estimator of the population slope coefficient. A hypothesis test is used to test whether a significant relationship exists between variables. The *t* statistic is used for evaluating the slope coefficient in a regression model.

***t* Test Statistic for Evaluating the Slope**

$$t = \frac{b_1 - \beta_1}{SE_{b_1}}$$

$$SE_{b_1} = \sqrt{\frac{s_{y|x}^2}{\sum(x_i - \bar{x})^2}} = \sqrt{\frac{\frac{1}{n-2}\sum(y_i - \hat{y})^2}{\sum(x_i - \bar{x})^2}}$$

$$= \sqrt{\frac{\frac{1}{n-2}\left[\sum(y_i - \bar{y})^2 - b_1\sum(x_i - \bar{x})(y_i - \bar{y})\right]}{\sum(x_i - \bar{x})^2}}$$

This *t* test statistic has $n - 2$ degrees of freedom under the assumptions of the regression model.

If the population parameter β_1 is set to 0 in the null hypothesis (i.e., $H_0{:}\beta_1 = 0$), the following mathematical expression involving the slope coefficient has a t distribution with $n-2$ degrees of freedom:

$$t = \frac{b_1 - 0}{SE_{b_1}}$$

The confidence interval for the slope can also be calculated in order to tell us about precision in our estimate and statistical significance.

Confidence Interval for the Slope in a Regression Model

$$b_1 \pm t_{1-\alpha/2,n-2} SE_{b_1}$$

Although we are generally interested in identifying whether the slope is significantly different than zero, we can also set the slope in the null hypothesis to be a different value. The t test statistic is then modified accordingly.

EXAMPLE 8.2

Data in the following table represent 2020 life expectancy and COVID-19 death rates as of August 18, 2020. The graph of these data shows that a linear line fits the data (**Figure 8.4**).

Country	Life Expectancy 2020	COVID-19 Death Rate per Million	$(x_i - \bar{x})$	$(y_i - \bar{y})$	$(x_i - \bar{x})(y_i - \bar{y})$	$(x_i - \bar{x})^2$	$(y_i - \bar{y})^2$
United States	79.11	531	3.17	117.60	372.56	10.04	13,829.76
Brazil	76.57	518	0.63	104.60	65.69	0.39	10,941.16
India	70.42	39	-5.52	-374.40	2067.44	30.49	140,175.36
Russia	72.99	110	-2.95	-303.40	895.64	8.71	92,051.56
South Africa	64.88	206	-11.06	-207.40	2294.26	122.37	43,014.76
Peru	77.44	807	1.50	393.60	589.61	2.24	154,920.96
Mexico	75.41	447	-0.53	33.60	-17.88	0.28	1,128.96
Colombia	77.87	307	1.93	-106.40	-205.14	3.72	11,320.96
Chile	80.74	553	4.80	139.60	669.80	23.02	19,488.16
Spain	83.99	616	8.05	202.60	1630.52	64.77	41,046.76
Mean	75.94	413.40		Total	8362.50	266.04	527,918.40

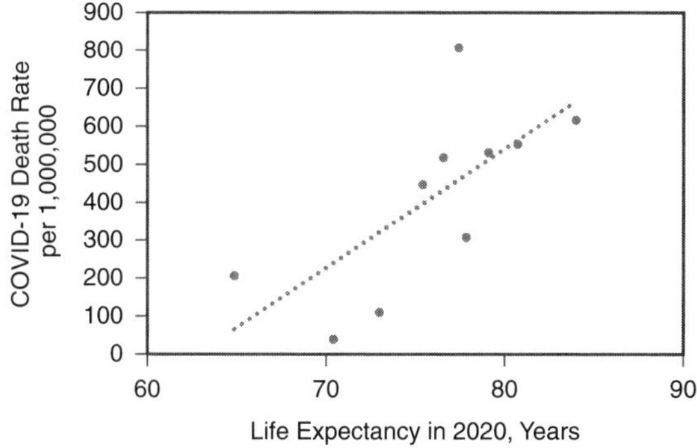

Figure 8.4 COVID-19 Death Rate by Life Expectancy
Data from References 7 and 8

Hence, we will proceed to calculate the regression line.

$$b_1 = \frac{\sum(x_i - \bar{x})(y_i - \bar{y})}{\sum(x_i - \bar{x})^2} = \frac{8362.50}{266.04} = 31.43$$

$$b_0 = \bar{y} - b_1\bar{x} = 413.4 - 31.43 \times 75.94 = -1973.39$$

$$SE_{b_1} = \sqrt{\frac{\frac{1}{n-2}\left[\sum(y_i - \bar{y})^2\right]}{\sum(x_i - \bar{x})^2}} = \sqrt{\frac{\frac{1}{n-2}\left[\sum(y_i - \bar{y})^2 - b_1\sum(x_i - \bar{x})(y_i - \bar{y})\right]}{\sum(x_i - \bar{x})^2}}$$

$$= \sqrt{\frac{\frac{1}{10-2}\left[527918.40 - 31.43 \times 8362.50\right]}{266.04}} = 11.16$$

Notice that we certainly do not want to extrapolate beyond the range of our observations of life expectancy. For example, if life expectancy was 0, then the COVID-19 death rate per million is –1973.39.

Now let us evaluate $H_0: \beta_1 = 0$ vs. $H_a: \beta_1 \neq 0$.

$$t = \frac{b_1 - \beta_1}{se_{b_1}} = \frac{31.43 - 0}{11.16} = 2.82$$

The corresponding *p*-value = 0.0225. The 95% confidence interval is

$$31.43 \pm 2.306 \times 11.16 \rightarrow 5.70 - 57.17.$$

Hence, we reject H_0 and conclude that there is a significant positive relationship between life expectancy and COVID-19 death rate.

Now refer to the Data Analysis option in Excel. If you do not have this feature, refer to Chapter 1, 1.5 for directions on adding it to Excel. Select it and choose Regression. For the input *Y* range, identify the array of data representing the dependent variable, and for the input *X* range, identify the array of data representing the independent variable. There are output options where the output range needs to be identified. Simply choose a cell where you would like this information to begin to appear. There are also options you can select for evaluating the model assumptions, like the residual plot, the line fit plot, and the normal probability plot.

Partial output from these steps appears as follows:

	Coefficients	Standard Error	t Stat	*p*-value	Lower 95%	Upper 95%
Intercept	–1973.7	849.441	–2.32353	0.048651	–3932.51	–14.8844
Life expectancy	31.43318	11.15968	2.816674	0.022609	5.698912	57.16746

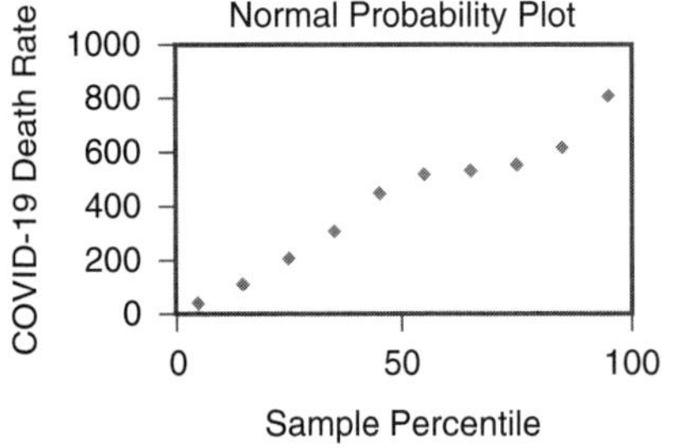

The normal probability plot is a type of graph that assesses whether the data set is normally distributed. The data are plotted against the theoretical normal distribution so that if the points form an approximate straight line, the normality assumption is satisfied.

The SAS data step and procedure code to obtain these results is as follows:

```
DATA COVLIFE;
  INPUT x y @@;
DATALINES;
  79.11 531 76.57 518 70.42 39 72.99 110 64.88 206
  77.44 807 75.41 447 77.87 307 80.74 553 83.99 616
;

PROC REG DATA=COVLIFE;
  MODEL y=x/CLB;
RUN;
```

Partial output from this SAS code is as follows:

Parameter Estimates							
Variable	DF	Parameter Estimate	Standard Error	t Value	Pr > |t|	95% Confidence Limits	
Intercept	1	-1973.69890	849.44104	-2.32	0.0487	-3932.51344	-14.88435
X	1	31.43318	11.15968	2.82	0.0226	5.69891	57.16746

The relationship between the slope and the correlation coefficient is shown as follows:

$$r = b_1 \frac{\sqrt{\sum (x_i - \overline{x})^2}}{\sqrt{\sum (y_i - \overline{y})^2}} = 31.43 \frac{\sqrt{266.04}}{\sqrt{527918.40}} = 0.71$$

Given that the slope coefficient is significant, the correlation coefficient is also significant. The 95% confidence interval for r is 0.15–0.93, based on Fisher's z-transformation (Chapter 7, Section 7.7). The confidence interval does not overlap 0, which also indicates statistical significance.

8.3.3 Confidence Interval for Mean *Y* Given a Value of *X*

The estimated regression equation is useful for predicting values for a group of subjects or for individual subjects. For example, it may be important to predict muscle mass according to age for a group of men, or muscle mass for a particular man. In both cases it is important for the variability associated with the regression line to reflect the prediction. The confidence interval for a mean value of Y given a value of X for a group of subjects is

$$\hat{y} \pm t_{1-\alpha/2, n-2} s_{y|x} \sqrt{\frac{1}{n} + \frac{(x - \overline{x})^2}{\sum (x_i - \overline{x})^2}},$$

where $s_{y|x} = \sqrt{\frac{1}{n-2}\left[\sum (y_i - \hat{y})^2\right]} = \sqrt{MSE}.$

8.3.4 Prediction Interval for an Individual Value *Y* Given a Value *X*

The predicted interval for an individual value of *Y* given *X* is

$$\hat{y} \pm t_{1-\alpha/2,n-2} s_{y|x} \sqrt{1 + \frac{1}{n} + \frac{(x-\bar{x})^2}{\sum (x_i - \bar{x})^2}}$$

The variance for predicting an individual value of Y_0 includes both the variance of individual points about the regression line and the variation attributed to many possible sample regression lines. Thus, the additional value 1 is included beneath the square root in the standard error. In addition, the numerator in the third term of the standard error is the square of the deviation from the given *x* value to the mean of the *x*'s. Therefore, how close the observation is to the mean influences the standard error. If *x* is closer to the mean, the prediction of Y_0 is more accurate.

The previous SAS program automatically produces the scatter plot of the data with the fitted regression line, the 95% confidence interval for the regression line, and the 95% predicted limits, as reproduced here.

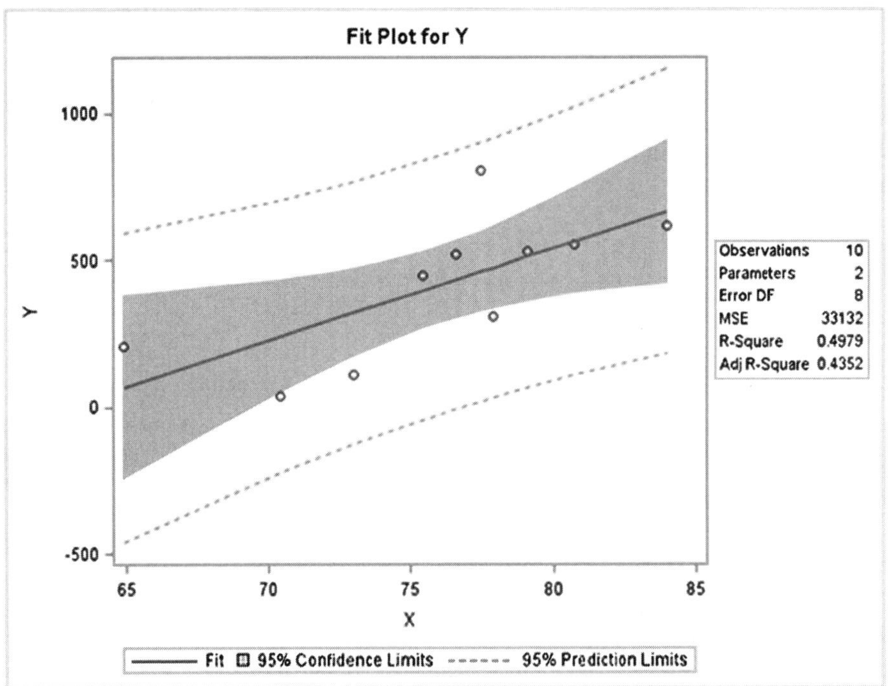

The confidence bands for the regression line and the individual observations are curved. They are narrowest at the mean of *X* and curve away from the line as we move in either direction of the mean of *X*. It should also be noted that if the mean value of *X* is used in the regression equation, the predicted value of *Y* is the mean of *Y*. In other words, the regression line goes through the mean of both *X* and *Y*.

Example 8.3

Continuing with Example 8.2, let's calculate the following:

1. The mean value of *y* given $x = 75$
2. The 95% confidence interval for mean *y* given $x = 75$
3. The 95% prediction interval for an individual value *y* given $x = 75$

Using Excel,[9] these statistics are calculated as follows:

	A	B	C	D	E	F	G	H
1	x	y						
2	79.11	531		n	10	=COUNT(A2:A11)		
3	76.57	518		df	8	=E2-2		
4	70.42	39		x-bar	75.94	=AVERAGE(A2:A11)		
5	72.99	110		x0	75			
6	64.88	206		y0	383.79	=FORECAST(E5,B2:B11,A2:A11)		
7	77.44	807		Sy|x	182.02	=STEYX(B2:B11,A2:A11)		
8	75.41	447		SSx	266.04	=DEVSQ(A2:A11)		
9	77.87	307		SE	58.51	=E7*SQRT((1/E2+(E5-E4)^2/E8))		
10	80.74	553		t-critical	2.31	=T.INV.2T(0.05,E3)		
11	83.99	616		Confidence Interval				
12				Lower	248.86	=E6-E10*E9		
13				Upper	518.72	=E6+E10*E9		
14								
15				SE	191.1963	=E7*SQRT((1+1/E2+(E5-E4)^2/E8))		
16				Predition Interval				
17				Lower	-57.11	=E6-E10*E15		
18				Upper	824.69	=E6+E10*E15		

8.4 Logistic Regression

Like linear regression, logistic regression is a useful technique for modeling the relationship between a dependent variable and an independent variable or variables. However, the difference is that the dependent variable is categorical, not continuous. This is a common occurrence in many situations encountered by researchers in the biological and medical sciences.

Logistic regression could be used to predict whether a tumor is malignant or not, the illness resulted in death or not, or a voice disorder was present or not. The application of logistic regression where the dependent variable is binary (two levels) requires the use of binomial logistic regression. When the categorical dependent variable is more than two levels, such as no pain, slight pain, or substantial pain, then ordinal logistic regression is used. In this book, we will focus on binomial logistic regression.

Logistic regression is used to describe the relationship between a categorical dependent variable and one or more independent variables, with different possible scales. **Binomial logistic regression** involves a binary dependent variable. **Ordinal logistic regression** involves an ordinal dependent variable with more than two levels.

Consider the simple linear regression model:

$$Y_i = \beta_0 + \beta_1 X_i + \epsilon_i$$

where the responses Y_i are binary 0 or 1.

$$E(Y_i) = \beta_0 + \beta_1 X_i$$

If Y_i is a Bernoulli random variable, the probability of $Y_i = 1$ is p_i and for $Y_i = 0$ is $1 - p_i$ as the probability of a failure in a single trial. Because $E(Y_i) = 1(p_i) + 0(1 - p_i) = p_i$,

$$E(Y_i) = p_i = \beta_0 + \beta_1 X_i.$$

There are three specific problems when the dependent variable is binary: (1) the error terms are not normally distributed, (2) the error variance is not constant, and (3) the response function $E(Y_i)$ is constrained between 0 and 1.

A nonlinear regression model that constrains the mean responses to the range 0 and 1 has the following form:

$$E(Y_i) = p_i = \frac{\exp(\beta_0 + \beta_1 X_i)}{1 + \exp(\beta_0 + \beta_1 X_i)}$$

This is called the logistic response function. A property of the logistic response function is that it is either monotonic increasing or monotonic decreasing, based on the sign of β_1. Another property of the logistic response function is that it can be linearized with the following transformation:

$$\log_e\left[\frac{p}{1-p}\right] = \beta_0 + \beta_1 X$$

This transformation is called the logit model. The expression on the left is called the logit response function or log-odds. We usually use log with the base of the mathematical constant e, or the natural log, expressed as ln. The relationship between the log-odds and X is linear.

When the regression equation is used to describe the relationship in a sample, it is written as follows:

$$\log_e\left[\frac{f}{1-f}\right] = b_0 + b_1 x$$

The slope b_1 is the change in the log-odds of the outcome per unit change in x.

Consider b_1 in a logistic model when x_1 is a binary variable that equals 1 if exposed and 0 if unexposed, as follows:

$$\log_e(\text{Odds})_{Exposed} = b_0 + b_1 \times 1$$

$$\log_e(\text{Odds})_{Unexposed} = b_0 + b_1 \times 0$$

$$b_1 = \log_e(\text{Odds})_{Exposed} - \log_e(\text{Odds})_{Unexposed} = \log_e(\text{Odds Ratio})$$

$$\text{Odds Ratio} = e^{b_1}$$

e^{b_1} is the odds ratio comparing exposed and unexposed groups. The odds ratio was presented in the previous chapter as a primary measure of association in case-control studies involving exposure and outcome variables, each involving two levels. Being able to derive the odds ratio from the estimated regression coefficient b_1 in a logistic regression model makes this model particularly important in biostatistics.

EXAMPLE 8.4

A psychologist investigated whether employee's emotional health (X) was associated with their ability to perform a task ($Y = 1$ if yes, 0 if no). If the emotional score was above the median for the group, the score is considered to be high (H), with H = 1, or 0 otherwise.

X	Y	Sex	X	Y	Sex	X	Y	Sex
376	0	M	523	1	M	421	0	M
333	0	F	442	1	M	510	1	F
352	0	M	400	0	F	498	0	F
383	1	M	550	1	M	391	0	F
419	1	M	453	1	M	516	0	M
584	0	M	325	0	F	521	1	M
295	0	F	463	1	F	473	0	M
482	1	M	448	0	F	462	1	F
538	1	F	398	1	F	405	0	F
395	0	M	300	0	F	500	1	M

Assuming the association between emotional health and performing a task is similar between males and females, a 2×2 table for these data collapsed over sex is as follows:

	Performs the Task	
High	**Yes**	**No**
Yes	10	5
No	4	11

Then, the odds of having high emotional health for those performing the task is 5.5 times greater than the odds of high emotional health for those not performing the task; that is,

$$\text{Odds Ratio} = \frac{10/4}{5/11} = 5.5.$$

Using SAS, a new variable (called H) is created, as follows:

```
DATA EX8_4;
   INPUT X Y Sex $;
   IF X GT 445 THEN H=1; ELSE H=0;
DATALINES;
   376  0  M
   ...
;
```

We can now use the logistic regression procedure in SAS to estimate the odds ratio, as follows:

```
PROC LOGISTIC DATA=EX8_4 DESC;
   MODEL Y=H;
RUN;
```

The DESC option is used because the dependent variable would otherwise be read 0 versus 1 instead of 1 versus 0. A portion of the SAS output is provided here:

Analysis of Maximum Likelihood Estimates					
Parameter	DF	Estimate	Standard Error	Wald Chi-Square	Pr > ChiSq
Intercept	1	-1.0116	0.5839	3.0018	0.0832
H	1	1.7047	0.8006	4.5344	0.0332

Odds Ratio Estimates			
Effect	Point Estimate	95% Wald Confidence Limits	
H	5.500	1.145	26.412

The relationship between the slope estimate and the odds ratio is

$$\text{Odds Ratio} = e^{1.7047} = 5.50.$$

The 95% confidence interval for the odds ratio can be computed from the estimated slope and standard error as

$$95\%\ CI\ (OR) = e^{(b_1 \pm 1.96 \times SE)} = e^{(1.7047 \pm 1.96 \times 0.8006)} \rightarrow 1.145 - 26.412.$$

The *p*-value for the odds ratio is 0.0332, which indicates statistical significance at the 0.05 level. The 95% confidence interval does not overlap 1, which also indicates statistical significance at the 0.05 level. Therefore, we may conclude that those with high emotional health have 5.5 times the odds of completing the task than those with low emotional health.

Another approach is to enter the data into SAS using the summary data:

```
DATA A;
INPUT H Y COUNT;
DATALINES;
   1 1 10
   1 0 5
   0 1 4
   0 0 11
;
```

Now, the following SAS procedure code gives the same result as before:

```
PROC LOGISTIC DATA=A;
   CLASS H (REF='0' PARAM=REF) Y (REF='0');
   MODEL Y=H;
   WEIGHT COUNT;
RUN;
```

A portion of the output from this SAS code is as follows:

Odds Ratio Estimates			
Effect	Point Estimate	95% Wald Confidence Limits	
X 1 vs 0	5.500	1.145	26.412

It may also be of interest to evaluate the task variable associates with the continuous emotional health variable. Using logistic regression, the SAS code is as follows:

```
PROC LOGISTIC DATA=EX8_4 DESC;
  MODEL Y = X;
RUN;
```

This produces the following output:

Analysis of Maximum Likelihood Estimates					
Parameter	DF	Estimate	Standard Error	Wald Chi-Square	Pr > ChiSq
Intercept	1	-6.5308	2.8740	5.1636	0.0231
X	1	0.0145	0.00640	5.1276	0.0235

Odds Ratio Estimates			
Effect	Point Estimate	95% Wald Confidence Limits	
X	1.015	1.002	1.027

The odds ratio is $e^{0.0145} = 1.015$, and the 95% confidence interval is $e^{(1.015 \pm 1.96 \times 0.0064)} \rightarrow 1.002 - 1.027$. The regression coefficient (0.0145) represents the change in log odds per unit change in X. The odds are 1.5% greater for a 1-unit change in X.

Logistic regression can be used as an alternative to the Wilcoxon rank sum test to estimate the ratio of cases to controls (odds ratio) according to exposure.

Example 8.5

Suppose we are interested in whether the odds of disease changes according to distance from a putative exposure. Bands of distance from the exposure must be selected prior to analysis. Let there be five bands, from 1 kilometer to 5 kilometers. Now consider the following hypothetical case-control data:

Distance from Site (kilometers)	Cases	Controls
1	40	100
2	35	100
3	30	100
4	15	100
5	12	100

A dose-response relationship is evident. That is, the odds of disease increases with closer proximity to the exposure. With a binary outcome variable (case versus control), logistic regression can be used to estimate the odds ratios and corresponding confidence intervals. SAS code for generating the odds ratios and 95% confidence intervals in the above table is as follows:

```
DATA EX8_5;
   INPUT Distance Case $ Count;
DATALINES;
   1 Yes 40
   1 No 100
   2 Yes 35
   2 No 100
   3 Yes 30
   3 No 100
   4 Yes 15
   4 No 100
   5 Yes 12
   5 No 100
;
PROC LOGISTIC DATA=EX8_5 DESC;
   CLASS Distance (REF='5');
   MODEL Case=Distance;
   WEIGHT Count;
   RUN;
```

A portion of the SAS output corresponding to this procedure code is:

Odds Ratio Estimates			
Effect	Point Estimate	95% Wald Confidence Limits	
Distance 1 vs 5	3.333	1.652	6.726
Distance 2 vs 5	2.917	1.431	5.943
Distance 3 vs 5	2.500	1.211	5.159
Distance 4 vs 5	1.250	0.557	2.804

So we see that the odds of being a case decreases with greater distance away from the site.

8.5 Poisson Regression

Another important regression model in biology and clinical medicine is Poisson regression. Poisson regression is appropriate when the dependent events occur infrequently, the events occur independently, and the events occur over some continuous medium such as area or time. The probability of a single event occurring is influenced by the extent of the area or the length of the time interval. Counts or rates of rare diseases are particularly well suited for modeling with Poisson regression.[10] Examples include the number of injuries reported to the emergency room on a given day, the number of car accidents occurring during a given storm, or the number of missed school days because of asthma during a week of poor air quality. When counts or rates do not represent a rare event, logistic regression or survival analysis should be considered.

Poisson regression is a type of generalized linear model where the random component specified by the Poisson distribution of the response variable is a count. Traditional regression assumes a symmetric distribution of errors, but the Poisson distribution is skewed. Traditional regression can produce negative predictive values, but the Poisson distribution is nonnegative. Traditional regression assumes constant variance, but the Poisson regression uses a log transformation that adjusts for skewness. Poisson regression also models the variance as a function of the mean.

Poisson regression is useful when the dependent variable *Y* has a Poisson distribution and the logarithm of its expected value is modeled as a linear combination of a set of parameters. We assume the observations are independent of one another and the mean of the Poisson random variable equals its variance.

The independent variable in a Poisson regression model is categorical. This is because the model uses total number of events or the total person–time rate per level of the categorical variable. If the independent variable is an indicator (dummy) variable, like obese (yes = 1, no = 0), then the exponential of the regression coefficient is an estimate of the rate ratio comparing the rate of the dependent variable for obese versus not obese subjects.

The following describes the meaning of the estimated regression coefficient b_1 in the Poisson regression model when x_1 is a binary variable equal to 1 if exposed and 0 if unexposed:

$$\log_e(\text{Rate})_{Exposed} = b_0 + b_1 \times 1$$

$$\log_e(\text{Rate})_{Unexposed} = b_0 + b_1 \times 0$$

$$b_1 = \log_e(\text{Rate})_{Exposed} - \log_e(\text{Rate})_{Unexposed} = \log_e(\text{Rate Ratio})$$

$$\text{Rate Ratio} = e^{b_1}$$

e^{b_1} is the estimated rate ratio comparing exposed and unexposed groups. If additional variables are included in the model, then e^{b_1} is adjusted for those variables.

Example 8.6

For the data in Table 7.5, the percentage of the population of India ≥ 60 years of age is (10.2%). In neighboring Pakistan, it is lower (6.9%). Because COVID-19 becomes more lethal with older age, we expect that the death rate from the disease to be greater in India than Pakistan. As of August 26, 2020, the number of deaths from COVID-19 was 60,629 (population = 1,382,048,762) in India and 6267 in Pakistan (population = 221,518,879).[11] The Poisson regression model can be estimated using SAS. Here is the data statement and procedure code for obtaining the COVID-19 death rate ratio for India versus Pakistan.

```
DATA EX8_6;
INPUT Country $ Death PYEARS;
LPYEARS=LOG(PYEARS);
DATALINES;
  1 60629 1382048762
  2 6267 221518879;
```

```
PROC GENMOD DATA=EX8_6;
  CLASS Country;
  MODEL DEATH=Country/DIST=POISSON LINK=LOG
  OFFSET=LPYEARS;
  ESTIMATE 'Country' Country 1 -1/EXP;
RUN;
```

A portion of the output from this procedure is as follows:

Contrast Estimate Results											
Label	Mean Estimate	Mean Confidence Limits		L'Beta Estimate	Standard Error	Alpha	L'Beta Confidence Limits		Chi-Square	Pr > ChiSq
Country	1.5506	1.5108	1.5915	0.4387	0.0133	0.05	0.4127	0.4647	1092.9	<.0001
Exp(Country)				1.5506	0.0206	0.05	1.5108	1.5915		

Therefore, the rate of COVID-19 death in India is 1.55 (55%) times higher than in Pakistan. The confidence interval and p-value both indicate statistical significance.

8.6 Log-Binomial Regression

Log-binomial regression is similar to logistic regression in that it is used when the outcome variable is binary. Both model the probability of the outcome given exposure status and possible confounders, and they both assume the error terms have a binomial distribution. However, they differ in the link between the independent variables and the probability of the outcome. Specifically, logistic regression involves the logit function, described earlier, whereas log-binomial regression uses the log function, as with Poisson regression. The log-binomial model gives an unbiased estimate of the risk ratio.[12]

Example 8.7

Previously, we referred to a study involving quality-of-life indicators for 94 patients with obstructive sleep apnea. Data are presented in Table 5.2. Suppose we are interested in identifying whether the risk of having a voice problem is similar between women and men. The data are summarized in the following 2 × 2 table.

	Voice Problem	No Voice Problem	Total
Women	24	17	41
Men	13	40	53

The risk of a voice problem is 0.585 (= 24/41) for women and 0.245 (= 13/53) for men. The risk ratio is 2.4. Now, based on the data in the form shown in Table 5.2, we can use SAS to compute the risk ratio using the following program:

```
PROC GENMOD DATA=T5_2 DESC;
  CLASS Sex;
  MODEL VP=Sex/DIST=BINOMIAL LINK=LOG;
  ESTIMATE 'Sex' Sex 1 -1/EXP;
RUN;
```

A portion of the SAS output is shown here:

Contrast Estimate Results											
		Mean			Standard		L'Beta			
Label	Mean Estimate	Confidence Limits		L'Beta Estimate	Error	Alpha	Confidence Limits		Chi-Square	Pr > ChiSq
Sex	2.3865	1.3936	4.0868	0.8698	0.2745	0.05	0.3319	1.4078	10.04	0.0015
Exp(Sex)				2.3865	0.6550	0.05	1.3936	4.0868		

Hence, we see that among patients with obstructive sleep apnea, women are almost 2.4 times more likely to have a voice problem than men. We are 95% confident that the true risk ratio of all adults with obstructive sleep apnea is bounded by the interval 1.39–4.09. This interval and the p-value both indicate statistical significance. Later in this chapter, this example will be expanded to provide an adjusted risk ratio.

8.7 Cox Proportional Hazard Model

Several statistical procedures are available for assessing survival data. In this book, we will focus on the Cox proportional hazard model, proposed by D. R. Cox in 1972.[13] This model is commonly used to analyze time-to-event (survival) data using the hazard (force of mortality or morbidity) scale. It is useful for evaluating the rate of an event (e.g., infection, injury, death) according to one or more factors at a given point in time.

The hazard function is denoted by $h(t)$ and is mathematically expressed as

$$h(t) = \lim_{\Delta t \to 0} \frac{P(t \le T < t + \Delta t \mid T \ge t)}{\Delta t} = \frac{f(t)}{S(t)}.$$

In words, the hazard function $h(t)$ is the probability that if you survive to time t, you will experience the event in the next instant. While the survival function $S(t) = P(T > t)$ focuses on the event not failing, the probability of a subject surviving past time t, the hazard function focuses on the event failing.

The Cox proportional hazards model equals a baseline hazard that involves survival time t, multiplied by the exponential that involves one or more independent variables. With one independent variable, the model is

$$h(t) = h_0(t)e^{b_1 x_1}.$$

The term $h_0(t)$ is referred to as the baseline hazard. It corresponds to the value of the hazard if $x_1 = 0$; $h_0(t)e^0 = h_0(t)$.

Taking the natural log of both sides of the equation yields the following model for a single independent variable:

$$\log_e(\text{Hazard}) = \beta_0 + \beta_1 X_1$$

The estimated model is

$$\log_e(\text{Hazard}) = b_0 + b_1 x_1.$$

The meaning of the estimated regression coefficient b_1 in the Cox proportional hazard model when x_1 is a binary variable equal to 1 if exposed and 0 if unexposed is as follows:

$$\log_e(\text{Hazard})_{Exposed} = b_0 + b_1 \times 1$$

$$\log_e(\text{Hazard})_{Unexposed} = b_0 + b_1 \times 0$$

$$b_1 = \log_e(\text{Hazard})_{Exposed} - \log_e(\text{Hazard})_{Unexposed} = \log_e(\text{Hazard Ratio})$$

$$\text{Hazard Ratio} = e^{b_1}$$

e^{b_1} is the estimated hazard ratio comparing exposed and unexposed groups. With additional variables in the model, e^{b_1} is adjusted for those variables. More will be said about the Cox proportional hazard model later in this chapter.

8.8 Multiple Regression

Thus far we have focused on simple regression, which involves a single independent variable in the model. However, rarely is the response function $E(Y)$ influenced by only one independent variable. Multiple independent variables may simultaneously affect the dependent variable, or confound or modify the relationship between dependent and independent variables. Multiple regression models are particularly useful for adjusting for possible confounding effects between variables and are more efficient than stratified simple regression models when data in the stratified combinations are sparse. Thus, application of the multiple regression model is very important in biological and medical research.

Extension of the regression models presented in this chapter and the interpretation of the slope coefficient for each model is shown in **Table 8.1**. The response variable in each model is a linear combination of the independent variables. The linear combination is a weighted average that yields a given

Table 8.1 Multiple Regression Models and Interpretation of the Slope Coefficient β_1

	Multiple Regression Model	Interpretation of β_1
Linear	$Y = \beta_0 + \beta_1 X_1 + \beta_2 X_2 + \cdots + \beta_k X_k + \epsilon$	Change in Y mean value per unit change in X_1, adjusted for the other variables in the model
Logistic	$\log_e(\text{Odds}) = \beta_0 + \beta_1 X_1 + \beta_2 X_2 + \cdots + \beta_k X_k$	Change in the log-odds of the outcome per unit change in X_1, adjusted for the other variables in the model
Poisson	$\log_e(\text{Rate}) = \beta_0 + \beta_1 X_1 + \beta_2 X_2 + \cdots + \beta_k X_k$	Change in the log rate of the outcome per unit change in X_1, adjusted for the other variables in the model
Log-binomial	$\log_e(\text{Risk}) = \beta_0 + \beta_1 X_1 + \beta_2 X_2 + \cdots + \beta_k X_k$	Change in the log risk of the outcome per unit change in X_1, adjusted for the other variables in the model
Cox	$\log_e(\text{Hazard}) = \beta_0 + \beta_1 X_1 + \beta_2 X_2 + \cdots + \beta_k X_k$	Change in the log hazard of the outcome per unit change in X_1, adjusted for the other variables in the model

number after the X's are multiplied by their corresponding β_1's and then summed.

As with simple linear regression, we use the method of least squares to fit the multiple linear regression model. This technique requires that we minimize the sum of squares of the residuals, which in this case is

$$\sum_i e_i^2 = \sum_i (y_i - \hat{y}_i)^2 = \sum_i (y_i - b_0 - b_1 x_{1i} - b_2 x_{2i} - \cdots - b_k x_{ki})^2.$$

Although the calculations of this model are more complicated than for just one independent variable, this is not a problem with the help of a computer.

The interpretation of the regression coefficients is different than with simple regression. With multiple regression, the slope coefficient represents change in the dependent variable per unit increase in the independent variable, adjusting for the other variables in the model. To adjust for the other variables in the model means to hold the values of the other variables in the regression equation constant (as if each subject had the same value for the other variables). This is an ideal approach for controlling for confounders.

Similar to the assumptions made when the regression model has a single independent variable, the multiple linear regression model has a set of analogous assumptions. Some of these assumptions can be checked in the computer diagnostic output associated with programs like SAS. For example, using PROC REG in SAS produces a residual plot, which displays the predicted values against residual values for a regression model. This plot is useful for checking the assumptions of linearity and constant variance. The assumption about normality can be assessed using a histogram or a normal probability plot.[14] In addition, highly correlated independent variables and small sample size can result in misleading results. In regression, multicollinearity refers to high correlation between two or more independent variables, which can increase the variance of the coefficient estimates and make the estimates unstable and difficult to interpret. As for sample size, a rule of thumb is that there should be at least 10 observations per independent variable.

Assumptions of Multiple Linear Regression

1. The X values of each independent variable are known (not random).
2. The residuals are normally distributed—multivariate normal.
3. The variance of the error terms is similar across the levels of the independent variables (homoscedasticity).
4. There is a linear relationship between the dependent variable and the independent variables.

8.8.1 Statistical Inference for Regression Coefficients

We are now interested in using the least-squares regression model to draw inferences about the population regression model. The estimated model is based on a sample drawn from the underlying population. If a different sample was taken from the population, the estimated model would be different. For this reason, standard errors of the estimators are needed to make inferences about the population.

Hypothesis testing of the intercept and slopes in the multiple regression model are conducted as with the simple regression model, except when testing $H_0: \beta_i = \beta_{i0}$ against $H_a: \beta_i \neq \beta_{i0}$ we make the assumption that the values of all other independent variables remain constant. In addition, if the null hypothesis is true, then

$$t = \frac{b_i - \beta_{i0}}{SE_{bi}}.$$

It follows a t distribution with $n-k-1$ degrees of freedom, where k represents the number of independent variables in the model. From this t distribution, we can find the p-value, which is the probability of observing an estimated slope as extreme or more so than b_i, given that true slope is β_{i0}.

Example 8.8

Data for 94 patients with obstructive sleep apnea appears in **Table 8.2**. The dependent variable is SF-36 component physical quality of life, which ranges from 0 (low) to 100 (high). Independent variables are a breathing symptom index (0 best, 40 worst), age, and body mass index (BMI). For these data, let us test the hypothesis that the breathing index score is associated with physical quality of life after adjusting for age and BMI.

SF-36 component physical quality of life (PHYS); breathing index (BI); age; and body mass index (BMI).

1. H_0: $\beta_{BI} = 0$
2. H_a: $\beta_{BI} \neq 0$
3. $\alpha = 0.05$, $n = 94$
4. t test statistic with 90 degrees of freedom.
5. Using Excel (the Regression option in the Data Analysis tab), we obtained the following, which represents a portion of the output. We will discuss the regression statistics in the next section. For now, the parameter estimates for the slope measuring the association between breathing and the component physical quality of life measure is –1.12 (SE = 0.21), with p-value <0.0001. The 95% confidence interval ranges from –1.53 to –0.71.

Regression Statistics	
Multiple R	0.623204
R Square	0.388384
Adjusted R Square	0.367997
Standard Error	18.95178
Observations	94

	Coefficients	Standard Error	t Stat	*p*-Value	Lower 95%	Upper 95%
Intercept	120.7801	11.94541	10.111	1.68E–16	97.04843	144.5117
BI	–1.11953	0.206595	–5.41895	4.97E–07	–1.52997	–0.70909
Age	–0.38262	0.155586	–2.45924	0.015835	–0.69172	–0.07352
BMI	–0.80347	0.196128	–4.09668	9.15E–05	–1.19312	–0.41383

6. Reject H_0: $\beta_{BR} = 0$ and conclude that as the breathing symptoms index increases by 1 (worsening), component physical quality of life decreases by −1.12.

Table 8.2 **Obstructive Sleep Apnea Patient Data**

#	PHYS	BI	AGE	BMI	#	PHYS	BI	AGE	BMI	#	PHYS	BI	AGE	BMI
1	83.2	2.0	67.4	31.9	32	72.7	4.0	44.7	39.2	63	63.9	3.0	67.5	35.9
2	80.0	4.0	43.5	37.7	33	53.2	9.0	60.7	34.1	64	38.2	0.0	57.3	35.9
3	66.1	29.0	24.0	33.4	34	70.9	2.0	78.1	21.3	65	85.7	10.0	45.4	28.5
4	81.1	0.0	68.5	35.0	35	89.8	6.0	63.0	23.1	66	22.5	4.0	54.5	41.6
5	65.7	4.0	53.2	48.1	36	78.9	0.0	49.6	28.5	67	75.0	2.0	41.6	30.1
6	80.0	7.0	40.4	33.9	37	53.9	1.0	32.4	37.7	68	84.3	6.0	62.6	31.4
7	92.0	31.0	38.1	28.9	38	63.2	17.0	76.2	34.4	69	84.1	16.0	45.7	25.3
8	60.0	12.0	53.7	32.3	39	75.5	0.0	45.7	29.3	70	40.0	6.0	67.6	35.6
9	17.7	27.0	33.5	80.1	40	95.5	0.0	61.7	26.4	71	89.8	9.0	48.4	27.7
10	48.0	17.0	58.2	30.3	41	80.9	10.0	36.0	25.8	72	59.8	15.0	80.1	36.1
11	37.5	26.0	53.9	26.6	42	73.2	3.0	45.3	38.0	73	75.7	11.0	53.5	26.2
12	48.2	9.0	38.2	28.5	43	80.7	5.0	77.3	28.9	74	52.7	5.0	67.3	30.4
13	36.1	2.0	38.4	34.2	44	49.5	4.0	58.2	23.7	75	84.3	5.0	34.9	38.4
14	84.1	0.0	38.7	52.9	45	82.5	2.0	66.8	29.8	76	57.7	1.0	45.3	34.3
15	48.4	20.0	64.6	46.2	46	25.0	10.0	63.9	30.0	77	63.2	20.0	53.9	53.0
16	91.4	0.0	68.8	23.7	47	24.5	25.0	55.1	31.1	78	16.6	31.0	55.2	75.6
17	73.9	4.0	77.7	35.9	48	39.1	24.0	73.5	27.8	79	31.4	20.0	66.1	36.3
18	84.5	6.0	63.5	29.2	49	70.0	2.0	67.1	30.2	80	74.3	17.0	58.7	32.9
19	86.8	0.0	59.2	27.0	50	76.6	14.0	48.5	29.2	81	11.4	36.0	57.5	37.9
20	20.2	16.0	68.2	42.9	51	84.3	2.0	23.4	32.3	82	50.7	17.0	44.8	27.2
21	90.0	5.0	46.0	25.1	52	59.3	10.0	59.9	48.2	83	16.8	35.0	61.3	27.4
22	29.5	10.0	69.5	43.5	53	84.5	0.0	47.9	23.2	84	15.5	0.0	56.0	37.8
23	79.5	2.0	62.3	26.2	54	55.2	6.0	59.4	34.5	85	62.7	0.0	51.9	31.7
24	92.5	0.0	54.8	31.2	55	37.3	29.0	47.4	30.6	86	70.5	0.0	64.2	36.6
25	74.3	3.0	60.6	29.6	56	88.2	0.0	45.9	29.1	87	73.0	4.0	33.8	55.4
26	74.3	0.0	55.0	40.3	57	25.0	18.0	40.9	30.0	88	93.2	0.0	50.6	30.7
27	90.9	0.0	62.9	33.4	58	68.9	9.0	42.0	30.3	89	57.3	15.0	68.5	38.5
28	58.6	20.0	59.5	34.9	59	75.5	3.0	33.4	42.0	90	64.1	17.0	42.3	54.8
29	71.4	0.0	77.1	33.1	60	70.9	1.0	67.0	35.1	91	55.5	9.0	68.7	36.6
30	26.8	2.0	54.5	38.4	61	4.5	0.0	64.9	62.1	92	13.2	33.0	61.0	34.7
31	18.9	15.0	58.9	38.0	62	74.1	3.0	32.5	43.5	93	50.2	6.0	46.9	35.4
										94	54.8	5.0	47.4	63.1

8.8.2 Evaluating the Model

Residual and other plots, as well as the coefficient of determination, are ways to assess how well a given least-squares model fits the observed data. In simple regression we can simply plot the dependent variable against the independent variable in a scatter plot to assess the model assumptions. With multiple regression where more than one independent variable is involved, it becomes necessary to evaluate the model assumptions by plotting the predicted versus the residual values. This is called a residual plot. By convention, we plot the predicted values on the *X*-axis and the residual values on the *Y*-axis. For example, the Excel Regression analysis tool used in Example 8.8 produced predicted physical values and model residuals (and standardized residuals). These plots are as follows:

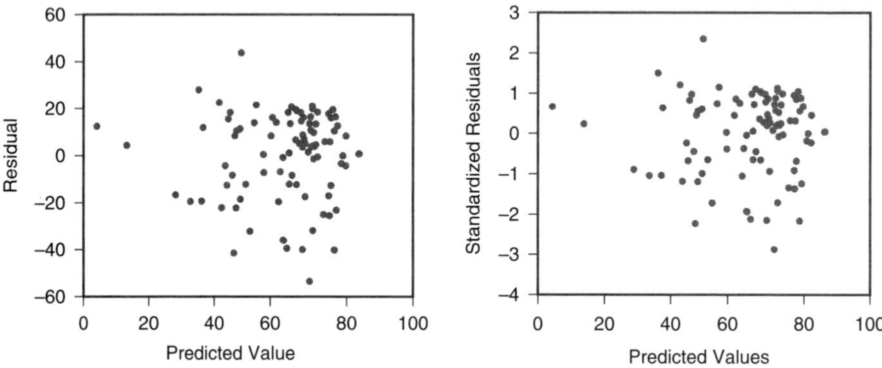

The advantage of the plot with the standardized residuals is that different plots with any model will have the same standardized *Y*-axis. Since a residual equals the observed minus the predicted, greater distance from the line at 0 indicates poorer prediction for that value. Values above the line at 0 mean the prediction was too low, and values below the line at 0 mean the prediction was too high. If the plot of residuals shows a random pattern, then a linear model is a good fit to the data.

A statistic called the multiple R from multiple-regression is analogous to the correlation coefficient r. It is the correlation between the actual and predicted values of the dependent variable. By squaring the multiple R (R^2) we get a measure that indicates the amount of variation in the dependent variable that is accounted for by the regression equation. As with r^2, the value ranges from 0 to 1, with 0 indicating no variation in the dependent variable is accounted for by the regression equation and 1 meaning all the variation is explained by the equation. The F test statistic is used instead of the t-test statistic for evaluating the significance of R^2.

It is important to note, however, that as variables are added to a model, the R^2 only increases. Thus, a model containing more variables than another model may appear superior for that fact alone, even if the additional variables are not statistically significant. The adjusted R^2 is a modified version of R^2 that accounts for the number of independent variables in the model. This statistic only increases if the additional variable improves the model fit more than expected by chance. It also can decrease if the independent variable improves the model fit less than expected by chance. To calculate the adjusted R^2, we first obtain R^2 and then use the following equation:

$$R_{adj}^2 = 1 - \frac{(1-R^2)(n-1)}{n-k-1}$$

Referring again to Example 8.8, the Excel summary output shows the computer derived R, R^2, and adjusted R^2. While the adjusted R^2 is useful for comparing models with different numbers of independent variables, it should not be interpreted as the proportion of variation in the dependent variable that is explained by the linear regression model.

8.8.3 Interaction Term

A regression model can be misleading if it does not include an interaction term when the association between a dependent variable and an independent variable differs among the levels of another variable. For example, modeling heart disease based on drug and alcohol use would have an interaction effect if the chemicals in these two substances interact to increase the chance of heart disease beyond the effect of either variable alone. Knowing your variables helps you determine whether or not to include an interaction term in the model. A test statistic can then be used to evaluate the significance of the interaction.

Statistical interaction can also be referred to as effect modification. In other words, an effect modifier is a third variable that causes the direction or magnitude of an association between two variables to differ. When using the Mantel-Haenszel method to obtain a summary statistic, an important assumption is that there is no statistical interaction (effect modification). If effect modification is present, we do not want to lose possibly very informative information by collapsing over the strata to achieve an overall summary measure. A valuable feature of regression analysis is being able to test possible interaction effects (effect modifiers) along with the main effects in the model.

Now let us consider the regression model with two independent variables X_1 and X_2:

$$Y_i = \beta_0 + \beta_1 X_{1i} + \beta_2 X_{2i} + \beta_3 X_{1i} X_{2i} + \epsilon_i$$

The cross-product $\beta_3 X_{1i} X_{2i}$ is referred to as the interaction term. Including the interaction term $\beta_3 X_{1i} X_{2i}$ in the model changes the interpretation of β_1 and β_2. Specifically, the change in the mean Y for a unit increase in X_1 given X_2 is held constant is $\beta_1 + \beta_3 X_2$. Similarly, the change in the mean Y for a unit increase in X_2 given X_1 is held constant is $\beta_2 + \beta_3 X_1$. Thus, the effect of X_1 on Y depends on X_2 and the effect of X_2 on Y depends on X_1. To illustrate the interaction term in the regression model, consider the following model without an interaction:

$$E(Y) = 5 + 2X_1 + 5X_2$$

The response function $E(Y)$ for $X_1 = 0$ through 10 and $X_2 = 1$ or $X_2 = 3$ is shown in **Figure 8.5**. The two response functions are parallel. In other words, mean response Y increases by β_1 with a unit increase in X_1, regardless of the value of X_2.

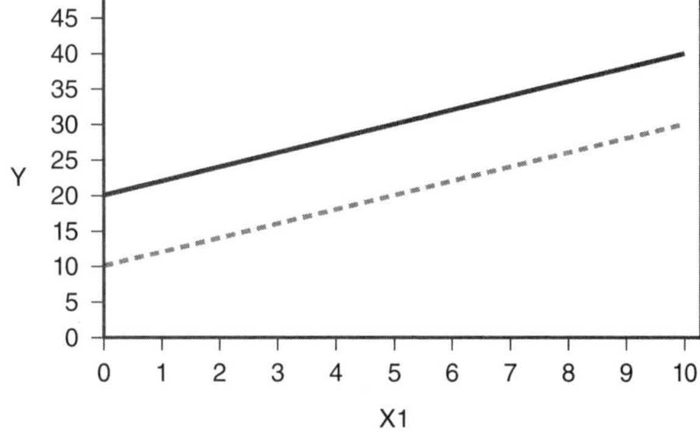

Figure 8.5 Model without Statistical Interaction

Now consider the extended model that includes the interaction term $1X_1X_2$.

$$E(Y) = 5 + 2X_1 + 5X_2 + 1X_1X_2$$

The response function $E(Y)$ when plotted against $X_1 = 0$ through 10 now has a different slope for $X_2 = 1$ versus $X_2 = 3$ (**Figure 8.6**). Note that the regression model with the interaction term is still a linear model. The term linear model indicates that the model is linear in the parameters.

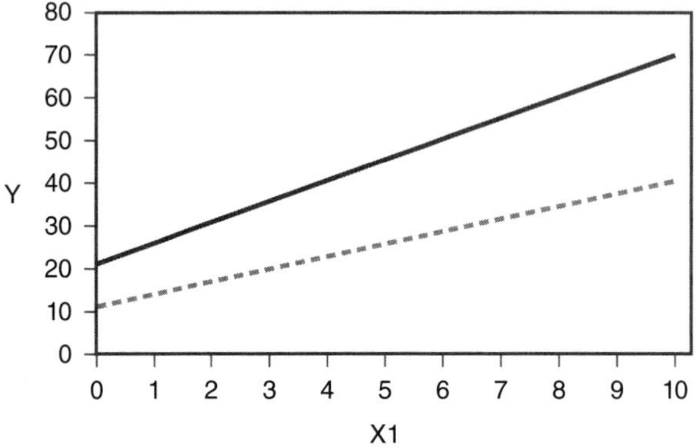

Figure 8.6 Model with Statistical Interaction

EXAMPLE 8.9

Hypothetical anxiety scores and average minutes of exercise per day were chosen for five women and five men. Of interest is whether anxiety is associated with exercise and if this association differs between women and men. Consider the following data:

Anxiety	Average Minutes of Exercise per Day	Sex
70	30	1
80	15	1
90	5	1
85	20	1
50	45	1
45	60	0
48	65	0
50	50	0
70	25	0
60	10	0

Women = 1, Men = 0

Partial output from Excel is shown here.

SUMMARY OUTPUT

Regression Statistics	
Multiple R	0.95451
R Square	0.91109
Adjusted R Square	0.86663
Standard Error	6.04208
Observations	10

	Coefficients	Standard Error	t Stat	*p*-Value	Lower 95%	Upper 95%
Intercept	69.59193	6.014924	11.56988	2.51E-05	54.87394	84.30992
Exercise	-0.35695	0.127948	-2.78981	0.031586	-0.67003	-0.04387
Sex	28.28442	8.01538	3.528768	0.012386	8.67148	47.89734
Exercise × Sex	-0.63767	0.23585	-2.70372	0.0354	-1.21478	-0.06057

The significant interaction term indicates that the association between exercise and anxiety differs between men and women. For men, as the exercise variable increases by 1, anxiety goes down by –0.357, on average. The corresponding estimate for women is –0.995. The average anxiety score for women is 28.28 greater for women than men.

8.9 Multiple Logistic Regression

The multiple logistic regression function has the same properties as the simple logistic regression function. It has the advantage in that more than one independent variable is often associated with the binary dependent variable. Multiple logistic regression also allows us to control for potential confounders and consider interaction effects. When an odds ratio is estimated from a multiple logistic regression model, it is adjusted for the other variables in the model. Homogeneity of odds ratios can be assessed by testing for interaction between independent binary variables in the logistic regression model. Homogeneity of odds ratios can be assessed by testing for interaction between independent binary variables in the logistic regression model. In addition, the independent variables should not be highly correlated with each other.

Assumptions of Multiple Logistic Regression

1. The dependent variable is binary in binary logistic regression or ordinal in ordinal logistic regression.
2. The observations are independent of each other (i.e., not coming from a repeated measures or matched pairs).
3. There is a linear relationship between the log odds and the independent variables.

The logistic response function is written as follows:

$$E(Y) = \frac{\exp(\beta_0 + \beta_1 X_1 + \beta_2 X_2 + \cdots + \beta_k X_k)}{1 + \exp(\beta_0 + \beta_1 X_1 + \beta_2 X_2 + \cdots + \beta_k X_k)}$$

The equation can be rewritten as the log of the odds being the dependent variable of a linear function:

$$\log_e(\text{Odds}) = \log_e\left(\frac{p}{1-p}\right) = \beta_0 + \beta_1 X_1 + \beta_2 X_2 + \cdots + \beta_k X_k$$

We can write the estimated model with the natural $\log_e$ of the odds as the dependent variable of a linear function:

$$\log_e(\text{Odds}) = \log_e\left(\frac{f}{1-f}\right) = b_0 + b_1 x_1 + b_2 x_2 + \cdots + b_k x_k$$

As shown with one independent variable, the antilog of the coefficient estimate e^{b_1} is the estimated odds ratio. This statistic is useful for comparing the odds of exposure among cases versus noncases. The odds ratio derived from multiple logistic regression is adjusted for the other variables in the model.

Example 8.10

In Example 7.8, we investigated the association between coffee drinking and osteoporosis for a group of women aged 30 years and older using a case-control study design. Stratifying the women by smoking status showed that smoking was a positive confounder. These data could similarly be evaluated using multiple logistic regression. The SAS Logistic procedure to obtain the crude odds ratio is:

```
PROC LOGISTIC DATA=EX7_8 DESC;
  MODEL Y = X;
  WEIGHT Count;
RUN;
```

The output from this SAS program is shown:

Odds Ratio Estimates			
Effect	Point Estimate	95% Wald Confidence Limits	
C	1.567	1.040	2.360

To control for smoking status, the program is modified by adding the smoking variable (S). The resulting output is as follows:

Odds Ratio Estimates			
Effect	Point Estimate	95% Wald Confidence Limits	
C	1.222	0.790	1.890
S	2.202	1.448	3.350

Thus, the odds of coffee drinking among women with osteoporosis is 1.57 (95% CI 1.04–2.36) times greater than the odds of coffee drinking among women without osteoporosis. However, after adjusting for smoking status, the odds ratio is 1.22 (95% CI 0.79–1.89), which is not statistically significant. Smoking, on the other hand, is significantly associated with osteoporosis. The model can further be extended with an interaction term, but it is insignificant (p-value = 0.9899).

8.10 Multiple Poisson Regression

Earlier we noted that the Poisson regression model is particularly suitable for studying rare health events in large populations. The independent variables are categorical. With multiple Poisson regression, the magnitude of the rate is an exponential function. The Poisson response function is

$$E(Y) = \exp(\beta_0 + \beta_1 X_1 + \beta_2 X_2 + \cdots + \beta_k X_k).$$

We can write the estimated model with the natural log of the rate as the dependent variable of a linear function:

$$\log_e(\text{Rate}) = b_0 + b_1 x_1 + b_2 x_2 + \cdots + b_k x_k$$

As shown with one independent variable, the antilog of the coefficient estimate e^{b_1} is the estimated rate ratio, but adjusted for the other variables in the model.

Example 8.11

Female breast cancer incidence rates are available in the United States from retrospective cohort data according to age, year, and race/ethnicity.[15] In this example, we will use Poisson regression to evaluate the effect of race/ethnicity on female breast cancer for women ages 50–79 years during the years 2013–2017. Using SAS, the data step and procedure code is as follows:

```
PROC FORMAT;

VALUE $Ethnicity '1'='Hispanic'
                 '2'='Non-Hispanic';
VALUE $Race '1'='American Indian or Alaska Native'
                 '2'='Asian or Pacific Islander'
                 '3'='Black'
                 '4'='White';
RUN;

DATA Cancer;
   INPUT Ethnicity $ Race $ Breast PYEARS;
   LPYEARS=LOG(PYEARS);
   FORMAT Ethnicity Ethnicity.;
   FORMAT Race Race.;
DATALINES;
   1 1 223 731451
   1 2 552 369631
   1 3 2125 1239103
```

```
    1 4 59338 24133648
    2 1 4833 1866190
    2 2 32612 13249003
    2 3 97219 29581143
    2 4 662647 186146317
;
RUN;

PROC GENMOD DATA=Cancer;
    CLASS Ethnicity Race;
    MODEL Breast=Ethnicity Race/DIST=POISSON LINK=LOG
    OFFSET=LPYEARS;
    ESTIMATE 'Ethnicity' Ethnicity 1 -1/EXP;
    ESTIMATE 'Race' Race 1 0 0 -1/EXP;
    ESTIMATE 'Race' Race 0 1 0 -1/EXP;
    ESTIMATE 'Race' Race 0 0 1 -1/EXP;
RUN;
```

Partial output from the program is:

Contrast Estimate Results										
		Mean					L'Beta			
Label	Mean Estimate	Confidence Limits		L'Beta Estimate	Standard Error	Alpha	Confidence Limits		Chi-Square	Pr > ChiSq
Ethnicity	0.6719	0.6664	0.6774	-0.3976	0.0042	0.05	-0.4058	-0.3894	9059.0	<.0001
Exp(Ethnicity)				0.6719	0.0028	0.05	0.6664	0.6774		
Race	0.6011	0.5847	0.6180	-0.5090	0.0141	0.05	-0.5367	-0.4813	1299.1	<.0001
Exp(Race)				0.6011	0.0085	0.05	0.5847	0.6180		
Race	0.6887	0.6811	0.6963	-0.3730	0.0056	0.05	-0.3840	-0.3620	4401.6	<.0001
Exp(Race)				0.6887	0.0039	0.05	0.6811	0.6963		
Race	0.9155	0.9095	0.9216	-0.0883	0.0034	0.05	-0.0949	-0.0816	677.26	<.0001
Exp(Race)				0.9155	0.0031	0.05	0.9095	0.9216		

The rate ratio for Hispanics compared with non-Hispanics adjusted by race is 0.6719. Thus, the adjusted rate of female breast cancer is 32.81% lower for Hispanics than non-Hispanics. The rate ratio for American Indians or Alaska Natives, Asian or Pacific Islanders, and Blacks compared with Whites adjusted by ethnicity is 0.6011 (39.89% lower), 0.6887 (31.13% lower), 0.9155 (8.45% lower), respectively. The low p-values corresponding to these estimates indicate statistical significance at the 0.05 level. Statistical significance is also evident from the 95% confidence intervals, which do not overlap 1.

8.11 Multiple Log-Binomial Regression

With multiple log-binomial regression, the magnitude of the risk is an exponential function. The response function

$$E(Y) = \exp(\beta_0 + \beta_1 X_1 + \beta_2 X_2 + \cdots + \beta_k X_k).$$

We can write the estimated model with the natural log of the rate as the dependent variable of a linear function:

$$\log_e(\text{Risk}) = b_0 + b_1x_1 + b_2x_2 + \cdots + b_kx_k$$

As shown with one independent variable, the antilog of the coefficient estimate e^{b_1} is the estimated rate ratio, but adjusted for the other variables in the model.

Example 8.12

In Example 8.7, the risk ratio of a voice problem for women versus men was 2.39 (95% CI = 1.39–4.09). We are now interested in obtaining a risk ratio adjusted for CPAP use. The SAS program is modified as follows:

```
PROC GENMOD DATA=T5_2 DESC;
   CLASS Sex CPAP;
   MODEL VP=Sex CPAP/DIST=BINOMIAL LINK=LOG;
   ESTIMATE 'Sex' Sex 1 -1/EXP;
   ESTIMATE 'CPAP' CPAP 1 -1/EXP;
RUN;
```

A portion of the SAS output is shown:

Contrast Estimate Results										
		Mean					L'Beta			
Label	Mean Estimate	Confidence Limits		L'Beta Estimate	Standard Error	Alpha	Confidence Limits		Chi-Square	Pr > ChiSq
Sex	2.4805	1.4338	4.2912	0.9085	0.2797	0.05	0.3603	1.4566	10.55	0.0012
Exp(Sex)				2.4805	0.6937	0.05	1.4338	4.2912		
CPAP	0.8603	0.5026	1.4726	-0.1504	0.2742	0.05	-0.6879	0.3870	0.30	0.5833
Exp(CPAP)				0.8603	0.2359	0.05	0.5026	1.4726		

So we see that adjusting for CPAP use had little influence on the risk ratio.

The data set also contained the SF-36 physical quality-of-life measure. Let's look at the risk of a voice problem according to sex and physical quality of life. The SAS code and a portion of the output is as follows:

```
PROC GENMOD DATA=T5_2 DESC;
   CLASS Sex;
   MODEL VP=Sex physical/DIST=BINOMIAL LINK=LOG;
   ESTIMATE 'Sex' Sex 1 -1/EXP;
   ESTIMATE 'Physical' Physical 1 -1/EXP;
RUN;
```

Contrast Estimate Results										
		Mean					L'Beta			
Label	Mean Estimate	Confidence Limits		L'Beta Estimate	Standard Error	Alpha	Confidence Limits		Chi-Square	Pr > ChiSq
Sex	1.8170	1.0616	3.1102	0.5972	0.2742	0.05	0.0597	1.1347	4.74	0.0294
Exp(Sex)				1.8170	0.4983	0.05	1.0616	3.1102		
Physical	0.9855	0.9763	0.9948	-0.0146	0.0048	0.05	-0.0240	-0.0052	9.29	0.0023
Exp(Physical)				0.9855	0.0047	0.05	0.9763	0.9948		

In this adjusted model both sex and physical quality of life are associated with a voice problem. An interaction term involving these variables was not significant (data not shown). Women have a greater risk of a voice problem than do men, and higher levels of physical quality of life are associated with lower risk of having a voice problem.

8.12 Multiple Cox Proportional Hazard Model

The Cox model is similar to the multiple regression model, except the response variable is the hazard function at a given time.

$$\log_e h_i(t) = \log_e h_0(t) + \beta_1 x_{1i} + \cdots + \beta_k x_{ki}$$

$$h_i(t) = h_0(t) e^{\beta_1 x_{1i} + \cdots + \beta_k x_{ki}}$$

The term $h_0(t)$ is the baseline hazard function. It represents the probability of reaching an event when the independent variables are 0. It is analogous to the intercept in a multiple regression model.

Following is the estimated model with the natural log of the hazard as the dependent variable of a linear function:

$$\log_e(\text{Hazard}) = b_0 + b_1 x_1 + b_2 x_2 + \cdots + b_k x_k$$

As seen with one independent variable, the antilog of the coefficient estimate e^{b_1} is the estimated hazard ratio, adjusted for the other variables in the model. It is useful for comparing the hazard of an event between exposed versus unexposed, or treatment versus no treatment, or a prognostic indicator being present versus not present.

The regression coefficients in the model represent the proportional change that is expected in the hazard that is related to a one-unit increase in the independent variable, with all other covariates held constant. The exponent to the power of the regression coefficient represents the hazard ratio for one-unit increase in the independent variable, with all other covariates held constant. A positive estimated regression coefficient is associated with higher risk (hazard) and shorter survival times. A negative estimated regression coefficient is associated with lower risk (hazard) and longer survival times. An important proportional hazards assumption is that the hazard ratio does not vary with time.

The name "proportional hazards" comes from the fact that we assume a constant relationship between the outcome variable and the independent variables. In other words, the covariate effects on the hazard rate (i.e., hazard ratios) are constant over time. For example, if group 1 has twice the hazard rate of group 2 one day after follow-up, the Cox model assumes this hazard rate will persist thereafter. If the proportional hazards assumption is violated, biased estimates and incorrect inferences about the effects can result.

Kaplan-Meier curves can be used to evaluate the proportional hazards assumption for categorical covariates with few levels. A graph of the survival function versus survival time can be used to evaluate the proportional hazards assumption. If the predictors satisfy the proportional hazard assumption, the shapes of the curves will be similar, and the separation between the curves will remain proportional across time. Similarly, a graph of the log(−log(survival)) versus log of the survival time should yield parallel curves if the predictor is proportional. Departure from the proportional hazards model can also be assessed with a time-dependent exploratory variable, which will be illustrated in the following example.

EXAMPLE 8.13

In this hypothetical data set, 40 individuals are in the late stages of leukemia. These patients are no longer receiving aggressive treatment but are considered to be terminal. The patients are randomly assigned to either receive a weekly blood transfusion or to not receive it. The survival time in days was recorded for the individuals in both groups. Four of the individuals died of other causes, so their survival times are censored. The data set contains the variables Days (survival time), Censor (0 = censored and 1 = not censored), Group (1 if receive the blood transfusions and 0 if not), Age, and Sex (1 = male, 0 = female).

```
DATA EX_8_13;
   INPUT Days Censor Group Age Sex $ @@;
DATALINES;
   3 1 0 84 M 64 1 0 87 M 8 1 0 97 F 88 1 0 72 M 20 1 0 69 F 112 1 0 27
   M 96 1 0 57 F 92 1 0 58 F 13 1 0 91 F 59 1 0 86 F 20 1 0 66 M 112 1
   0 66 M 30 1 0 51 M 34 1 0 45 F 46 1 0 77 M 12 1 0 78 M 78 1 0 79 M
   16 0 0 86 F 44 0 0 69 M 17 1 0 83 F 56 1 1 93 F 63 1 1 78 M 98 1 1 75
   F 39 1 1 89 F 132 1 1 45 F 98 1 1 84 M 33 1 1 18 F 84 1 1 87 F 48 1 1
   87 M 76 1 1 79 F 109 1 1 87 M 104 1 1 66 M 61 1 1 80 M 80 1 1 80 F
   80 1 1 48 M 96 1 1 84 F 126 1 1 26 F 123 1 1 82 M 18 0 1 90 F 59 0 1
   88 M
;
```

In the MODEL statement, Days is crossed with the censoring variable, and the value representing censoring is in the parentheses. The value for DAYS is considered censored if the value of Censor is 0; otherwise, they will be treated as event times.

```
PROC PHREG DATA = EX_8_13;
CLASS Sex;
MODEL Days*Censor(0)=Group Sex Age;
RUN;
```

A portion of the SAS output appears as follows:

Model Fit Statistics		
Criterion	Without Covariates	With Covariates
-2 LOG L	194.711	179.392
AIC	194.711	185.392
SBC	194.711	190.143

Testing Global Null Hypothesis: BETA=0			
Test	Chi-Square	DF	Pr > ChiSq
Likelihood Ratio	15.3188	3	0.0016
Score	13.9670	3	0.0030
Wald	13.1796	3	0.0043

Analysis of Maximum Likelihood Estimates								
Parameter		DF	Parameter Estimate	Standard Error	Chi-Square	Pr > ChiSq	Hazard Ratio	Label
Group		1	-1.24534	0.39405	9.9880	0.0016	0.288	
Sex	F	1	0.53293	0.37581	2.0109	0.1562	1.704	Sex F
Age		1	0.03547	0.01256	7.9784	0.0047	1.036	

The model fit statistics display information that are useful for model comparison and selection. Because this is our first model, we do not have another model to compare it. These statistics explain how much unexplained variation there is in the model, such that the lower the value, the more accurate the model. The three tests in the Testing Global Null Hypothesis: BETA = 0 are asymptotically equivalent but can differ for small samples. The likelihood ratio is usually the test of choice. In this example, however, the tests agree that at least one of the regression coefficients in the model is significantly different than 0. The Analysis of Maximum Likelihood Estimates table shows model coefficients, tests of significance, and hazard ratios. The hazard ratio for a group of 0.288 indicates that the hazard function for those receiving the weekly blood transfusion is smaller than that for those not receiving the weekly blood transfusion, after adjusting for Sex and Age. In other words, those receiving the weekly blood transfusion are living longer. Sex is not significant but age is significant.

Notice that there is no intercept; in Cox regression, the intercept is absorbed into the baseline hazard function, which remains unspecified.

The test to evaluate the validity of the proportional hazard's assumption is simple. For two groups, the ratio of hazards is $e^{\beta_1} = e^{-1.24534} = 0.28$, which is independent of time. The proportional hazards model assumption is not valid if the hazards ratio changes with time. We can investigate departure of the proportional hazards model by considering the time-dependent covariate:

$$X = \text{Group} \times (\log_e(\text{Days}));$$

When this variable is included in the model, the hazard ratio becomes $e^{\beta_1} t^{\beta_2}$, where β_2 is the regression parameter coefficient for the time-dependent variable X. If $\beta_2 > 0$, then the hazard ratio increases with time, whereas if $\beta_2 < 0$, the hazard ratio decreases with time. In the MODEL statement, X is defined within the procedure.

```
PROC PHREG DATA = EX_8_13;
  CLASS Sex;
  X = Group*(LOG(Days));
  MODEL Days*Censor(0)=Group X Sex Age;
RUN;
```

In the output from this program, the χ^2 statistic for testing the null hypothesis that $\beta_2 = 0$ is 2.2770, which is not significant when compared with a χ^2 distribution with 1 degree of freedom (p-value = 0.1313). Therefore, there is no evidence of an increasing or decreasing trend over time in the hazard ratio. The same approach can be taken to assess the proportional hazards assumption for the other two variables in the model, neither of which were significant (data not shown).

Analysis of Maximum Likelihood Estimates								
Parameter		DF	Parameter Estimate	Standard Error	Chi-Square	Pr > ChiSq	Hazard Ratio	Label
Group		1	-5.24466	2.74870	3.6407	0.0564	0.005	
X		1	1.00849	0.66832	2.2770	0.1313	2.741	
Sex	F	1	0.48869	0.37320	1.7146	0.1904	1.630	Sex F
Age		1	0.03303	0.01224	7.2834	0.0070	1.034	

To use the Kaplan-Meier survival function to evaluate proportional hazards for categorical covariates, plots can be obtained using the LIFETEST procedure in SAS. For example, consider the following code:

```
PROC LIFETEST DATA=EX_8_13 PLOTS = (S, LLS);
   STRATA Group;
   TIME Days*Censor(0);
   RUN;
```

The SAS generated plots are shown here, which indicate that the proportional hazards assumption holds.

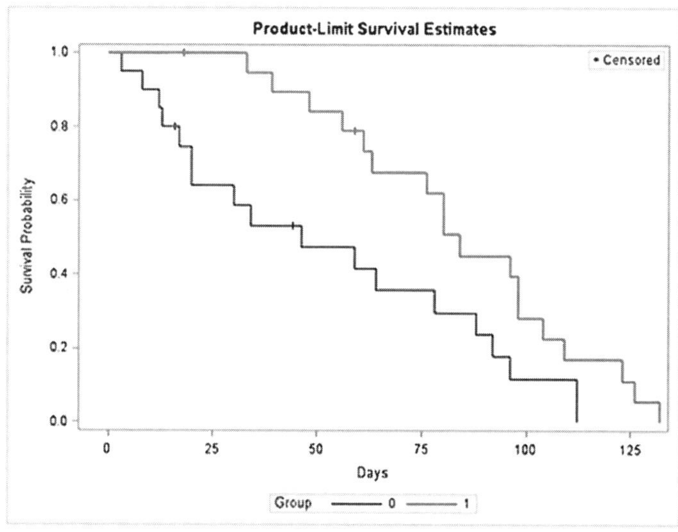

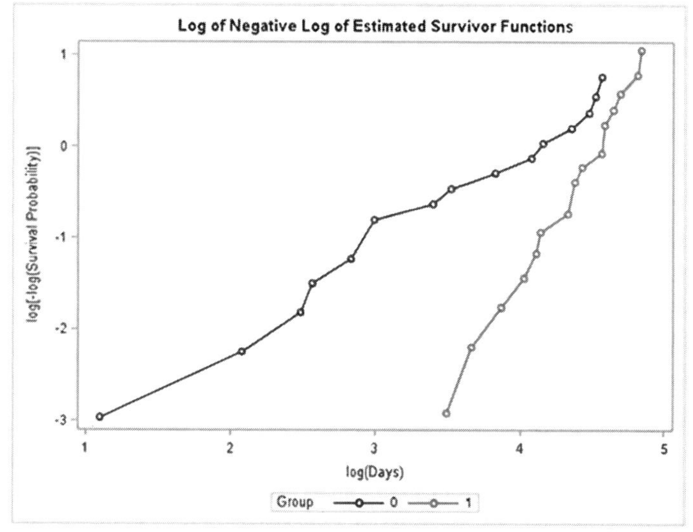

News File

It is well established that cigarette smoking is a risk factor for cardiovascular disease (CVD). Smoking cessation also lowers the risk of CVD. However, the time course of CVD following smoking cessation has been unclear until a recent study.[16] In a sample of 8770 retrospectively assessed individuals from the Framingham Heart Study, researchers used Poisson regression to estimate incidence rates per 1000 person years and Cox proportional hazards regression to estimate cause-specific hazard ratios. Quitting within 5 years compared with current heavy smoking (≥ 20 pack-years) was associated with significantly lower rates of CVD (−4.51, 95% CI = −5.90–2.77; 11.56, 95% CI = 10.30–12.95 for current heavy smokers and 6.94, 95% CI = 5.61–8.59 for those who quit within 5 years). The hazard ratio for those who quit smoking within 5-years versus current heavy smokers was 0.61, 95% CI = 0.49–0.76. However, compared with never smokers, the risk CVD for former smokers remained significantly higher beyond 5 years following smoking cessation.

8.13 Polynomial Regression

When a linear regression line does not adequately fit the data, a polynomial regression line may be an appropriate choice. In Excel, a graph can be constructed with the data fit using a polynomial line graph. For example, consider the data 5, 3, 5, 9, 20, and 35. Type this data into a column in an Excel spreadsheet. Highlight the data, and choose the Insert tab and the line graph option with markers. In the graph, click the line a couple times until on the right of the page, the Format Data Series appears. Choose "No line." Select the "+" to the upper right of the graph, check the Trendline box, and then choose More Options. Choose the Polynomial option, Order 2, and select the bottom two boxes to display the equation on the chart and the R^2 value.

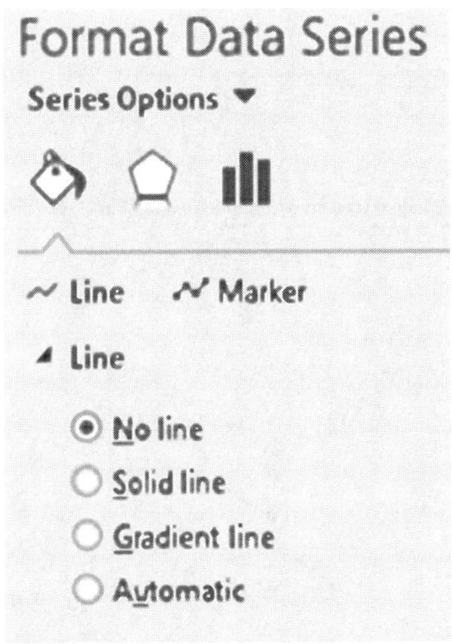

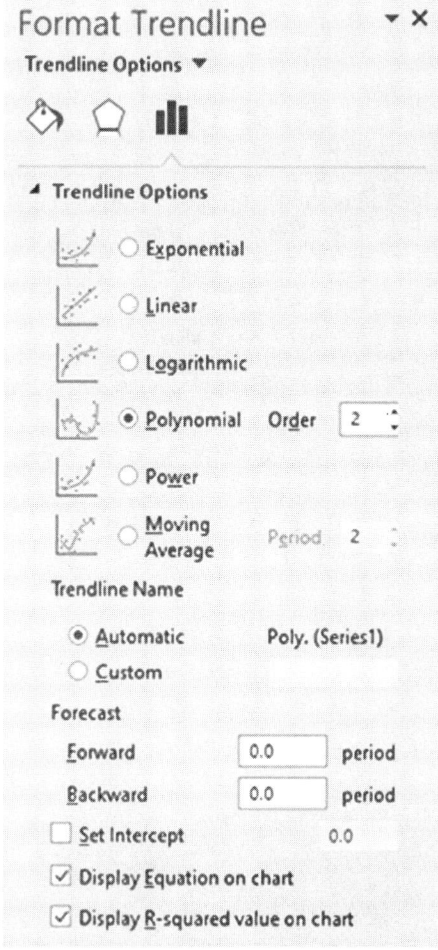

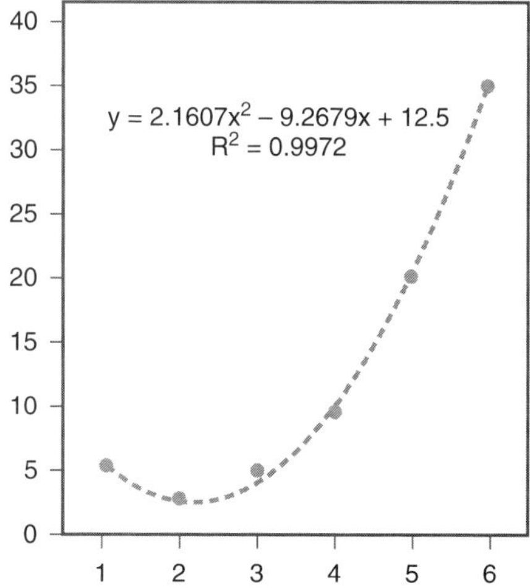

Using data from CDC Wonder, a system for disseminating public health data, and the U.S. Geological Survey,[15,17] county-level average daily precipitation was associated with altitude (**Figure 8.7**). In this graph, a second-order polynomial fit the data well. Further, using data from the CDC COVID data tracker,[18] a line graph was constructed of the number of cases reported to the CDC by states and territories over time (**Figure 8.8**). A third-order polynomial model fit this data well.

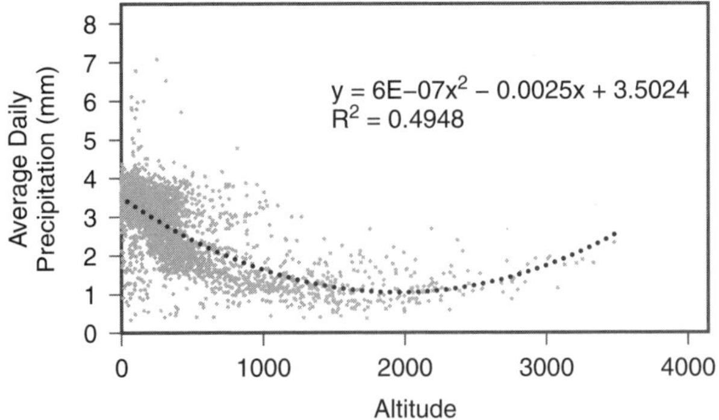

Figure 8.7 County-Level Data in the Contiguous United States Showing Precipitation by Altitude

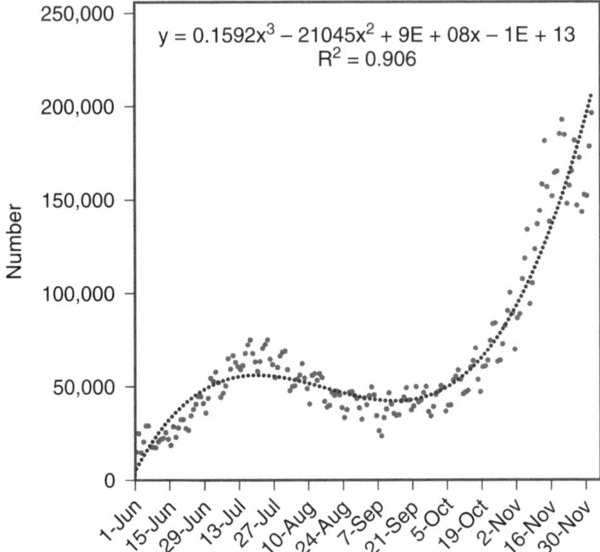

Figure 8.8 Trend in Number of COVID-19 Cases in the United States, June 1–December 2, 2020

8.14 Summary

The focus of this chapter was on measuring the association between a dependent variable and one or more independent variables. The value of the dependent variable is predicted as a function of one or more independent variables. A regression function describes this relationship. Each type of regression model considered in this chapter has a linear function in which the expected value of Y given X is linear in the unknown parameters that are estimated from the data.

The most common form of regression analysis is linear regression. The word "linear" refers to the parameters, not the independent variables. Simple linear regression has one dependent variable and one independent variable. Assumptions for applying simple linear regression are (1) the values of X are known (not random); (2) for each value of X, the distribution of Y is normally distributed; (3) the standard deviation of the Y does not change over X; (4) the Y variables are independent; and (5) a linear relationship exists between X and Y. Multiple linear regression involves one dependent variable and two or more independent variables. Assumptions for multiple linear regression and other linear models were presented in this chapter. For regression models in general, the decision as to which variable is treated as dependent and which variable is treated as independent is determined by the researcher, based on observation and experience.

The method of least squares was presented as an approach to obtain the intercept and slope of the regression line. The standard error of the estimated intercept or slope is used to test hypotheses and also to construct confidence intervals for the population intercept or slope. Confidence bands for the regression line and the individual observations are curved. They are narrowest at the mean of X and curve away from the line as we move in either direction from the mean of X. If the mean value of X is used in the regression equation, the predicted value of Y is the mean of Y.

If the association between a dependent variable and an independent variable varies according to the level of a third variable, an interaction term involving this independent and third variable should be included in the model.

Logistic regression involves describing the relationship between a categorical dependent variable and one or more independent variables, with different possible scales. Poisson regression is useful when the dependent variable Y has a Poisson distribution, representing a count or rate, and the logarithm of its expected values is modeled as a linear combination of a set of parameters.

Log-binomial regression is used when the outcome variable is binary and gives an unbiased estimate of the risk ratio.

The Cox proportional hazard model allows us to evaluate the effect of one or more risk factors on the hazard rate. The hazard rate is the risk of failure (i.e., probability of experiencing an event) given the subject has survived to a point in time.

Multiple regression models are important because variables may simultaneously affect a dependent variable or confound or modify the relationship between dependent and independent variables. The residual is the difference between the observed and predicted values. Residual plots are an effective way to evaluate the assumptions of multiple linear regression. The coefficient of determination r^2, multiple R^2, and adjusted R^2 are also useful statistics for evaluating models.

Important formulas have been shown in this chapter. These are summarized in **Table 8.3**.

Table 8.3 Summary of Selected Formulas Involving Association

Statistic	Equation
Simple linear regression model	$$Y_i = \beta_0 + \beta_1 X_i + \epsilon_i$$ Y_i = value of the dependent variable for observation i X_i = value of the independent variable for observation i ϵ_i = value of random fluctuation or error for observation i β_0 = a parameter that represents the population regression line intercept; mean of Y when $X = 0$ β_1 = a parameter that represents the slope of the population regression line; mean value of Y for a unit increase in X
Mean of the expected value of Y	$$E(Y_i) = E(\beta_0 + \beta_1 X_i + \epsilon_i) = \beta_0 + \beta_1 X_i + E(\epsilon_i) = \beta_0 + \beta_1 X_i$$ Assume $\epsilon_i \sim N(0, \sigma^2)$, independent, and the relationship between X and Y is linear in the parameter β_1. If X is fixed, then $Y_i \sim N(\mu_i, \sigma^2)$.
Residual	$$e_i = y_i - \hat{y}_i$$ If y_i is the observed outcome of Y_i for a particular value x_i, $\hat{y}_i$ is the corresponding predicted value.

(Continues)

Table 8.3 Summary of Selected Formulas Involving Association (*Continued*)

Statistic	Equation
Estimated simple linear regression model	$\hat{y}_i = b_0 + b_1 x_i$
Estimated slope coefficient	$b_1 = \dfrac{\sum(x_i - \bar{x})(y_i - \bar{y})}{\sum(x_i - \bar{x})^2}$
Estimated intercept coefficient	$b_0 = \bar{y} - b_1\bar{x}$
Relationship between the estimated slope and the correlation coefficient	$b_1 = r\dfrac{\sqrt{\sum(y_i - \bar{y})^2}}{\sqrt{\sum(x_i - \bar{x})^2}}; \quad r = b_1\dfrac{\sqrt{\sum(x_i - \bar{x})^2}}{\sqrt{\sum(y_i - \bar{y})^2}}$
t test statistic for evaluating slope	$t = \dfrac{b_1 - \beta_1}{SE_{b_1}}$ $SE_{b_1} = \sqrt{\dfrac{s^2_{y\mid x}}{\sum(x_i - \bar{x})^2}} = \sqrt{\dfrac{\frac{1}{n-2}\sum(y_i - \hat{y})^2}{\sum(x_i - \bar{x})^2}} = \sqrt{\dfrac{\frac{1}{n-2}\left[\sum(y_i - \bar{y})^2 - b_1\sum(x_i - \bar{x})(y_i - \bar{y})\right]}{\sum(x_i - \bar{x})^2}}$ Degrees of freedom: $n-2$
Confidence interval for β_1	$b_1 \pm t_{1-\alpha/2,n-2} SE_{b_1}$
Logistic response function	$E(Y_i) = p_i = \dfrac{\exp(\beta_0 + \beta_1 X_i)}{1 + \exp(\beta_0 + \beta_1 X_i)}$
Logit model	$\log_e\left[\dfrac{p}{1-p}\right] = \beta_0 + \beta_1 X$
Estimated logit model	$\log_e\left[\dfrac{f}{1-f}\right] = b_0 + b_1 x$ Odds Ratio $= e^{b_1}$
Estimated Poisson regression model	$\log_e(\text{Rate}) = b_0 + b_1 x_1$ Rate Ratio $= e^{b_1}$
Estimated log-binomial model	$\log_e(\text{Risk}) = b_0 + b_1 x_1$ Risk Ratio $= e^{b_1}$
Estimated Cox proportional hazard model	$\log_e(\text{Hazard}) = b_0 + b_1 x_1$ Hazard Ratio $= e^{b_1}$
Confidence interval for mean Y given a value of X	$\hat{y} \pm t_{1-\alpha/2,n-2}\, s_{y\mid x}\sqrt{\dfrac{1}{n} + \dfrac{(x - \bar{x})^2}{\sum(x_i - \bar{x})^2}}$
Predicted interval for an individual value of Y given X	$\hat{y} \pm t_{1-\alpha/2,n-2}\, s_{y\mid x}\sqrt{1 + \dfrac{1}{n} + \dfrac{(x - \bar{x})^2}{\sum(x_i - \bar{x})^2}}$
Multiple linear regression	$Y = \beta_0 + \beta_1 X_1 + \beta_2 X_2 + \cdots + \beta_k X_k + \epsilon$

Table 8.3 Summary of Selected Formulas Involving Association (*Continued*)

Statistic	Equation
Estimated multiple linear model	$\hat{y}_i = b_0 + b_1x_{1i} + b_2x_{2i} + \cdots + b_kx_{ki}$ b_1 adjusted for the other variables in the model
Estimated multiple logistic regression model	$\log_e(\text{Odds}) = b_0 + b_1x_{1i} + b_2x_{2i} + \cdots + b_kx_{ki}$ Odds Ratio $= e^{b_1}$ adjusted for the other variables in the model
Estimated multiple Poisson regression model	$\log_e(\text{Rate}) = b_0 + b_1x_{1i} + b_2x_{2i} + \cdots + b_kx_{ki}$ Rate Ratio $= e^{b_1}$ adjusted for the other variables in the model
Estimated log-Binomial regression model	$\log_e(\text{Risk}) = b_0 + b_1x_{1i} + b_2x_{2i} + \cdots + b_kx_{ki}$ Risk Ratio $= e^{b_1}$ adjusted for the other variables in the model
Estimated multiple Cox proportional hazard model	$\log_e(\text{Hazard Ratio}) = b_0 + b_1x_{1i} + b_2x_{2i} + \cdots + b_kx_{ki}$ Hazard Ratio $= e^{b_1}$ adjusted for the other variables in the model

Exercises

1. A student was asked to state the simple linear regression model. The following was written:

$$E(Y_i) = \beta_0 + \beta_1 X_i + \epsilon_i.$$

   Do you agree?

2. Why is $Y_t = \beta_0 + \beta_1 t + \beta_2 t^2 + \epsilon_i$ considered a linear regression model?
3. Suppose the regression function relating high-density lipoprotein (HDL) and typical servings of fruit and vegetables per day is $E(Y_i) = 45 + 0.5X_i$, where X ranges from 0 to 10. A friend concludes that fruit and vegetable consumption is significantly associated with HDL on average because the slope coefficient is greater than 0. Do you agree or disagree? Explain why.
4. The accompanying pairs of values give X, advertising expense (in thousands) during a period of the importance of getting vaccinated for the coronavirus, and Y, the percent of the population getting vaccinated.

x	8	9	7	5	2	4	9	4	11	3
y	65	72	90	35	25	55	68	50	90	25

   a. Estimate the regression equation: $\hat{y}_i = b_0 + b_1 x_i$
   b. Calculate the predicted value of Y given $X = 5$.
   c. Calculate the 95% confidence interval for the mean Y given $X = 5$.
   d. Calculate the 95% prediction interval for an individual value Y given $X = 5$.
   e. Calculate the standard error of the slope of the regression line.
   f. Test the hypothesis $H_0: \beta_1 = 0$ versus $H_a: \beta_1 > 0$ by using the t statistic. Let $\alpha = 0.05$.

g. Test the hypothesis $H_0: \beta_1 = 0$ versus $H_a: \beta_1 > 0$ by using the F statistic. Let $\alpha = 0.05$.
h. Calculate and interpret the coefficient of determination r^2.

5. Muscle mass is expected to decrease with age. Suppose you are interested in studying this relationship in a group of 20 women aged 30 through 79. You choose four women to represent each 10 year age range. Assume a simple linear regression model is appropriate.
   a. Calculate and interpret the estimated regression function.
   b. What is a point estimate of the mean muscle mass for a women aged $X = 60$?
   c. Calculate and interpret the coefficient of determination?
   d. Evaluate the model assumptions by computing the residual plot. Is the assumption of simple linear regression satisfied?

i	1	2	3	4	5	6	7	8	9	10
X_i	34	36	32	38	45	43	45	49	56	56
Y_i	109	118	132	122	116	100	98	89	98	112
i	11	12	13	14	15	16	17	18	19	20
X_i	58	53	64	67	68	65	71	73	76	78
Y_i	82	73	91	81	78	85	64	74	65	77

6. A hospital administrator is interested in the relation between patient satisfaction (Y), severity of illness (X_1, index measure), anxiety (X_2, index measure), age (X_3, in years), and sex (X_4, $1 =$ Male and $0 =$ Female). Larger index measures are associated with more patient satisfaction, severity of illness, and more anxiety. The data appear as follows:

i	1	2	3	4	5	6	7	8	9	10
X_{1i}	40	45	66	75	65	70	80	75	48	60
X_{2i}	54	63	46	66	54	58	70	73	40	50
X_{3i}	50	56	72	94	65	78	83	89	46	29
X_{4i}	1	1	0	1	0	0	1	0	0	0
Y_i	67	55	54	40	64	43	44	52	64	47
i	11	12	13	14	15	16	17	18	19	20
X_{1i}	35	50	72	74	53	60	69	76	58	63
X_{2i}	39	46	67	68	45	60	63	72	55	38
X_{3i}	48	43	92	65	40	72	83	80	71	53
X_{4i}	0	1	1	1	0	0	1	1	1	0
Y_i	82	75	57	46	68	56	60	40	59	55
i	21	22	23	24	25	26	27	28	19	30
X_{1i}	56	74	80	75	60	50	53	67	70	78

X_{2i}	53	60	73	74	45	46	41	60	74	69
X_{3i}	56	73	79	67	39	55	49	89	90	78
X_{4i}	1	0	1	0	1	1	0	1	1	0
Y_i	73	66	40	50	59	78	68	54	53	60

a. Describe the distributions for each continuous scaled variable.
b. Fit a regression model to the data, drop variables not significant, one at a time, and state the final estimated regression function.
c. Construct a plot of the residuals and discuss whether the model assumptions are satisfied.

7. A dietary program was designed to increase high-density lipoprotein (HDL) and lower low-density lipoprotein (LDL). HDL was recorded at two time periods, 6 months apart. The following data represent whether 50 subjects participated or not in the dietary program and their HDL levels at baseline and follow-up.

ID	Diet	HDL1	HDL2	Change	ID	Diet	HDL1	HDL2	Change
1	Y	54	66	12	26	Y	51	60	9
2	Y	62	80	18	27	Y	57	91	34
3	N	55	64	9	28	Y	51	48	-3
4	N	56	55	-1	29	N	45	46	1
5	Y	55	72	17	30	Y	44	55	11
6	Y	57	62	5	31	Y	47	76	29
7	Y	61	85	24	32	Y	37	58	21
8	Y	83	87	4	33	Y	44	45	1
9	N	85	88	3	34	Y	49	58	9
10	Y	59	61	2	35	N	44	47	3
11	Y	58	62	4	36	Y	51	53	2
12	Y	74	87	13	37	N	42	55	13
13	N	44	48	4	38	Y	54	62	8
14	N	45	55	10	39	Y	61	63	2
15	Y	53	65	12	40	Y	54	59	5
16	N	98	85	-13	41	Y	70	82	12
17	Y	77	96	19	42	N	48	40	-8
18	Y	62	67	5	43	Y	50	44	-6
19	Y	69	60	-9	44	Y	48	47	-1
20	Y	69	86	17	45	Y	41	36	-5
21	N	45	48	3	46	Y	50	64	14
22	Y	66	66	0	47	Y	64	59	-5
23	Y	69	85	16	48	N	45	36	-9

ID	Diet	HDL1	HDL2	Change	ID	Diet	HDL1	HDL2	Change
24	Y	50	65	15	49	Y	68	69	1
25	Y	68	76	8	50	Y	53	62	9

a. Estimate the regression equation with HDL2 as the dependent variable and HDL1 as the independent variable.
b. Plot the residual plot. What do you conclude about the assumptions for simple linear regression?
c. Plot the graph of HDL2 against HDL1, along with the estimated regression line and the confidence interval for the mean HDL2 given HDL1 and the prediction interval for an individual value HDL2 given HDL1.
d. Create a dummy variable for Diet (1 for "Yes" and 0 for "No"). Note that PROC REG does not take CLASS variables but PROC GLM does.
e. Estimate the regression equation with HDL2 as the dependent variable and HDL1 and diet as independent variables.
f. Is diet significantly associated with HDL2 after adjusting for HDL1?
g. What is the adjusted R^2 and discuss its meaning?
h. Is there a significant interaction term between HDL1 and diet?
i. If the interaction term is not significant, is it good practice to leave it in the model anyway?
j. If the interaction term is significant, but one of the main effects that makes up the interaction term is not significant, should the main effect be dropped from the model?
k. Estimate a new regression equation with the change in HDL regressed on diet.
l. Calculate the 95% confidence interval for the variable diet.
m. What do you conclude from the model with change in HDL as the dependent variable and diet as the independent variable?

8. Refer to the data in Exercise 8.4. Compute a logistic regression model with the dependent variable (performing the task) regressed on the independent variables (dichotomized emotional score and sex). Include an interaction term in the model. Is it appropriate to retain the interaction term?

9. The local health department sent fliers to its community to encourage people to get a flu shot. In a pilot follow-up study, 30 individuals were randomly selected and asked if they received a flu shot ($Y = 1$ yes versus $Y = 0$ no). The data were combined with reported health awareness (X_1, an index where higher indicates greater awareness), age (X_2, in years), and sex (X_3, 1 = Male and 0 = Female).

i	1	2	3	4	5	6	7	8	9	10
X_{1i}	55	75	35	66	75	50	55	40	43	75
X_{2i}	67	82	36	44	65	33	49	23	27	60
X_{3i}	0	0	1	0	0	1	0	1	1	0
Y_i	1	1	0	1	1	0	1	0	0	1
i	11	12	13	14	15	16	17	18	19	20
X_{1i}	46	65	43	46	70	46	73	65	65	43
X_{2i}	42	30	36	28	47	22	50	46	55	40

X_{3i}	0	1	1	1	0	1	0	1	1	0
Y_i	0	1	0	0	1	0	1	0	1	0
i	21	22	23	24	25	26	27	28	29	30
X_{1i}	63	47	50	58	55	35	51	65	38	69
X_{2i}	27	26	39	44	43	27	52	49	30	74
X_{3i}	0	0	1	0	1	1	0	0	1	0
Y_i	1	0	0	1	0	0	1	1	0	1

a. Assess the association among the independent variables.
b. Construct a logistic regression model for each of these variables separately.
c. Should a logistic regression model be constructed with each of the independent variables included simultaneously in the model?
d. Comment on the assumptions of the logistic regression model.

10. Suppose a researcher was interested in identifying the ratio of observed to expected counts of disease X, in relation to the distance (kilometers) lived from a chemical plant. A Poisson regression model produced an estimated intercept of 0.7666 and distance coefficient of –0.0729. Calculate the ratio of observed to expected counts for each kilometer increase in distance from the plant. Interpret your result for living 10 kilometers from the plant.

11. Female breast cancer death among diagnosed cases was assessed using a Cox model. The variables and estimated coefficients are shown as follows:

Variable	Cox Regression Coefficient	Standard Error
Local stage	Reference	
Regional stage	1.258	0.064
Distant stage	3.088	0.089
Unknown stage	1.639	0.135
Grade I	Reference	
Grade II	0.811	0.184
Grade III	1.471	0.181
Unknown grade	1.158	0.180
Age (1 year)	0.007	0.002

Calculate hazard ratios and 95% confidence intervals for each estimate.

12. One of the first cohort studies to identify a link between smoking and increased risk of death was conducted by Doll and Hill (1966) where they followed a group of British doctors.[19] They classified these doctors according to age and smoking status and then followed them over time. Data from this study are shown in the following table.

Age	Smoker	Count	Population
35–44	Yes	32	52,407
45–54	Yes	104	43,248

(Continues)

Age	Smoker	Count	Population
55–64	Yes	206	28,612
65–74	Yes	186	12,663
75–84	Yes	102	5317
35–44	No	2	18,790
45–54	No	12	10,673
55–64	No	28	5710
65–74	No	28	2585
75–84	No	31	1462

a. Estimate a Poisson regression model for these data.
b. Evaluate the significance of the rate ratio for death among smokers compared with nonsmokers, adjusted for age.
c. Describe how the rate of death changes with older age, after adjusting for smoking.

13. Refer to Example 8.4. Calculate an odds ratio and 95% confidence interval that adjusts for sex.
14. For the following data, evaluate whether the risk of illness (1 = Yes, 2 = No) is associated with vaccination, adjusting for sex.

Subject	Vaccinated	Ill	Sex	Subject	Vaccinated	Ill	Sex
1	1	2	B	14	1	1	B
2	1	2	B	15	2	1	G
3	2	2	G	16	1	2	B
4	2	1	G	17	1	2	B
5	2	1	G	18	1	2	B
6	1	2	B	19	1	2	B
7	2	1	B	20	2	2	G
8	2	1	G	21	1	2	B
9	1	2	G	22	1	2	B
10	2	2	B	23	2	1	G
11	1	2	B	24	1	1	B
12	1	2	B	25	1	2	G
13	1	2	G	26	1	2	G

15. The following data involves age-specific death rates (per 100,000) from COVID-19 in the United States (weeks ending 2/1/2020 to 12/19/2020).[20] Construct a line chart of the death rates by age. Fit the data using a polynomial model.

<1	1–4	5–14	15–24	25–34	35–44	45–54	55–64	65–74	75–84	85+
0.82	0.11	0.12	1.10	4.44	12.72	34.55	82.37	197.82	499.22	1404.35

References

1. Sato K, Amemiya AA, Haseda M, et al. Postdisaster changes in social capital and mental health: A natural experiment from the 2016 Kumamoto earthquake. *Am J Epidemiol.* 2020;*189*(9):910–921.
2. Ice E, Ang S, Greenberg K, Burgard S. Women's work-family histories and cognitive performance in later life. *Am J Epidemiol.* 2020;*189*(9):922–930.
3. Ekheden I, Yang X, Chen H, et al. Associations between gastric atrophy and its interaction with poor oral health and the risk for esophageal squamous cell carcinoma in a high-risk region of China: A population-based case-control study. *Am J Epidemiol.* 2020;*189*(9):931–941.
4. Mok Y, Ballew SH, Sang Y, et al. Albuminuria, Kidney function, and cancer risk in the community. *Am J Epidemiol.* 2020;*189*(9):942–950.
5. Unkart JT, Allison MA, Araneta MRG, Ix JH, Matsushita K, Criqui MH. Burden of peripheral artery disease on mortality and incident cardiovascular events: The multi-ethnic study of atherosclerosis. *Am J Epidemiol.* 2020;*189*(9):951–962.
6. Prentice RL, Aragaki AK, Chlebowski RT, et al. Dual-outcome intention-to-treat analyses in the women's health initiative randomized controlled hormone therapy trials. *Am J Epidemiol.* 2020;*189*(9):972–981.
7. Life expectancy by state 2020. https://worldpopulationreview.com/state-rankings/life-expectancy-by-state. August 18, 2020.
8. Worldometer. COVID-19 coronavirus pandemic. https://www.worldometers.info/coronavirus/?utm_campaign=instagramcoach1?. August 18, 2020.
9. Zaiontz C. Real statistics using excel. Confidence and prediction intervals for forecasted values. https://www.real-statistics.com/regression/confidence-and-prediction-intervals/. Accessed August 18, 2020.
10. Frome EL, Checkoway H. Use of Poisson regression models in estimating incidence rates and ratios. *Am J Epidemiol.* 1985;*212*:309–323.
11. Worldometer. Coronavirus cases. https://www.worldometers.info/coronavirus/?utm_campaign=instagramcoach1? August 26, 2020.
12. McNutt LA, Wu C, Xue X, Hafner JP. Estimating the relative risk in cohort studies and clinical trials of common outcomes. *Am J Epidemiol.* 2003:*157*(10):940–943.
13. Cox DR. Regression models and life tables. *J Roy Statist Soc B.* 1972;*34*:187–220.
14. Wilk MB, Gnanadesikan R. Probability plotting methods for the analysis of data. *Biometrika.* 1968;*55*(1):1–17.
15. Centers for Disease Control and Prevention. CDC Wonder. https://wonder.cdc.gov/ Accessed April 3, 2021.
16. Duncan MS, Freiberg MS, Greevy RA Jr, Kundu S, Vasan RS, Tindle HA. Association of smoking cessation with subsequent risk of cardiovascular disease. *JAMA.* 2019;*322*(7):642–650.
17. U.S. Geology Survey. https://www.usgs.gov/faqs/how-do-i-find-average-elevation-a-county?qt-news_science_products=0#qt-news_science_products. Accessed April 3, 2021.
18. Centers for Disease Control and Prevention. CDC COVID Data Tracker. https://covid.cdc.gov/covid-data-tracker/#trends_dailytrendscases. Accessed December 2, 2020.
19. Doll R, Hill AB. Lung cancer and other causes of death in relation to smoking: A second report on mortality or British doctors. *BMJ.* 1956;2:1071.
20. Centers for Disease Control and Prevention. COVID-19 Death Data and Resources. https://www.cdc.gov/nchs/nvss/vsrr/covid_weekly/index.htm. Accessed December 20, 2020.

CHAPTER 9

Nonparametric Methods

KEY CONCEPTS

- Parametric statistics assume that sample data are derived from a population that can be modeled by a probability distribution with a specific set of parameters.
- A parametric family consists of a set of probability distributions uniquely identified by a parameter or collection of parameters.
- Nonparametric statistical methods are appropriate when parametric assumptions do not hold, when the underlying distribution is not known, and the sample size is small.
- Nonparametric statistical tests are used for nominal or ordinal scaled data, for non-normally distributed data, or for data with heterogeneous variance.
- The Kolmogorov-Smirnov test is one of several methods for assessing whether or not data are normally distributed. Tests like this calculate the probability that the sample was taken from a normal population.
- The sign test is a nonparametric procedure to evaluate the null hypothesis about the median in a single population or to test for the median of paired differences, which uses data from two dependent samples.
- The Wilcoxon signed-rank test evaluates whether matched pair samples are drawn from populations that have different mean ranks.
- The Mood's test evaluates whether two samples are drawn from distributions with the same medians.
- The Mann-Whitney U test (or Wilcoxon rank-sum test) evaluates whether two independent samples are drawn from the same distribution.
- The Kruskal-Wallis test is an extension of the Mann-Whitney U test to allow for comparisons of more than two independent groups.
- The Friedman test is used to assess the differences among three or more repeated (matched) samples.
- The Kendall's tau-b correlation coefficient measures the direction and strength of association between two variables measured on an ordinal or higher scale. It is preferred to the Pearson correlation coefficient when the data fail to meet that measure's assumptions. It is also better than the Spearman correlation coefficient when the sample size is small and there are several tied ranks.

Statistical inference often makes assumptions about the nature of the population from which data are drawn. **Parametric statistics** involve the area of statistics that assumes that sample data derives from a population that can be modeled by a probability distribution, with a specific set of parameters. In general, a parametric family consists of a set of probability distributions uniquely identified by a parameter or collection of parameters. A parameter for a distribution is a number that describes characteristics of the probability distribution. For example, the distribution parameters for a binomial are the probability of success and number of trials; for the Poisson, it is the expected value; for the chi square, it is the degrees of freedom; for the normal, they are the mean and standard deviation; and for the *t*, they are the mean, standard deviation, and degrees of freedom.

Well-known statistical methods like **Pearson correlation coefficient**, analysis of **variance**, and the *t* test provide valid information only when the population upon which the data analysis is based meets certain assumptions. A common assumption is that the population data are normally distributed. If the data are from a **normal distribution**, sample data can be used to estimate the distribution parameters (mean and standard deviation) and evaluate hypotheses about their possible values.

When the assumptions for parametric statistics do not hold, **nonparametric statistics** may be an appropriate alternative. This chapter presents some nonparametric (distribution-free) inferential statistical methods for testing hypotheses where assumptions are not made about the probability distribution of the variables under consideration.

9.1 What Is Nonparametric Statistics?

Nonparametric statistics do not require that the population data meet the assumptions for parametric statistics, such as normality, linearity, homogeneity of variance, and so on. For this reason, nonparametric statistics are sometimes referred to as distribution free. Nonparametric statistical methods are often used when parametric assumptions are invalid, when the underlying distribution is not known, and when examining small sample sizes.

Some nonparametric methods are ranking tests or order tests, and involve nominal and ordinal data. As already discussed, the levels of nominal variables have no numerical values (e.g., **exposure** status [yes, no] or disease status [yes, no]). The levels of ordinal data also have no numerical values, but instead comprise ranking or order. For example, when studying population data that have a preference rating and no clear numerical interpretation is evident, application of nonparametric statistics is appropriate. Thus, parametric tests are sometimes used to focus on the order or ranking of scores, not their numerical values. While a parametric test may focus on assessing difference in means, nonparametric tests may focus on difference in medians. While nonparametric procedures are more powerful when the parametric assumptions do not hold, especially for small sample size, they generally have less power than parametric tests if the parametric assumptions hold. Nevertheless, for many of the nonparametric methods commonly used, the decrease in power is small.[1]

9.2 Reasons to Use Nonparametric Statistical Tests

Many of the same types of research questions already presented for employing statistics apply here. However, evaluating inferences about these questions will require nonparametric tests if the parametric test assumptions are violated. In addition, nonparametric tests are used when nominal or ordinal data are analyzed and when small sample sizes are involved.

Each parametric test has an alternative nonparametric test. Parametric tests have more power than nonparametric tests and should be used unless their assumptions are violated. For example, if a distribution of data is skewed, then the median is a better representation of central tendency. Hence, a nonparametric test that evaluates the **null hypothesis** about the median is preferred.

In general, parametric tests deal with continuous data and are highly sensitive to outliers. On the other hand, nonparametric tests involve ordinal data, ranked data, and are not sensitive to outliers. Further, if the normality assumption is not satisfied and the sample size is small, use of a nonparametric test may be the only option.

9.3 Choosing an Appropriate Statistical Test

A nonparametric statistical test involves a model that may require that certain assumptions be satisfied, such as the observations be independent and the variable be continuous. However, these assumptions do not say anything about the specific form of the distribution from which the sample was taken, and the assumptions are fewer and weaker than found with parametric statistical tests. In contrast to such tests, nonparametric statistical tests often involve different hypotheses about the population and are applied to data measured on a nominal or ordinal scale.

Of the many statistical tests available, the question is which test is valid (uses the data in the sample appropriately)? This depends on whether the data are nominal, ordinal, interval, or ratio, as well as knowledge about the population. Nonparametric statistical tests are used for nominal or ordinal (instead of interval or ratio) scaled data. They are also used for non-normally distributed data or for data with heterogeneous variance, despite being interval or **ratio data**.

Whether the assumptions underlying a given statistical test are satisfied requires a thorough assessment of the data and consideration of the realistic basis of the research question. If the assumptions for a parametric statistical test are met, the parametric test is as effective as a nonparametric test, but with a sample that is 10% smaller. In addition, the tables required with nonparametric tests may be less widely available than those used with parametric tests.[2]

To conclude this section, consider some situations where choosing a nonparametric statistical test is appropriate. These are summarized in **Table 9.1**.

Table 9.1 **When to Consider Using a Nonparametric Test[2]**

The sample size is small, and the nature of the population distribution is not known exactly.
The hypothesis tested by a nonparametric test may be better suited for the research question.
The assumptions for parametric tests are not realistically met.
The data are measured on a nominal scale, and no parametric method applies.
The data are inherently in ranks such that it is unrealistic to make assumptions about the underlying distribution.
The non-parametric test is sometimes easier to apply and more directly interpreted than a parametric test.

Table 9.2 Common Nonparametric Statistical Tests

Measurement Scale	One Sample	Two Related Samples	Two Independent Samples	Three or More Related Samples	Three or More Independent Samples	Measures of Association
Nominal	Binomial test **(4.3.1)** Chi-square goodness-of-fit test **(5.7.1)**	McNemar test **(5.5.4)**	Chi-square test for $r \times 2$ tables **(5.7.2, 6.7.1)** Fisher's exact test **(5.7.3)**	Cochran-Armitage trend test **(6.7.2)**	Chi-square test for $r \times k$ tables **(5.7.2, 6.7.1)**	Cohen's kappa coefficient of agreement, k **(5.5.4)**
Ordinal or ordered	Kolmogorov-Smirnov test **(9.5)** Sign test **(9.6)**	Sign test **(9.6)** Wilcoxon signed-rank test **(9.7)**	Mood's median test **(9.8)** Mann-Whitney U test (also called the Wilcoxon rank-sum test) **(9.9)**	Friedman test **(9.9)**	Extension of the median test Kruskal-Wallis test **(9.10)**	Spearman correlation coefficient, r_s **(7.4)** Kendall tau-b correlation coefficient **(9.11)**
Interval or ratio	Test for distribution symmetry	Permutation test for paired replicates	Permutation test for two independent samples			

9.4 Nonparametric Statistical Tests

Several nonparametric statistical tests are available for assessing data. Some of these have already been presented. Others will be covered in this chapter. A summary of some of the more common nonparametric tests are shown in **Table 9.2**.

9.5 Kolmogorov-Smirnov Test

The Kolmogorov-Smirnov test examines if data values follow some distribution in a given population. The "given" distribution of interest is typically normal, but other distributions may also be considered. Various statistical software packages are useful for generating graphs and tests for assessing normality. In SAS, PROC Univariate (with the options Plot and Normal) provides graphs and tests (Shapiro-Wilk, Kolmogorov-Smirnov, Cramér-von Mises, Anderson-Darling) for assessing the assumption of normality. For example, suppose we are interested in assessing the data appearing in the following SAS program, but first want to check whether it is normally distributed:

```
DATA Example;
INPUT X @@;
DATALINES;
75 72 85 65 67 55 20 28 67 81 79 85 44 81 30 67 66 50
;
```

```
PROC UNIVARIATE DATA=Example PLOT NORMAL;
VAR X;
RUN;
```

A portion of the SAS output shows four different tests of normality, including the Kolmogorov-Smirnov test.

Tests for Normality				
Test	Statistic		p Value	
Shapiro-Wilk	W	0.891891	Pr < W	0.0416
Kolmogorov-Smirnov	D	0.22477	Pr > D	0.0172
Cramer-von Mises	W-Sq	0.122869	Pr > W-Sq	0.0497
Anderson-Darling	A-Sq	0.730133	Pr > A-Sq	0.0472

Since p-value $= 0.0172 < 0.05 = \alpha$, we reject the null hypothesis that the data come from a normal distribution. Hence, we will want to consider a nonparametric option for assessing the data. The PLOT option generates a horizontal histogram, a box plot, and a normal probability plot.

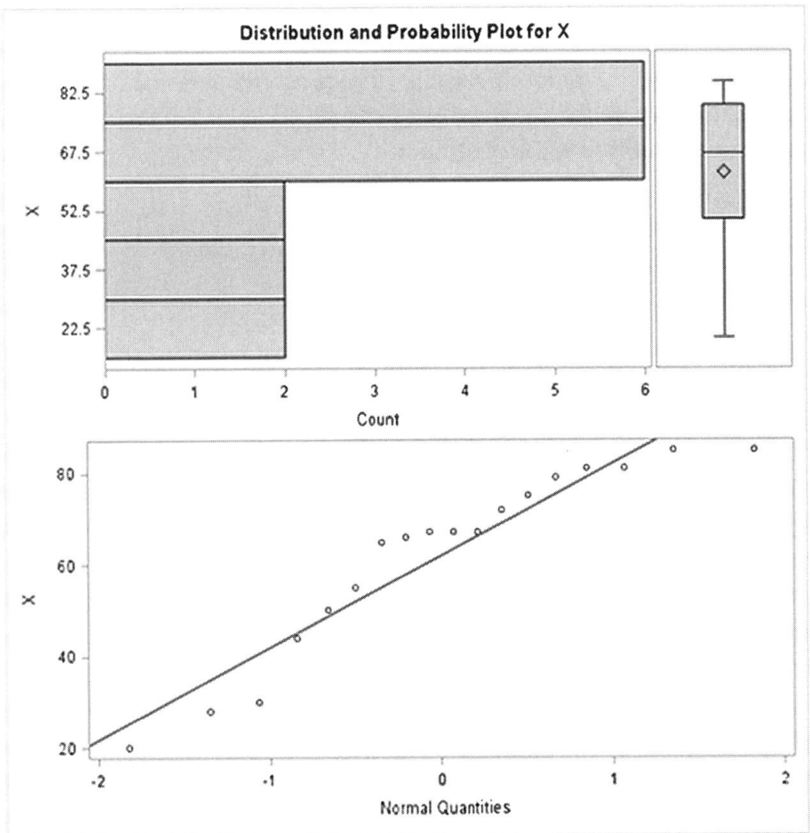

The normal probability plot indicates whether or not the data are normally distributed. If the data are normally distributed, the dots will fall along the diagonal line. There are different types of departure from the standard normal distribution (**Figure 9.1**).

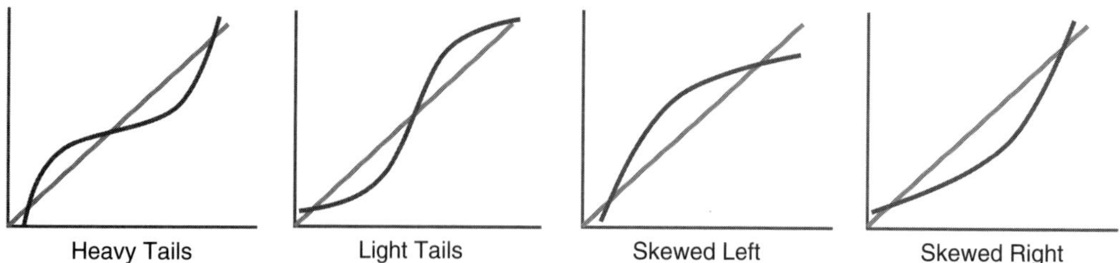

Figure 9.1 Departures from Normality Indicated by the Normal Probability Plot

9.6 Sign Test

The sign test is a simple nonparametric procedure to evaluate the null hypothesis that the median of a distribution is equal to a standard value. The one-sample sign test may be thought of as the nonparametric equivalent of the one-sample *t* test. The test is not based on numerical information but on plus and minus signs, wherein its name is derived. The test may be used to (1) evaluate the median in a single population (one-sample sign test) or to (2) conduct a test for the median of paired differences, which uses data from two dependent samples. Like the *t* test, it may be a left-, right-, or **two-tailed test**.

The assumptions of the one-sample sign test are summarized as follows:

1. The data have at least an ordinal scale.
2. The data reflect a random sample of independent measurements from a population where the median is not known.
3. The variable of interest is continuous.

The sign test is performed using the following steps:

1. Assess whether the data are normally distributed, based on visual inspection and consideration of the sample size. If they are, use the *t* test.
2. The test involves comparing the total number of observations that are greater than (+) or less than (–) the hypothesized median value or 0 if paired data are involved. If the value is the same, assign it a 0.
3. Count the number of positives and the number of negatives.
4. Sum the number of items in the sample and subtract any equal to 0.
5. The test simply involves performing a binomial test or the normal approximation to the binomial if the sample size is sufficiently large on the signs. The probability under the null hypothesis is 0.5 (an equal number of positives and negatives). The number of "successes" is the smaller of either the number of positive or negative signs from Step 2.
6. When the sign test is applied to paired data and the null hypothesis is that the median difference is 0 (i.e., a two-tailed test is involved), then the *p*-value obtained from the binomial test is computed as $2 \times P(X \leq \text{Smaller number of the + or – sign})$. For a **one-tailed test** do not multiply by 2.

Example 9.1

The National Health and Nutrition Examination Survey says that among alcohol drinkers, the median calories consumed from alcohol beverages is 105 per day. We think it may be different in our community. To test this, a random sample of 15 alcohol drinkers is taken, with the results shown in **Figure 9.2**.

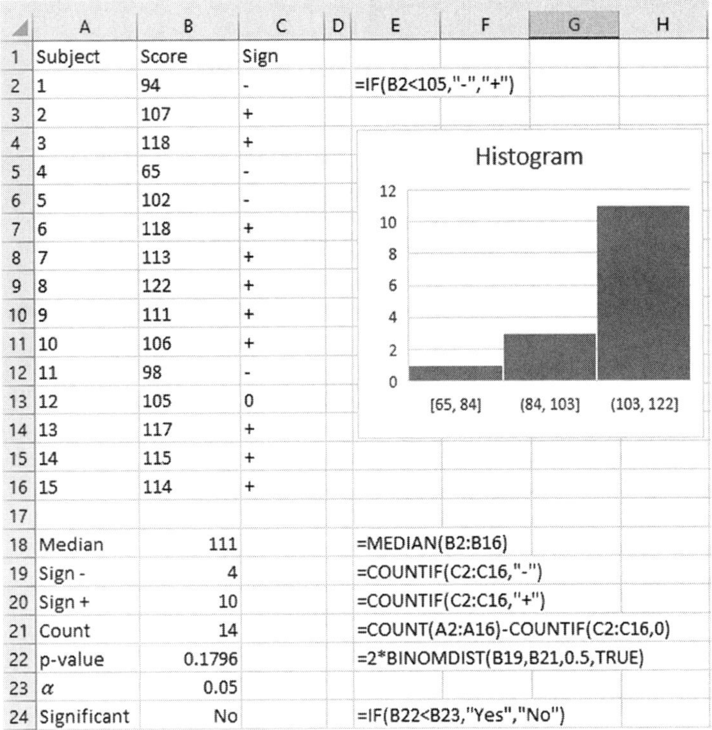

	A	B	C	D	E
1	Subject	Score	Sign		
2	1	94	-		=IF(B2<105,"-","+")
3	2	107	+		
4	3	118	+		
5	4	65	-		
6	5	102	-		
7	6	118	+		
8	7	113	+		
9	8	122	+		
10	9	111	+		
11	10	106	+		
12	11	98	-		
13	12	105	0		
14	13	117	+		
15	14	115	+		
16	15	114	+		
17					
18	Median	111			=MEDIAN(B2:B16)
19	Sign -	4			=COUNTIF(C2:C16,"-")
20	Sign +	10			=COUNTIF(C2:C16,"+")
21	Count	14			=COUNT(A2:A16)-COUNTIF(C2:C16,0)
22	p-value	0.1796			=2*BINOMDIST(B19,B21,0.5,TRUE)
23	α	0.05			
24	Significant	No			=IF(B22<B23,"Yes","No")

Figure 9.2 Sign Test for Example 9.1

Now we will go through the steps of hypothesis testing.

1. H_0: Median = 105
2. H_a: Median ≠ 105
3. Let $\alpha = 0.05$, $n = 15$
4. Binomial test
5. If the null hypothesis is true, then the probability that the median calories is < 105 is 0.5. Hence, we will test the probability that 4 out of 14 observations are less than the median given that the probability of any trial is 0.5; *p*-value = 2 × BINOMDIST(4, 14, 0.5, TRUE) = 0.1796.
6. Since the *p*-value > 0.05 = α, we fail to reject the null hypothesis and cannot conclude with 95% confidence that the median calories consumed from alcohol beverages is different than 105.

Example 9.2

In a group of 15 overweight or obese adult males, their body mass index (BMI) was recorded before and after a weight loss intervention. We are interested in testing whether BMI decreased significantly between baseline and follow-up. **Figure 9.3** shows the BMI scores before and after the intervention, along with the difference scores, the corresponding signs, and other statistical results.

The steps of hypothesis testing for this example follow:

1. H_0: Median difference is 0.
2. H_a: Median difference is not 0.
3. Let $\alpha = 0.05$, $n = 15$
4. Binomial test
5. The two-sided *p*-value is $2 \times P(X \leq 3)$, which is equivalent to $P(X \leq 3) + P(X \geq 12)$. *p*-value = 2 × BINOMDIST(3, 15, 0.5, TRUE) = 0.035.
6. We reject the null hypothesis (since *p*-value = 0.035 < 0.05 = α) and conclude with 95% confidence that there is a difference in BMI after the intervention compared with before.

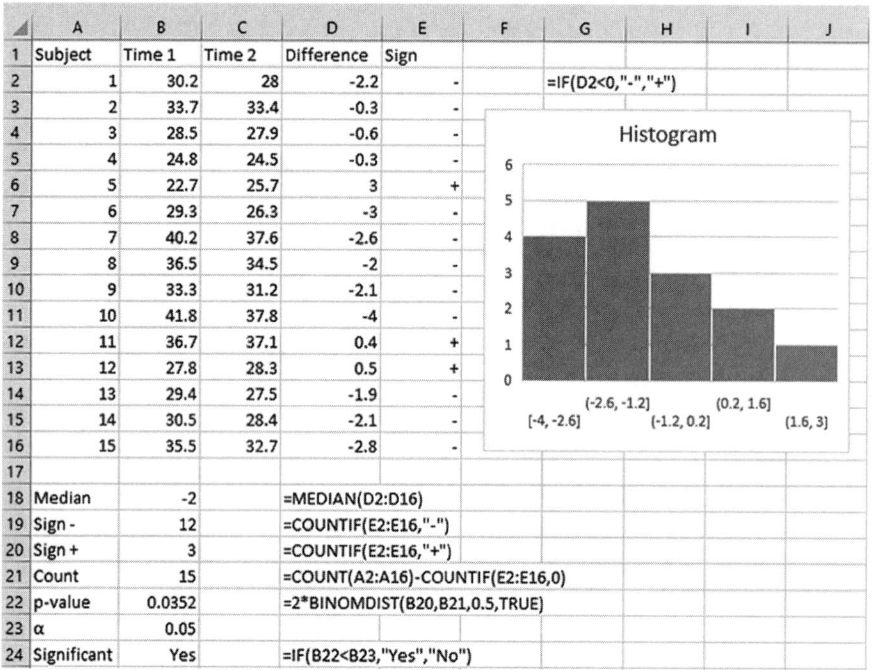

	A	B	C	D	E	F	G
1	Subject	Time 1	Time 2	Difference	Sign		
2	1	30.2	28	-2.2	-		=IF(D2<0,"-","+")
3	2	33.7	33.4	-0.3	-		
4	3	28.5	27.9	-0.6	-		
5	4	24.8	24.5	-0.3	-		
6	5	22.7	25.7	3	+		
7	6	29.3	26.3	-3	-		
8	7	40.2	37.6	-2.6	-		
9	8	36.5	34.5	-2	-		
10	9	33.3	31.2	-2.1	-		
11	10	41.8	37.8	-4	-		
12	11	36.7	37.1	0.4	+		
13	12	27.8	28.3	0.5	+		
14	13	29.4	27.5	-1.9	-		
15	14	30.5	28.4	-2.1	-		
16	15	35.5	32.7	-2.8	-		
17							
18	Median	-2		=MEDIAN(D2:D16)			
19	Sign -	12		=COUNTIF(E2:E16,"-")			
20	Sign +	3		=COUNTIF(E2:E16,"+")			
21	Count	15		=COUNT(A2:A16)-COUNTIF(E2:E16,0)			
22	p-value	0.0352		=2*BINOMDIST(B20,B21,0.5,TRUE)			
23	α	0.05					
24	Significant	Yes		=IF(B22<B23,"Yes","No")			

Figure 9.3 Sign Test with Paired Data for Example 9.2

9.7 Wilcoxon Signed-Rank Test

For paired designs, the nonparametric procedure called the Wilcoxon signed-rank test is appropriate when the assumptions for the t test for two paired samples are not satisfied. While the sign test can also be used for paired data, the Wilcoxon signed-rank test is recommended because it has greater power (to correctly reject the null hypothesis when it is false), unless the distribution of the differences deviates considerably from symmetry; that is, the sign test for paired data does not require symmetry. The Wilcoxon-signed rank test assumes the following:

1. Each difference is symmetric about 0.
2. The paired observations are randomly and independently drawn.
3. The data are measured on an ordinal or continuous level.

To conduct the Wilcoxon signed-rank test, we proceed with the following steps:

1. Select a random sample of n pairs of observations.
2. Calculate the difference for each pair of observations.
3. Ignoring the signs of the difference scores, rank their absolute values from smallest to largest.
4. Do not rank differences of 0, but reduce the sample size by eliminating this pair.
5. Tied differences are assigned an average rank.
6. Assign each rank a plus (+) or minus (–) sign according to the sign of the difference.
7. Compute the sum of the positive ranks and sum of the negative ranks.
8. Let the smaller sum be denoted T.
9. Evaluate the null hypothesis that the underlying population of differences for the pairs of observations has a median difference of 0. This means we should have approximately equal numbers of positive and negative ranks. The sum of positive ranks should be similar to the sum of the negative ranks.

10. Evaluate the data with the statistic

$$Z_T = \frac{T - \mu_T}{\sigma_T}.$$

The mean of the sum of ranks is

$$\mu_T = \frac{n(n+1)}{4}.$$

The standard deviation is

$$\sigma_T = \sqrt{\frac{n(n+1)(2n+1)}{24}}.$$

If the null hypothesis is true and the sample size > 15, then Z_T is an approximate normal distribution with mean 0 and standard deviation 1. Otherwise, Z_T cannot be assumed to follow a standard normal distribution, and the nonparametric table for the Wilcoxon signed-rank test (**Table 9.3**) should be used.[2] If T < the table value, then reject the null hypothesis.

Example 9.3

The Wilcoxon signed-rank test will now be applied to the data in Example 9.2. The steps to conduct the Wilcoxon signed-rank test appear in the figure. We evaluated the data using both the critical value from Table 9.3 and also using the z statistic.

1. H_0: Median difference is 0.
2. H_a: Median difference is not 0.
3. Let $\alpha = 0.05$, $n = 15$
4. Wilcoxon signed-rank test. The critical value for a two-tailed test from Table 9.3[25]. The critical value for z is ±1.96.
5. The sum of the smaller value T is 20.5 (**Figure 9.4**). The calculated test statistic is −2.24.

Table 9.3 Critical Values of the Wilcoxon Signed-Rank Test

	Two-Tailed Test		One-Tailed Test	
n	$\alpha = 0.05$	$\alpha = 0.01$	$\alpha = 0.05$	$\alpha = 0.01$
8	3	0	5	1
9	5	1	8	3
10	8	3	10	5
11	10	5	13	7
12	13	7	17	9
13	17	9	21	12
14	21	12	25	15
15	25	15	30	19
16	29	19	35	23
17	34	23	41	27
18	40	27	47	32

	A	B	C	D	E	F	G	H	I	J	K	L	M	N	O	P
1	Subject	Time 1	Time 2	Diff	Sign	|Diff|	Rank	Signed Rank								
2	1	30.2	28	-2.2	-1	2.2	10	-10		=C2-B2 for column D						
3	2	33.7	33.4	-0.3	-1	0.3	2	-2		=IF(D2>0,1,-1) for column E						
4	3	28.5	27.9	-0.6	-1	0.6	5	-5		=ABS(D2) for column F						
5	4	24.8	24.5	-0.3	-1	0.3	1	-1		=RANK.AVG(F2,$F$2:$F$16,1) for column G						
6	5	22.7	25.7	3	1	3	13.5	13.5		=E2*G2 for column H						
7	6	29.3	26.3	-3	-1	3	13.5	-13.5								
8	7	40.2	37.6	-2.6	-1	2.6	11	-11								
9	8	36.5	34.5	-2	-1	2	7	-7								
10	9	33.3	31.2	-2.1	-1	2.1	8	-8								
11	10	41.8	37.8	-4	-1	4	15	-15								
12	11	36.7	37.1	0.4	1	0.4	3	3								
13	12	27.8	28.3	0.5	1	0.5	4	4								
14	13	29.4	27.5	-1.9	-1	1.9	6	-6								
15	14	30.5	28.4	-2.1	-1	2.1	9	-9								
16	15	35.5	32.7	-2.8	-1	2.8	12	-12								
17																
18	Sum +	20.5		=SUMIF(H2:H16,">0",H2:H16)						n	15		=COUNT(A2:A16)-COUNTIF(H2:H16,0)			
19	Sum -	-99.5		=SUMIF(H2:H16,"<0",H2:H16)						μ_T	60		=K18*(K18+1)/4			
20	T	20.5		=IF(ABS(B18)<ABS(B19),ABS(B18),ABS(B19))						σ_T	17.61		=SQRT(K18*(K18+1)*(2*K18+1)/24)			
21	α	0.05								Z_T	-2.24		=(B20-K19)/K20			
22	Table	25								p-value	0.0249		=2*NORMDIST(B20,K19,K20,TRUE)			
23	Significant	Yes		=IF(B20<B22,"Yes","No")						Significant	Yes		=IF(K22<B21,"Yes","No")			

Figure 9.4 Wilcoxon Signed-Rank Test for Example 9.3

6. We reject the null hypothesis (since $T <$ table value, or because p-value $= 0.0249 < 0.05 = \alpha$) and conclude with 95% confidence that BMI differs after the intervention is received compared with before.

The sign test and the Wilcoxon signed-rank test used to assess the null hypothesis that the median difference in paired data is 0 can also be evaluated using SAS with PROC UNIVARIATE.

```
DATA Example;
INPUT Time1 Time2;
Diff=Time2-Time1;
DATALINES;
...
;

PROC UNIVARIATE DATA=Example PLOT NORMAL;
VAR Diff;
RUN;
```

The Kolmogorov-Smirnov test result shown in the output indicates that the distribution of difference scores is not normally distributed; that is, because p-value $= 0.0399 < 0.05 = \alpha$, we reject the null hypothesis of normally distributed difference scores with 95% confidence.

Tests for Normality				
Test	Statistic		p Value	
Shapiro-Wilk	W	0.924828	Pr < W	0.2281
Kolmogorov-Smirnov	D	0.22517	Pr > D	0.0399
Cramer-von Mises	W-Sq	0.089757	Pr > W-Sq	0.1433
Anderson-Darling	A-Sq	0.508279	Pr > A-Sq	0.1744

The SAS output also shows results from the *t* test, sign test, and the Wilcoxon signed-rank test, with the null hypothesis that the difference scores equal 0.

Tests for Location: Mu0=0				
Test	Statistic		p Value	
Student's t	t	-2.90781	Pr > |t|	0.0115
Sign	M	-4.5	Pr >= |M|	0.0352
Signed Rank	S	-39.5	Pr >= |S|	0.0219

In this example, all three tests indicate that we have sufficient evidence at the 0.05 level to reject the null hypothesis that the median difference in paired scores is 0. The *p*-value is slightly different than we found using Excel because SAS uses a continuity correction.

9.8 Mood's Median Test

The Mood's median test is used to determine whether the median of two independent samples are drawn from the sample population or from populations with different medians. This test can be used with more than two samples, but it is less powerful than the Kruskal-Wallis test. It is a nonparametric alternative to the one-way ANOVA. The Mood's median test has certain assumptions:

Observations are independent within and between samples.
Observations reflect a population with a continuous distribution function.
The populations from which the samples are drawn have the same shape.

This test involves the following steps:

1. For the combination of the two samples, calculate the median.
2. Create a 2 × 2 contingency table with the group assignment on the top and in the first row if the score is above the median, but in the second row if less than or equal to the median.
3. Evaluate independence using the χ^2 test.
4. If the *p*-value < α, then reject the null hypothesis that the medians are equal.

Example 9.4

We are interested in evaluating a drug that was designed to reduce pain. Patients with a certain average level of back pain were randomly assigned to the drug or placebo arm of the study. After 4 weeks of the experiment, the pain scores appear as shown in **Figure 9.5**.

	A	B	C	D	E	F	G	H	I	J	K	L	M
1		Treatment	Placebo		Median	21.7			=MEDIAN(B2:C13)				
2		23.4	29										
3		17.8	26.4		Observed 2x2 table								
4		13.5	22.7			Treatment	Placebo						
5		19.8	27.2		> Median	3	8		=COUNTIF(B2:B13,">"&$F$1)				
6		15.8	25.1		≤ Median	9	4		=COUNT(B2:B13)-F5				
7		22.1	21.7										
8		24	24		Expected 2x2 table				=SUM(F5:F6)*SUM(F5:G5)/SUM(F5:G6) for F11				
9		18.8	21.8			Treatment	Placebo		=SUM(F5:G5)*SUM(G5:G6)/SUM(F5:G6) for G11				
10		17.6	25.3		> Median	5.5	5.5		=SUM(F5:F6)*SUM(F6:G6)/SUM(F5:G6) for F12				
11		20.8	21.7		≤ Median	6.5	6.5		=SUM(F6:G6)*SUM(G5:G6)/SUM(F5:G6) for G12				
12		21.2	20										
13		18.3	20.5		Chi-square	4.20			=CHISQ.INV.RT(F15,1)				
14					p-value	0.0405			=CHISQ.TEST(F5:G6,F11:G12)				
15	Mean	19.4	23.8		α	0.05							
16	Median	19.3	23.4		Significant	Yes			=IF(F15<F16,"Yes","No")				

Figure 9.5 Mood's Median Test for Example 9.4

1. H_0: There is no difference in the median pain score between treatment and placebo groups.
2. H_a: Otherwise
3. Let $\alpha = 0.05$, $n = 12$ per group
4. Mood's median test
5. The median value for the treatment group is 19.4 and for the placebo group is 23.4. The χ^2 value is 4.20.
6. Since p-value $= 0.0405 < 0.05 = \alpha$, we reject the null hypothesis and conclude that there is a significant difference between the treatment and placebo population medians.

In practice, the Wilcoxon rank-sum test (also called Mann-Whitney U test) is preferred to the Mood's median test because the former has more power.

9.9 Mann-Whitney U Test (Also Called Wilcoxon Rank-Sum Test)

The Mann-Whitney U test is a nonparametric procedure used to test the null hypothesis that the distribution of an ordinal or continuous scaled response variable is the same in two independently sampled populations. The nonparametric test does not require that the underlying population be normally distributed or that their variances be equal. However, it does assume that the two distributions have a similar shape. The specific null hypothesis is that the medians from two independent populations are the same.[3, 4]

The Mann-Whitney U test is an alternative to the two-sample t test when the underlying populations are not normally distributed, their variances are not equal, and sample sizes are small ($n < 30$). Under these conditions, the Mann-Whitney U test has much greater power than the two-sample t test. The Mann-Whitney U test is usually more powerful than Mood's median test because, where the median test considers just the position of each observation relative to the overall median, the Mann-Whitney test takes the ranks of each observation into account. The Mann-Whitney U test has four assumptions:

1. The samples are drawn from the population at random.
2. Observations are independent of each other.
3. The measurement scale of the response variable is ordinal or continuous.
4. Both groups have the same shape distribution.

To carry out the Mann-Whitney U Test, take the following steps:

1. Select an independent random sample from each of two populations of interest.
2. Order the observations from smallest to greatest, irrespective of sample.
3. Assign a rank to each subject's score.
4. For tied ranks, assign an average rank to all measurements with the same rank.
5. Separately sum the ranks for each sample, R_1 for sample 1 and R_2 for sample 2.
6. Calculate the U statistic for both samples as follows:

$$U_1 = R_1 - \frac{n_1(n_1 + 1)}{2}$$

$$U_2 = R_2 - \frac{n_2(n_2 + 1)}{2}$$

   where n_1 is the sample size for sample 1 and n_2 is the sample size for sample 2. It does not matter which sample is considered 1 or 2.
7. The smaller U_1 or U_2 is then selected and compared with the critical value found in the table.
8. Report the results.

For a large sample, U has an approximate normal distribution, such that

$$Z = \frac{U - \mu_T}{\sigma_W},$$

$$\sigma_W = \sqrt{\frac{n_1 n_2 (n_1 + n_2 + 1)}{12}},$$

$$\mu_T = \frac{n_1 n_2}{2}.$$

n_1 = number of observations in the sample with the smaller sum of ranks.
n_2 = number of observations in the sample with the larger sum of ranks.[2]

Example 9.5

We are interested in evaluating a drug that was designed to reduce pain. Patients with a certain average level of back pain were randomly assigned to the drug or placebo arm of the study. After 4 weeks of the experiment, the pain scores are as shown in **Figure 9.6**.

These results can also be obtained in SAS using PROC NPAR1WAY and the program, as follows:

```
DATA Example;
INPUT Score Group $ @@;
DATALINES;
23.4 T 17.8 T 13.5 T 19.8 T 15.8 T 22.1 T 24.0 T 18.8 T 17.6 T 20.8
T 21.2 T 18.3 T 29.0 C 26.4 C 22.7 C 27.2 C 25.1 C 21.7 C 24.0 C
21.8 C 25.3 C 21.7 C 20.0 C 20.5 C
;
```

	A	B	C	D	E	F	G	H	I	J	K	L	M	N
1	Treatment	Control		Treatment	Control									
2	23.4	29		17	24		=RANK.AVG(A2,SAS2:SBS13,1)							
3	17.8	26.4		4	22									
4	13.5	22.7		1	16		R_1	99.5		=sum(D2:D13)				
5	19.8	27.2		7	23		R_2	200.5		=SUM(E2:E13)				
6	15.8	25.1		2	20									
7	22.1	21.7		15	12.5		n_1	12		=COUNT(D2:D13)				
8	24	24		18.5	18.5		n_2	12		=COUNT(E2:E13)				
9	18.8	21.8		6	14									
10	17.6	25.3		3	21		U_1	21.5		=E15-E18*(E18+1)/2				
11	20.8	21.7		10	12.5		U_2	122.5		=E16-E19*(E19+1)/2				
12	21.2	20		11	8									
13	18.3	20.5		5	9		U	21.5		=MIN(E21:E22)				
14														
15							Z	-2.92		=(E24-E18*E19/2)/SQRT(E18*E19*(E18+E19+1)/12)				
16							p-value	0.0035		=2*NORMDIST(E26,0,1,TRUE)				
17							α	0.05						
18							Significant	Yes		=IF(E27<E28,"Yes","No")				

Figure 9.6 Mann-Whitney U Test for Example 9.5


```
PROC NPAR1WAY DATA=Example WILCOXON;
CLASS Group;
VAR Score;
RUN;
```

Partial SAS output is shown:

Wilcoxon Two-Sample Test	
Statistic	99.5000
Normal Approximation	
Z	-2.8880
One-Sided Pr < Z	0.0019
Two-Sided Pr > |Z|	0.0039
t Approximation	
One-Sided Pr < Z	0.0041
Two-Sided Pr > |Z|	0.0083
Z includes a continuity correction of 0.5.	

Note that the Z includes a continuity correction of 0.5, which is why SAS shows a different p-value than Excel.

News File

One study found that women who underwent mastectomy for breast cancer had a higher risk of developing depressive symptoms (≤ 3 years of surgery) than women in the general population.[5] Middle- and older-age breast cancer patients had greater risk than younger patients for longer-term depression following mastectomy. Some of the higher levels of depression in the older women may be because these women tend to experience more co-morbidities, which also associates with depression. The authors of this study suggest that breast cancer patients undergoing hysterectomy may benefit from early psychiatric referrals in order to facilitate provision of appropriate psychosocial support and medical aid.

Because the number of depressive symptoms was not normally distributed, the Mann-Whitney U test was used to analyze differences between breast cancer patients receiving a mastectomy and the general population.

9.10 Kruskal-Wallis Test

The Kruskal-Wallis test was developed in the early 1950s as a generalization of the two sample Wilcoxon rank sum test to three or more groups.[6] This non-parametric test is used to assess the hypothesis that the distribution of a response variable is the same in multiple independently sampled populations; it is used to determine if a difference among the medians of three or more independent groups is statistically significant. The Kruskal-Wallis test is used in place of the one-way ANOVA if the assumptions for ANOVA (i.e., normality and equal variance) are not met. In this situation, it is a more powerful test than the conventional ANOVA. Otherwise, ANOVA is the more powerful test. Specific assumptions are required for the Kruskal-Wallis test:

1. The samples are drawn from the population at random.
2. Observations are independent of each other.
3. The measurement scale of the response variable is ordinal or continuous.
4. All groups have the same shape distribution.

When each group being compared has at least five observations, the test statistic approximates a χ^2 distribution, with k (#groups) – 1 degree of freedom.[1]

To perform the Kruskal-Wallis test, the following steps are taken:

1. Select an independent random sample from each of three or more populations of interest.
2. Assign a rank to each subject's score.
3. For tied ranks, assign an average rank to all measurements with the same rank.
4. Separately sum the ranks for each sample, R_1 for sample 1, R_2 for sample 2, etc.
5. Calculate R^2/n for each sample.
6. Calculate the test statistic:

$$H = 12/(n(n+1)) * \Sigma R_j^2/n_j - 3(n+1)$$

where n is the total sample size and j is the jth group.

Under the null hypothesis, the H statistic follows a χ^2 distribution with degrees of freedom = $k - 1$.

7. Report the results.

Example 9.6

Consider three independent groups of people whose general quality of life was classified as high, medium, and low. Ten people were randomly sampled in each of these groups. We then measured their voice-related quality of life (1 poor and 10 high). We are interested in evaluating whether the voice-related quality of life varied according to their general quality-of-life classification.

The steps of hypothesis testing are as follows:

1. H_0: The distribution of voice-related quality of life is the same for independently sampled high, medium, and low general quality-of-life populations.
2. H_a: Otherwise
3. Let $\alpha = 0.05$, $k = 3$, $n = 30$
4. Kruskal-Wallis H test: $df = k - 1 = 2$. $\chi^2_{Critical} = 5.991$
5. The Kruskal-Wallis H test statistic = 6.682 (see **Figure 9.7**).
6. Since p-value = $0.035 < 0.05 = \alpha$, we reject the null hypothesis and conclude that voice-related quality of life differs significantly among the high, medium, and low quality-of-life population medians.

	A	B	C	D	E	F	G	H	I	J	K	L	M	N	O
1	High	Medium	Low		Rank (H)	Rank (M)	Rank (L)								
2	8.2	6.9	6.5		16.5	8	6		=RANK.AVG(A2,$A$2:$C$11,1)						
3	9.3	9.1	8		28.5	24.5	13.5		=RANK.AVG(B2,$A$2:$C$11,1)						
4	9.2	8.5	8		26.5	18	13.5		=RANK.AVG(C2,$A$2:$C$11,1)						
5	8	8	9.1		13.5	13.5	24.5								
6	8.8	7.5	5.5		19.5	9	3		n	30		=COUNT(A2:C11)			
7	9	7.6	4.8		22	10	1		K	3		=COUNTA(A1:C1)			
8	7.8	9	5.2		11	22	2		H	6.682		=12/(J2*(J2+1))*SUM(E15:G15)-3*(J2+1)			
9	9.5	5.6	6.7		30	4	7		p-value	0.0354		=CHIDIST(J4,J3-1)			
10	9.2	5.9	9.3		26.5	5	28.5		α	0.05					
11	8.8	8.2	9		19.5	16.5	22		Significant	Yes		=IF(J5<J6,"Yes","No")			
12															
13				R	213.5	130.5	121		=SUM(E2:E11)						
14				n	10	10	10		=COUNT(E2:E11)						
15				R^2/n	4558.225	1703.025	1464.1		=E13^2/E14						

Figure 9.7 Kruskal-Wallis One-Way Analysis of Variance for Example 9.6

These results can also be obtained in SAS using PROC NPAR1WAY and the program, as follows:

```
DATA Example;
INPUT VRQOL GQOL $ @@;
DATALINES;
8.2 H 9.3 H 9.2 H 8.0 H 8.8 H 9.0 H 7.8 H 9.5 H 9.2 H 8.8 H 6.9 M
9.1 M 8.5 M 8.0 M 7.5 M 7.6 M 9.0 M 5.6 M 5.9 M 8.2 M 6.5 L 8.0 L
8.0 L 9.1 L 5.5 L 4.8 L 5.2 L 6.7 L 9.3 L 9.0 L
;

PROC NPAR1WAY DATA=Example WILCOXON;
```

```
CLASS GQOL;
VAR VRQOL;
RUN;
```

Partial SAS output is shown:

Kruskal-Wallis Test	
Chi-Square	6.7103
DF	2
Pr > Chi-Square	0.0349

9.11 Friedman Test

The Friedman test is a nonparametric alternative to the one-way ANOVA for testing repeated measures. It is similar to the Kruskall-Wallis test, but it is used with repeated measures. The test does not require that the outcome measure be normally distributed. The Friedman test has the following assumptions:

1. A single group is measured three or more times.
2. The samples are drawn from the population at random.
3. The measurement scale of the response variable is ordinal or continuous.

The test statistic is defined as follows:

$$Q = \frac{12}{nk(k+1)} \sum_{j=1}^{k} R_j^2 - 3n(k+1).$$

where n = the number of subjects, k = the number of groups, and R_j is the sum of the ranks for the subjects in group j. Under the null hypothesis that the sum of the ranks of each group are the same, then

$$Q \sim \chi^2(k-1)$$

when $k \geq 5$ or $n > 15$. Reject the null hypothesis if $Q > \chi^2_{Critical}$.

Example 9.7

A voice quality index was designed to identify various forms of voice quality, with scores ranging from 0 (poor) to 10 (excellent). Researchers were interested in whether the index would capture changes in voice quality between morning, midday, and evening among individuals who regularly used their voice through the day. They recruited 12 adult women with "normal" voices who satisfied the criterion for participation. The voice quality index was self-reported by each woman, three times during the day, with the scores appearing in columns B through D of **Figure 9.8**.

The steps of hypothesis testing are as follows:

1. H_0: The distribution of voice quality index is the same at all times of the day.
2. H_a: Otherwise
3. Let $\alpha = 0.05$, $k = 3$, $n = 12$
4. Friedman's Test, $df = k - 1 = 2$. $\chi^2_{Critical} = 5.991$
5. Friedman's Q statistic = 14

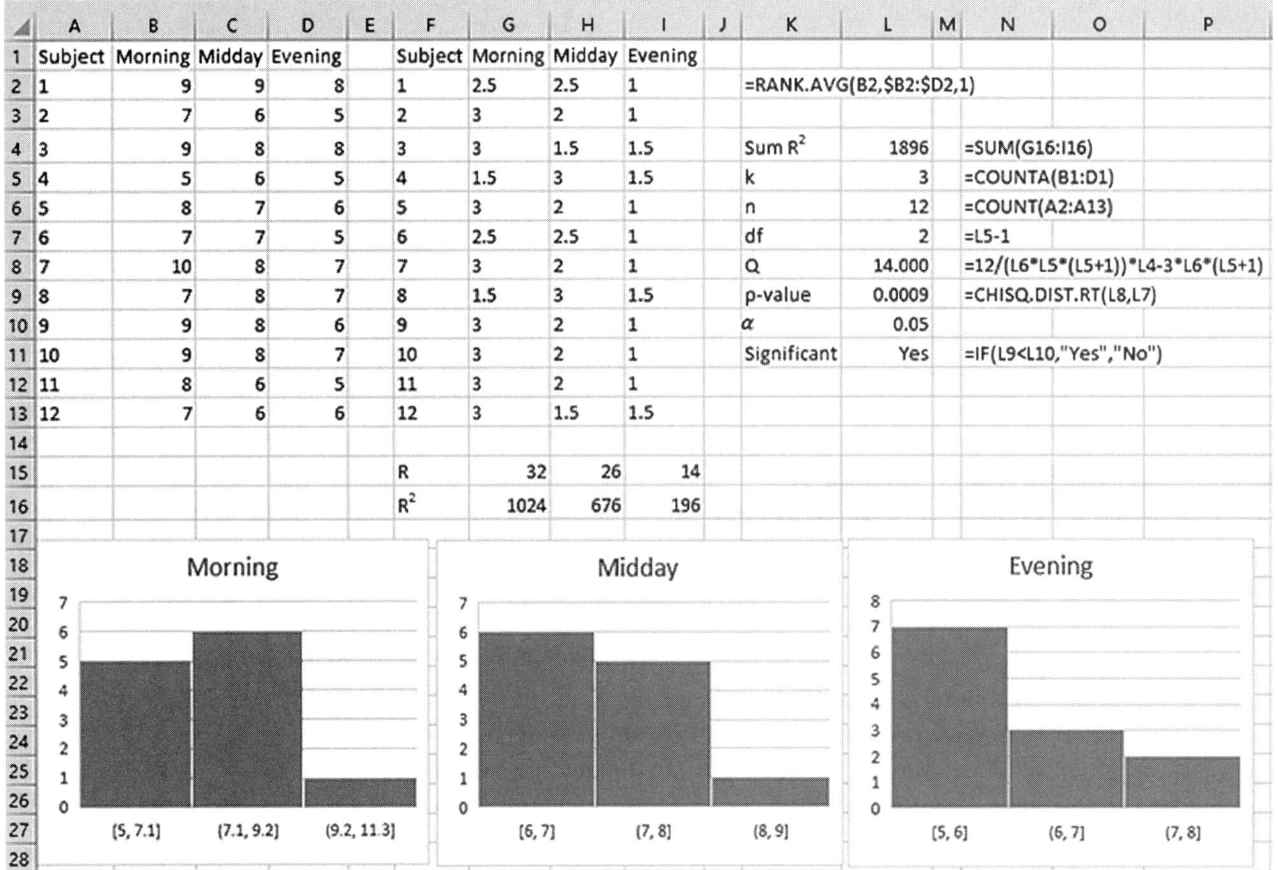

	A	B	C	D	E	F	G	H	I	J	K	L	M	N
1	Subject	Morning	Midday	Evening		Subject	Morning	Midday	Evening					
2	1	9	9	8		1	2.5	2.5	1		=RANK.AVG(B2,$B2:$D2,1)			
3	2	7	6	5		2	3	2	1					
4	3	9	8	8		3	3	1.5	1.5		Sum R^2	1896		=SUM(G16:I16)
5	4	5	6	5		4	1.5	3	1.5		k	3		=COUNTA(B1:D1)
6	5	8	7	6		5	3	2	1		n	12		=COUNT(A2:A13)
7	6	7	7	5		6	2.5	2.5	1		df	2		=L5-1
8	7	10	8	7		7	3	2	1		Q	14.000		=12/(L6*L5*(L5+1))*L4-3*L6*(L5+1)
9	8	7	8	7		8	1.5	3	1.5		p-value	0.0009		=CHISQ.DIST.RT(L8,L7)
10	9	9	8	6		9	3	2	1		α	0.05		
11	10	9	8	7		10	3	2	1		Significant	Yes		=IF(L9<L10,"Yes","No")
12	11	8	6	5		11	3	2	1					
13	12	7	6	6		12	3	1.5	1.5					
14														
15						R	32	26	14					
16						R^2	1024	676	196					

Figure 9.8 Freidman's Test for Example 9.7

6. Since p-value $= 0.001 < 0.05 = \alpha$, we reject the null hypothesis and conclude that the voice-quality index measure differs significantly between morning, midday, and evening.

9.12 Kendall Tau-b Correlation Coefficient

The Kendall tau-b correlation coefficient (or just Kendall tau-b) is a nonparametric statistic. It measures the direction and strength of association between two variables measured on an ordinal or higher scale. It is used instead of the Pearson correlation coefficient when the data fail to meet the assumptions of that test. It is also an alternative to the Spearman correlation coefficient when the sample size is small and has several tied ranks. For example, Kendall's tau-b could be used to assess the association between health classification (excellent, good, fair, poor) and education (less than high school, high school, some college, college, college plus).

The following assumptions are required to appropriately use Kendall's tau-b:

1. Both variables are measured on an ordinal or continuous (interval or ratio) scale.
2. A monotonic relationship is desired, but this is not a strict assumption. A monotonic relationship helps make the results more meaningful.

Kendall's tau-b correlation coefficient can be estimated in various statistical software packages. For example, PROC CORR in SAS produces this statistic by adding the option Kendall.

Example 9.8

Suppose we are interested in evaluating the association between education and health. The following SAS code can be applied to measurements taken on 17 subjects:

```
/*Excellent=4, Good=3, Fair=2, Poor=1 and <HS=1, HS=2, Some
College=3, College=4, College+=5*/

DATA Example;
INPUT EDU Health @@;
DATALINES;
1 3 1 1 2 4 2 3 2 3 2 2 3 4 3 3 3 3 3 2 4 2 4 4 4 4 4 4 5 4 5 4 5 4
;

PROC CORR DATA=Example KENDALL;
VAR EDU Health;
RUN;
```

The steps of hypothesis testing are as follows:

1. H_0: There is no association between health and education.
2. H_a: Otherwise
3. Let $\alpha = 0.05$, $n = 17$
4. Kendall's tau-b correlation coefficient
5. The Kendall's tau-b correlation coefficient is 0.5093.
6. Since p-value $= 0.0156 < 0.05 = \alpha$, we reject the null hypothesis and conclude that there is a significant positive association between increasing education and better health.

Kendall Tau b Correlation Coefficients, N = 17 Prob > |tau| under H0: Tau=0		
	EDU	HEALTH
EDU	1.00000	0.50929 0.0156
HEALTH	0.50929 0.0156	1.00000

9.13 Other Selected Tests

One sort of hypothesis is about the shape of a distribution. We can infer that a set of data comes from an unknown but symmetrical distribution. The null hypothesis is that the observations are from the same symmetrical distribution, with an unknown median value. The alternative hypothesis is that the observations are not from a symmetrical distribution. To assess this, we can apply the test for distributional symmetry. This test will not be covered in this text. Two other nonparametric tests that will not be covered here are the permutation test for paired replicates and the permutation test for two independent samples.

9.14 Summary

Many techniques of inference do not require stringent assumptions about the population from which the data are sampled. These techniques represent a branch of statistics that is not based on parameterized families of probability distributions. Nonparametric tests are useful in situations where the parametric test assumptions are violated, when nominal or **ordinal data** are analyzed, and when small sample sizes are involved. Nonparametric tests for **nominal data** have been covered in earlier chapters. In this chapter, we focused on nonparametric tests for assessing ordinal and continuous data. Each of these nonparametric tests has a parametric version.

The Kolmogorov-Smirnov test is one of several methods for determining the probability that a sample was drawn from a normal population. The sign test assesses the null hypothesis about the median in a single population. It is also used to test the value of the median of paired differences. However, the Wilcoxon signed-rank test has more power and is preferred to the sign test for assessing whether the median difference is 0. Mood's test is used to assess the equality of medians from two or more independent populations. The Kruskal-Wallis test is preferred when more than two independent samples are considered. The Mann-Whitney U test (or Wilcoxon rank-sum test) evaluates whether two independent samples come from the same distribution. The Kruskal-Wallis test is a rank-based test that compares three or more independent groups. On the other hand, the Friedman test is used to assess more than two related samples. Kendall's tau-b measures the direction and strength of association between two variables measured on an ordinal or higher scale.

Nonparametric tests may also be used for assessing interval or ratio data, such as test for distribution symmetry for one sample, permutation test for paired replicates, and permutation test for two independent samples.

Exercises

1. Match the nonparametric tests on the left to the alternative parametric tests on the right.

___ Sign test	A. Pearson correlation coefficient
___ Wilcoxon signed-rank test	B. One-way ANOVA test for repeated measures
___ Mood's median test	C. One-way ANOVA
___ Mann-Whitney U test	D. One-sample t test
___ Kruskal-Wallis test	E. Two-sample t test with independent groups
___ Friedman test	F. t test for two-paired samples
___ Kendall tau-b	

2. A local hospital administrator indicates that the median number of hospitalizations for COVID-19 per day is 12. A doctor from the same hospital believes it is more than 12. From hospital admission records, the doctor identified the number of hospitalizations for COVID-19 on 10 random days in the past month. Use the sign test to evaluate whether we can respect the hospital administrators claim at the 0.05 level of significance.

Day	1	2	3	4	5	6	7	8	9	10
Number Admitted	6	14	12	14	10	9	10	13	15	9

3. You would like to test the hypothesis that a significant decrease in depression scores on the Beck Depression Inventory occurred because of an intervention. A random sample of 10 of the 348 Beck Depression Inventory change scores produced –8, –2, –1, 1, –5, 0, –5, 0, –3, and 0. Use the sign test to evaluate whether a significant change in scores occurred for these data.

4. Repeat the previous problem, only use the Wilcoxon signed-rank test. Describe whether your conclusion changes. Which test is preferred?

5. We are interested in evaluating a drug designed for patients with cystic fibrosis. The drug is designed to improve air flow in the lungs and slow loss of pulmonary function that is frequently associated with the disease. The following data reflect a reduction in forced vital capacity (FVC), which is the volume of air that can be expelled from the lungs in 6 seconds, in patients over 25 weeks of placebo (Y_{1i}) compared with 25 weeks of treatment with the drug (Y_{2i}) for the same patients. We do not assume the differences in reduction of FVC (milliliters) are normally distributed. The null hypothesis is that the median difference is equal to 0. Use the Wilcoxon signed-rank test to evaluate the null hypothesis.

i	1	2	3	4	5	6	7
Y_{1i}	225	75	80	540	73	84	292
Y_{2i}	214	94	32	441	-35	-29	344
i	8	9	10	11	12	13	14
Y_{1i}	-22	524	-39	507	255	526	1020
Y_{2i}	-177	377	142	333	9	66	342

6. A study of older adults found that healthy minimum squeeze measurements (grip strength) were approximately 72.6 pounds for men and 44 pounds for women.[1] Poorer grip strength has been associated with poorer mobility and higher risk of cardiovascular death, heart attack, stroke, and death for all causes.[7–9] Suppose you design an intervention aimed at improving hand-grip strength. Grip strength was measured on 15 males, aged 60 years (T_{1i}). After 8 weeks of the intervention, their grip strength was measured a second time (T_{2i}). The results are summarized here.

i	1	2	3	4	5	6	7	8
T_{1i}	68	73	80	58	80	75	82	65
T_{2i}	72	75	81	80	78	78	81	70
i	9	10	11	12	13	14	15	
T_{1i}	78	59	54	80	84	75	74	
T_{2i}	84	55	60	76	92	80	78	

Apply the Wilcoxon signed-ranks test to determine if there is a significant change in grip strength. Present your results using the six steps of hypothesis testing.

7. Among high school seniors from four schools who indicated on a survey that they had previously smoked marijuana, we want to know whether the age when they first smoked marijuana (Y_{1i}) differed between Hispanics and non-Hispanics (Y_{2i}). The school (Y_{3i}) was also identified.

i	1	2	3	4	5	6	7	8	9	10	11	12	13	14	15	16	17	18	19
Y_{1i}	17	17	17	17	12	16	17	17	17	17	17	14	14	14	17	16	16	17	13
Y_{2i}	No	No	No	Yes	Yes	No	Yes	No	No	No	No	Yes	No	No	No	No	Yes	No	No
Y_{3i}	1	1	1	1	1	1	1	1	1	1	1	1	1	2	2	2	2	2	2
i	20	21	22	23	24	25	26	27	28	29	30	31	32	33	34	35	36	37	38
Y_{1i}	17	16	16	17	14	14	15	10	16	17	17	17	16	17	17	16	17	15	14
Y_{2i}	No	No	Yes	Yes	No	Yes	Yes	No	No	No	No	No	No	No	No	No	No	Yes	Yes
Y_{3i}	2	2	2	2	2	2	2	2	2	3	3	3	3	3	3	3	3	3	3
i	39	40	41	42	43	44	45	46	47	48	49	50	51	52	53	54	55	56	
Y_{1i}	15	17	10	17	15	16	14	12	17	10	17	16	14	14	17	16	13	16	
Y_{2i}	No	No	No	No	No	No	No	Yes	No	Yes	No	No	No	No	No	Yes	No	Yes	
Y_{3i}	3	3	3	3	3	4	4	4	4	4	4	4	4	4	4	4	4	4	

a. Assess whether age is normally distributed.
b. Use the Mann-Whitney U test to evaluate whether median age when marijuana was first smoked differed between Hispanics and non-Hispanics.

8. Suppose three medications are available for treating back pain. Of interest is whether they have different effects on reducing pain. Thirty adults who recently visited a pain clinic because of back pain were randomly assigned one of the three medications. After 6 weeks of using the medication, each individual completed a questionnaire, with an index pain score derived, on a scale from 1 to 30 (most severe).

Drug 1	23	18	17	28	14	18	11	8	19	20
Drug 2	10	6	14	8	16	5	11	20	8	15
Drug 3	18	17	25	22	17	16	19	4	20	14

Apply the Kruskal-Wallis test using a 0.05 level of significance to determine if the three drugs have different effects on pack pain. Present your results using the six steps of hypothesis testing.

9. Statewide mandatory mask use in public and social gathering restrictions were put in place to reduce the spread of SARS-CoV-2. Positive test rates (%) were gathered for 12 counties in a state prior to the requirements and then again at 3 weeks and 6 weeks after the requirements began.

County	1	2	3	4	5	6	7	8	9	10	11	12
Before	17.6	14.5	16.4	21.2	15.0	16.8	11.1	15.3	18.1	17.3	20.5	14.3
Week 3	17.4	14.8	12.2	13.6	15.1	15.1	10.4	13.9	16.8	17.2	17.0	11.7
Week 6	14.3	14.0	8.7	9.8	14.8	14.7	11.0	13.8	11.9	14.9	15.3	10.7

Apply Friedman's test using a 0.05 level of significance to determine if the state's mandatory coronavirus prevention measures had an effect on the positive test rate. Present your results using the six steps of hypothesis testing.

10. Suppose we are interested in evaluating the association between CPAP use (1 = nightly, 2 = weekly, 3 = less than weekly) and daytime sleepiness (1 = never, 2 = sometimes, 3 = always) among a group of 12 individuals with obstructive sleep apnea. Evaluate the null hypothesis that there is no association between CPAP use and daytime sleepiness.

Subject	1	2	3	4	5	6	7	8	9	10	11	12
CPAP use	1	1	1	2	1	3	3	2	1	3	2	1
Daytime sleepiness	2	1	1	3	1	3	2	2	2	3	2	1

References

1. Stokes ME, Davis CS, Koch GG. *Categorical Data Analysis Using the SAS System*. 2nd ed. Cary, NC: SAS Institute Inc.; 2000.
2. Siegel S, Catellan NJ. *Nonparametric statistics for the behavioral sciences*. 2nd ed. New York, NY: McGraw-Hill; 1988.
3. Wilcoxon F. Individual comparison by ranking methods. *Biometrics*. 1945;*1*:80–83.
4. Mann HB, Whitney DR. On a test of whether one of two random variables is stochastically larger than the other. *Ann Math Statist*. 1947;*18*:50–60.
5. Kim M-S, Kim SY, Kim J-H, Park B, Choi HG. Depression in breast cancer patients who have undergone mastectomy: A national cohort study. *PLoS ONE*. 12(4):e0175395. https://doi.org/10.1371/journal.pone.0175395
6. Kruskal WH, Wallis WA. Use of ranks in one-criterion variance analysis. *J Am Stat Assoc*. 1952;*47*:583–621.
7. Sallinen J, Stenholm S, Rantanen T, Heliövaara M, Sainio P, Koskinen S. Hand-grip strength cut points to screen older persons at risk for mobility limitation. *J Am Geriatr Soc*. 2010;58(9):1721–1726.
8. Celis-morales CA, Welsh P, Lyall DM, et al. Associations of grip strength with cardiovascular, respiratory, and cancer outcomes and all cause mortality: prospective cohort study of half a million UK Biobank participants. *BMJ*. 2018;*361*:k1651.
9. Gale CR, Martyn CN, Cooper C, Sayer AA. Grip strength, body composition, and mortality. *Int J Epidemiol*. 2007;*36*(1):228–235.

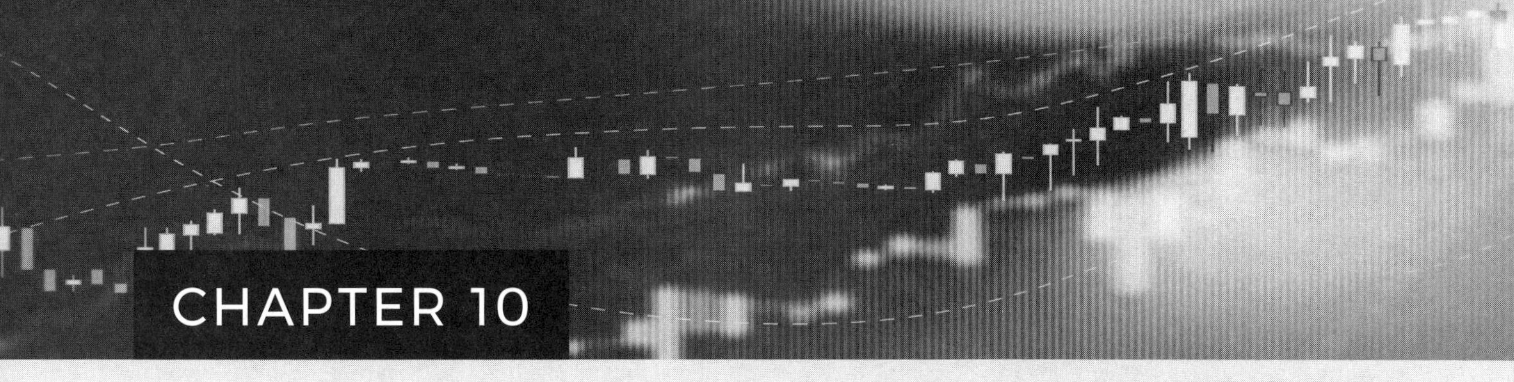

CHAPTER 10

Survey Research

KEY CONCEPTS

- A survey is a research method used to collect data by asking individuals questions in order to obtain information on selected topics.
- Health surveys can be useful for monitoring and assessing health-related information, which can then inform strategies to prevent and control health problems.
- A census survey involves the entire population. A sample survey accesses a subset of the population.
- A survey proposal is a written document that contains an abstract, administrative aspects involving the budget, budget justification, timeline, description and qualifications of the research team, and the study plan (protocol).
- A protocol describes the study design for the survey and consists of a statement of purpose and identification of the survey population; the sample size; the type of survey used; the content, questions, and layout; the steps to validate and pretest the instrument; the process of conducting the survey and cleaning the data; the analysis plan; and who will be informed of the survey results.
- A statement of the purpose for the survey should be supported by a description of what is already known about the topic and why new information is important. A review of the literature and focus groups can help in formulating survey questions that support the study objectives.
- The sample size should be large enough to meet the purpose and objectives of the survey.
- Types of surveys include questionnaires (mail, online/email) and interviews (telephone, face to face). A survey may be cross-sectional or longitudinal, based on probability or nonprobability sampling, and questions may be open- or closed-ended, factual or attitudinal.
- Rating scales typically involve asking respondents to rate abstract concepts, such as pain level, satisfaction, or level of agreement. Rating scales may be linear numerical, Likert, frequency, forced ranking, pick some, paired comparison, comparative scale/comparative intensity, semantic differential, adjective checklist, semantic distance, pictorial/graphic, visual analog/slider, and more.
- Cronbach's alpha is a measure of internal consistency—an indicator of scale reliability.
- Component analysis and common factor analysis are methods used to reduce dimensionality of a dataset to fewer unobserved constructs than variables.
- It is good practice to begin constructing a survey by writing a detailed list of information to be collected and the concepts to be measured. A list of variables and their classification (i.e., independent, dependent, confounder, moderator, and mediator) should be constructed.
- Survey questions should be answerable, unambiguous, and appropriately phrased. Avoid loaded questions, double-barreled questions, and questions with hidden assumptions.
- A new survey instrument requires pilot testing to assess its validity. Validity indicates how accurately a method measures something. Measures of validity include face validity, content validity, construct validity, and criterion validity.
- A response rate represents the number of completed surveys divided by the number of people making up the total sample. A completion rate is the number of completed surveys among respondents who entered the survey.
- Careful construction of the survey instrument can help avoid coverage error, sampling error, measurement error, nonresponse error, and data processing error.

KEY CONCEPTS (*Continued*)

- After the analysis is complete, a report should be prepared describing purpose, methods, results, discussion, and conclusions.
- Existing data are available to researchers from alternative sources rather than from their own original data collection. It is classified as secondary data, ancillary data, or systematic reviews.
- A meta-analysis is a statistical examination of data from a group of independent studies covering the same subject, with the intent of providing an overall summary measure.

A survey is a flexible method for collecting data from a specified group of respondents in order to gain information about selected topics of interest. For example, the National Health Interview Survey was used in 2019 to identify 9.5%, 3.4%, and 2.7% of adults who experienced mild, moderate, or severe anxiety in the previous 2 weeks, respectively.[1] The percentage of adults experiencing anxiety was greatest among those aged 18–29 years and decreased with older age. Women experienced higher levels of mild, moderate, or severe anxiety than did men. The percentage of adults experiencing any level of anxiety was greatest among non-Hispanic whites (16.5%), followed by non-Hispanic blacks (14.6%), Hispanics (14.5%), and then non-Hispanic Asians (8.5%).

A variety of survey methods are available, with application in a number of domains. Survey research can help us learn about knowledge, beliefs, attitudes, behaviors, traits, facts, etc. A health survey can enable us to identify health status, health behavior, health risk factors, health awareness, health knowledge, healthcare access, and healthcare quality. Health survey results can then be used to inform disease prevention and control efforts. In general, a health survey can help us assess, monitor, and formulate strategies to improve the health status of individuals, communities, and populations.

A survey may involve an entire population (census) or be carried out using a sample of the target population. Most surveys involving community, state, and national level data are sample surveys. The U.S. Census Bureau is currently carrying out several sample surveys, like the Household Pulse Survey, which is a new survey designed to efficiently collect data on how individual's lives are impacted by the COVID-19 pandemic.[2] Other examples of large-scale sample surveys will be presented later in this chapter.

The best scenario is to use an existing, validated instrument without modification to collect data and answer your research questions, if appropriate. For example, the RAND Corporation provides several validated health-related surveys, which are free and easily accessible from the public domain.[3] The advantage of using existing instruments is that it saves time, money, and makes results comparable. The disadvantage is that there may not be an existing instrument that is relevant to your study objectives. Sometimes research questions can be answered using secondary data, sometimes adding one or more questions to an existing survey instrument may be adequate, and sometimes a set of completed studies addressing a particular question can be summarized and conclusions made about a body of research.[4]

When existing data to address a research topic are not available, conducting your own survey may be necessary. Creating a survey instrument can be simple but is generally complex and time consuming and should only be done if an existing, relevant, and validated instrument is not available.

A certain process should be taken when carrying out a survey, which begins with a proposal—a document that contains a detailed study plan (protocol), researcher qualifications, budget, and timeline. It is a written document used for obtaining research funds. The portion of the proposal that is the study plan involves several steps, which will be covered in this chapter. In some cases, where funding is not necessary, it is still important to write a protocol in order to direct and focus the survey research and to acquire ethical approval.

The purpose of this chapter is to present the steps for conducting a survey. Types of existing data will be introduced. Some statistical methods used in creating and assessing survey data will also be presented.

10.1 Write a Proposal

Writing a proposal can take time and several iterations. It is an expanded version of a detailed written study protocol. Writing a proposal in the context of survey research forces the investigator to organize, clarify, and refine the elements of the survey. It guides the work and is important for obtaining funding and ethical approval from the institutional review board.

When biological and medical research funding is sought, it is typically obtained from one of four sources: the National Institutes of Health, foundations and societies, manufacturers of drugs and devices, or intramural funds. Proposals should be formatted according to the specific guidelines of the funding agency. Working with representatives from these funding agencies in preparing the proposal is strongly encouraged.

Major elements of a proposal are the abstract, administrative aspects involving the budget, budget justification, timeline, description and qualifications of the research team, and the study protocol.[5] The major elements of the written protocol consist of the survey's purpose; target population; sample size; type; content, questions, and layout; pretesting; conducting and cleaning the data; analyzing the data; and reporting the findings.[6] These items are interconnected. For example, the budget will influence the type of survey used and the length of the survey; the survey questions will influence the type of data obtained and the statistical procedures used for assessment; and the sample size and sampling method will influence the extent to which the sample results are generalizable to the target population.

10.2 Purpose of the Survey

The research process should begin with a clear understanding of the purpose of the survey. For example, the primary purpose of a health survey may be to monitor and assess health-related information, which can be used to formulate strategies to prevent and control health problems. Objectives should be specified, along with the information sought from the questions related to the objectives. For example, an objective may be to assess individuals' attitudes toward wearing face masks during the COVID-19 pandemic. Possible questions may be, "Do you wear a mask while in public?" If yes: "Does wearing a mask protect you from infection?" If no: "Wearing a mask is not effective at slowing the spread of SARS-COV-2." (Agree – Neutral – Disagree). "People do not wear masks because they are uncomfortable to wear." (Agree – Neutral – Disagree). "People do not wear masks because being required to do so violates civil liberties." (Agree – Neutral – Disagree).

The purpose of the study should be supported by a description of what is already known about the topic and, then, a mention of how the survey results will advance current knowledge and why it is important. Previous research should be cited and mention given to what uncertainties still remain. It needs to be clear as to how the survey will help resolve uncertainties and contribute to improved practice guidelines and health decisions.

A thorough review and synthesis of the literature often helps the investigator to refine and improve the rationale for the study. Sometimes focus groups representing the intended study population are helpful in focusing the purpose of a survey. They can also assist in formulating and interpreting questions in a survey.

A **focus group** is a group interview, generally conducted with a homogeneous collection of six to ten individuals whose responses can provide insights.

10.3 Survey Population

The survey population consists of those who are best suited to help address the purpose of the study. It should consist of those who can provide information and insights into a situation related to our topic of interest. The population may consist of healthcare workers, the elderly, Hispanics, workers, and so on. For example, one study conducted a survey of U.S. adults to learn about the prevalence, severity, and utilization of health care in relation to food allergies.[7] The International Public Opinion Survey on Cancer 2020 assessed what people currently feel, think, and believe about cancer, based on a sample of 15,427 people across 20 countries.[8] Another survey investigated the mental health impact of COVID-19 among healthcare workers in the United States.[9] The Pew Research Center Religious Landscape Study survey of religious groups in the United States identified information on demographic characteristics, religious beliefs, and frequency of faith-based practices.[10]

Population refers to a collection of individuals who share one or more personal or observational characteristics from which data may be collected and evaluated. Social, economic, family (marriage, and divorce), work and labor force, and geographic factors may characterize a population.

The **target population** is a large set of people to whom the results will be generalized. The **accessible population** is a geographically and temporally defined subset of the target population. These are the subjects who are available for study. A **survey sample** reflects a subset of the accessible population and comprises the participants in a study. The goal is to recruit a sample from the accessible population that represents the target population. It is very important to avoid nonresponse bias (nonrepresentative sample) and systematic sources of error (reoccurring inaccuracies in the same direction) in the survey. It is also critical that the number of subjects satisfy the sample size requirement. Having a sufficiently large sample size will control for spurious findings and random sources of error.

Nonresponse bias leads to a sample that is not representative of the target population.

Systematic errors are predictable, reoccurring inaccuracies in the same direction attributed to the instrument or process for measurement.

10.4 Sample Size

Sample size for a survey is based on the desired reliability of the estimates. However, large sample sizes are expensive, so sometimes the ideal sample size may be difficult to attain because of high survey costs. Yet, the sample size needs to be large enough to satisfy the purpose of the survey. The sample size should not exceed what is necessary to satisfy the desired precision (margin of error) and confidence level. Excessive sample size is wasteful in terms of time and money.

10.4.1 Sample Size Calculation

Sample size is determined by three things, the desired margin of error, the confidence level (typically 90%, 95%, or 99%), and variability of the characteristic being measured. The desired margin of error is the amount of error that is tolerated. A common margin of error is 5%. The margin of error is inversely related to sample size; that is, as sample size goes up, the margin of error goes down.

The confidence level refers to the amount of uncertainty that is tolerated. Consider a survey consisting of 20 "Yes" or "No" questions. A confidence level of 95% means that we would expect that for one of the questions, the percentage answering "Yes" would exceed the margin of error away from the truth. A true answer is what would occur if everyone in the population was interviewed.

Greater variance in the sample size calculation equates to a larger required sample size. When the sample size involves a proportion, 0.5 gives the largest sample size. When the proportion is not known, use 0.5. The process of calculating sample size for a proportion and mean are shown in **Table 10.1**.[11]

Table 10.1 Sample Size Calculations

Proportion	Formula	Example
	$n = \frac{z_{1-\alpha/2}^2 p(1-p)}{d^2}$ p = estimated proportion d = desired margin of error	$n = \frac{1.96^2 \times 0.5(1-0.5)}{0.05^2} = 384$
Mean	**Formula**	**Example**
	$n = \frac{z_{1-\alpha/2}^2 \sigma^2}{d^2}$ σ = standard deviation d = desired margin of error	$n = \frac{1.96^2 \times 2.5^2}{1^2} = 24$

If the sample fraction is greater than 0.05 (or 5%), then an adjustment to the sample size calculation is needed, which is

$$n' = \frac{n}{1 + n / N}$$

where,

n' = the final adjusted sample size
n = the sample size based on the formula in Table 10.1
N = the size of the total population from which the sample is drawn
n / N = the sampling fraction; ratio of the sample size to the population size

Example 10.1

Suppose you are interested in calculating the required sample size for a survey in which you are evaluating several "Yes" or "No" questions regarding attitudes around preventive measures for COVID-19 (e.g., masks should be worn any time while in public). The population from which the sample will be drawn is 5000. The desired margin of error is 5%, and the confidence level is 95%. You do not know the response distribution so use 50%. What is the required sample size?

$$n' = \frac{n}{1 + \frac{n}{N}} = \frac{384}{1 + \frac{384}{5000}} = 357$$

Therefore, if 50% of the people in a population of 5000 agree that masks should be worn while in public, and if the survey of 357 was repeated several times, then 95% of the time we would expect to find 45% to 55% of people in the survey to answer "Yes." For the remaining 5% of the time, we would expect the survey response to be greater than 0.05 away from the truth. In other words, we are 95% confident that the response is within 0.05 of the true answer.

If our experience indicates that 90% agree that masks should be worn in public, then the required sample size is 135; that is,

$$n' = \frac{138}{1 + 138 / 5000} = 135.$$

If we further changed the confidence level to 90%, then the required sample size is 96; that is,

$$n' = \frac{97}{1 + 97 / 5000} = 96.$$

Example 10.2

Suppose that you are interested in conducting a survey in which the primary variable of interest is mean IQ among a group of individuals who have been diagnosed with depression. What is the required size of the survey using a 99% confidence level, a margin of error of 3, and a standard deviation of 15? Assume the standard deviation of IQ was obtained from a study involving a similar group of people. The population size from which the sample is drawn is 2500.

$$n = \frac{2.576^2 \times 15^2}{3^2} = 166$$

$$n' = \frac{166}{1 + 166 / 2500} = 156$$

Therefore, the required sample size for a 99% confidence level within ±3 points, with a standard deviation for IQ of 15 points, is 156.

The equations presented are used for simple random sampling in which every member of the population has an equal chance of being included in the sample. Simple random sampling requires a sampling frame. Although this is a theoretically simple approach, it may not be feasible to obtain representation from subgroups of the population like race/ethnicity, and often a sampling frame may not be available.

10.4.2 Sample Size Calculation for Strata

In some cases, a simple random sample may not be effective at including adequate representation from all groups desired to be in the sample. Stratified random sampling is an alternative to simple random sampling that can help ensure representation of population subgroups. With this approach, the target population is divided into suitable, nonoverlapping strata. Each stratum should be homogeneous but heterogeneous with other strata. There are two types of stratified sampling: proportionate stratified sampling (the sample size drawn from each stratum is proportionate to the relative size of that stratum in the total population) and disproportionate stratified sampling (an equal sample size is drawn from each stratum). For proportionate stratified sampling, the strata sample sizes are determined as follows:

$$n_h = (N_h / N) \times n$$

where,
n_h = the sample size for stratum h
N_h = the population size for stratum h
N = the total population size
n = the total sample size

For disproportionate stratified samples, calculate a sample size for each stratum.

10.4.3 Sample Size Calculation for Clusters

Cluster sampling is useful when the population is geographically dispersed or when a sampling frame is not available. In cluster sampling, the population is divided into existing clusters (naturally forming externally homogeneous but internally heterogeneous groups from the population). A sample of the clusters is selected at random from the population. Then, those in the sampled clusters are included in the survey. For example, to sample a population of senior residents in assisted-living facilities, a sample of facilities can be selected, and then all the residents within each facility are sampled. This sampling approach would require less travel and time than simple random sampling.

Now suppose we are interested in sampling a group of school children where a sampling frame is not available. We can take a random sample of classrooms and then all of the children in each selected classroom are included in the survey. Because precision is lost with this approach, to maintain the same level of precision as in simple random sampling, double the sample size that would have been used for a simple random sample.[6]

10.5 Survey Method

A number of survey methods are available, producing different types of data. The data collection process may involve observation, measurement, evaluation, and judgment. Observation is a systematic way of obtaining data where subjects are observed in their natural situations or settings. Survey data may be measured on a categorical (nominal, ordinal) or continuous (interval, ratio) scale, and the type of data collected determines the method of evaluation. Judgmental (purposive) sampling is where the researcher selects subjects to be sampled based on their knowledge and professional expertise.

10.5.1 Questionnaire or Interview

There are two broad types of surveys: questionnaire and interview. The questionnaire consists of a list of questions that are administered through mail, online/email, telephone, or face to face. Much has been written about these various survey methods, their strengths, weaknesses, and areas of application.[12]

Mail surveys are becoming less common because of cost and poor response rates. Online/email surveys are becoming more popular than mail surveys because they are less expensive, more easily standardized, and the responses are fairly accurate. However, complicated questions may confuse respondents. Emailed questionnaires are a relatively easy way to collect data, which can be directly entered into a database. However, they can only be sent to people who have access to or familiarity with the internet. Questionnaires on websites or handheld devices are efficient and inexpensive, producing very clean data that can be automatically checked for missing or out-of-range values. Telephone surveys are still widely used, particularly with large-scale surveys. However, several factors have made telephone surveys more challenging to conduct, including caller identification and cell phones.

An interview is where the investigator asks a series of questions by phone or in person. Face-to-face interviews are useful in some situations, where the researcher is trying to understand more complex issues. However, this medium tends to be more costly, time consuming, and interviews may be inconsistently conducted.

Some important issues related to interviewing need mentioning. The interviewers need to be thoroughly trained so that the interviews are conducted in a standardized fashion. Interviewers also need to be taught how to locate the appropriate respondents and how to encourage them to participate and complete the survey. Standardizing the interview procedure is key to reproducibility. This involves using uniform wording or nonverbal signals. The interviewer should avoid changing words or tones in order to avoid introducing bias into the data. Probing (following-up to unclear answers) is an important part of the interview process, but it should be standardized, with phrases below each question. With computer-assisted telephone interviewing (CATI), the interviewer should follow a script, with the computer recording the data. If a study requires direct observation/examination (or if the participants do not have phones or if they are homeless), it may be necessary to conduct an in-person interview.

It should be emphasized that each survey method is susceptible to imperfect recall and respondents trying to give socially acceptable answers. There are ways to minimize these problems, such as making the survey anonymous in order to minimize respondents giving more socially correct responses.

10.5.2 Cross-Sectional or Longitudinal

A survey may involve a cross-sectional or a longitudinal assessment. A cross-sectional survey collects information from an accessible population at a given point in time. The researcher depends on cross-sectional research methods when interested in descriptive assessment of the respondents. Repeated cross-sectional surveys are called serial surveys. Longitudinal survey research is conducted with cohorts over a continuum of time, sometimes months or years. Behaviors, preferences, attitudes, knowledge, and beliefs are often observed and measured over time in order to identify change. For example, suppose you want to learn about the dietary practices of college students. Perhaps a cohort of college freshman could be followed over their college experience to identify patterns and trends.

10.5.3 Probability or Nonprobability Sampling

The selection of participants in a survey may be based on probability or nonprobability sampling, depending on the research objective. Probability sampling, defined as a random sampling technique used to create a sample, was presented in Chapter 3. Nonprobability sampling techniques include convenience sampling, snowball sampling, consecutive sampling, judgmental sampling, and quota sampling.

Nonprobability Sampling

Convenience sampling is where the researcher uses subjects who are readily available to participate in the study. **Snowball sampling** is where existing study subjects recruit other subjects from among their network of associates. **Consecutive sampling** is where each subject meeting the criteria for inclusion is selected into the study until the required sample size is met. **Judgmental sampling** is where the researcher chooses a sample from which the most can be learned (analogous to calling in the experts for their advice). **Quota sampling** is where the population is divided into exclusive subgroups that represent certain characteristics, the proportion of these subgroups in the population is identified, and samples are taken from these subgroups according to the proportions. It is a nonprobabilistic version of stratified sampling.

10.5.4 Question Types

Survey questions may be classified as open-ended or closed-ended. Open-ended questions open a conversation that provides more feedback (e.g., How do you feel about being vaccinated?). Closed-ended questions provide a nice way to collect information on a single response. Closed-ended questions can be classified as multiple-choice questions or rating scales. Multiple-choice questions are usually straightforward and involve concrete selections. They may involve a single response (e.g., Have you ever been told by a doctor that you have arthritis?), or a small set of possible responses (e.g., What is your marital status?). Sometimes "Yes" or "No" questions are appropriate, which are a way to segment your respondents. For example, say we are interested in understanding what barriers or objections are stopping individuals from being vaccinated. We can ask if something is stopping them from being vaccinated, and follow up with those who said "Yes" by asking them to either explain why in an open-ended question, or giving them some reasons to choose from in a closed-ended question.

Definitions

Open-ended questions are unstructured and solicit answers that are not suggested, wherein individuals respond in their own words.

Close-ended questions ask respondents to select from a list of predefined choices.

"Yes" or "No" questions are a quick way to segment respondents.

If the researcher wants to know about the frequency and pattern of a health problem, closed-ended multiple-choice questions may be best. If the researcher wants to explore how people feel about certain things, open-ended questions may be useful. Closed-ended questions have the advantage of being quicker and easier to answer, and analysis of the responses is straightforward, but they can limit respondents to answer a certain way. When constructing closed-ended questions, it is important that the answer choices be mutually exclusive and exhaustive. Open-ended questions can provide more information and have fewer limits but require qualitative methods or special systems to code and analyze the responses, and results may be more subjective. Surveys should include an appropriate balance of closed-ended and open-ended questions.

Survey questions may also be classified as factual (objective) or attitude (subjective). Factual questions require fact-based answers. These questions gather data that categorize or quantify subjects or events and can be independently verified according to correctness. For example, "What is your age?" "What is your sex?" "What is your race/ethnicity?" "Were you exposed?" "Did you manifest clinical symptoms?" "Was there a positive diagnosis?" "When did the event occur?" "What was the incubation period?" On the other hand, attitude questions are subjective and measure judgments, feelings, and perceptions. They are based on how individuals think, or what they experience. For example, "Why did you choose to start smoking?" or "How do you feel about retiring?" The type of question asked depends on the objective of the survey.

10.5.5 Rating Scales

Rating scales typically involve asking respondents to rate abstract concepts, such as pain level, satisfaction, or level of agreement. The types of rating scales include linear numerical, Likert, frequency, forced ranking, pick some, paired comparison, comparative scale/comparative intensity, semantic differential, adjective checklist, semantic distance, pictorial/graphic, and visual analog/slider (**Table 10.2**).[13]

Table 10.2 Types of Scale Measures

<table>
<tr><th>Scale</th><th>Definition</th><th>Example</th></tr>
<tr><td>Linear Numeric</td><td>Numeric response provided to a question or statement</td><td>How likely are you to recommend a dietary program?

Never Neutral Extremely likely
0 1 2 3 4 5 6 7 8 9 10</td></tr>
<tr><td>Likert</td><td>Special case of linear numeric–agreement to multiple statements</td><td>
<table>
<tr><th></th><th>No Problem</th><th>Mild</th><th>Moderate</th><th>Severe</th></tr>
<tr><td>Sleep apnea</td><td>0</td><td>1</td><td>2</td><td>3</td></tr>
<tr><td>Snoring</td><td>0</td><td>1</td><td>2</td><td>3</td></tr>
<tr><td>Daytime sleepiness</td><td>0</td><td>1</td><td>2</td><td>3</td></tr>
</table></td></tr>
<tr><td>Multiple Rating Matrix</td><td>Way to present multiple linear numeric items and is a typical method for presenting Likert items</td><td>Rate your attitude toward each of the following contributing to voice problems.
<table>
<tr><th></th><th>Not at All</th><th></th><th></th><th></th><th></th><th></th><th></th><th></th><th></th><th></th><th>Major Cause</th><th>N/A</th></tr>
<tr><td>Exercise</td><td>0</td><td>1</td><td>2</td><td>3</td><td>4</td><td>5</td><td>6</td><td>7</td><td>8</td><td>9</td><td>10</td><td>___</td></tr>
<tr><td>Cold weather</td><td>0</td><td>1</td><td>2</td><td>3</td><td>4</td><td>5</td><td>6</td><td>7</td><td>8</td><td>9</td><td>10</td><td>___</td></tr>
<tr><td>Fumes or odors</td><td>0</td><td>1</td><td>2</td><td>3</td><td>4</td><td>5</td><td>6</td><td>7</td><td>8</td><td>9</td><td>10</td><td>___</td></tr>
<tr><td>Stress</td><td>0</td><td>1</td><td>2</td><td>3</td><td>4</td><td>5</td><td>6</td><td>7</td><td>8</td><td>9</td><td>10</td><td>___</td></tr>
<tr><td>Acid reflux</td><td>0</td><td>1</td><td>2</td><td>3</td><td>4</td><td>5</td><td>6</td><td>7</td><td>8</td><td>9</td><td>10</td><td>___</td></tr>
<tr><td>Allergies</td><td>0</td><td>1</td><td>2</td><td>3</td><td>4</td><td>5</td><td>6</td><td>7</td><td>8</td><td>9</td><td>10</td><td>___</td></tr>
</table></td></tr>
<tr><td>Frequency</td><td>How often actions are performed or events occur</td><td>How often do you experience ___________?
<table>
<tr><th></th><th>Never</th><th>Yearly</th><th>Monthly</th><th>Weekly</th><th>Daily</th></tr>
<tr><td>Hoarseness</td><td>0</td><td>1</td><td>2</td><td>3</td><td>4</td></tr>
<tr><td>Tired voice</td><td>0</td><td>1</td><td>2</td><td>3</td><td>4</td></tr>
<tr><td>Change in voice quality</td><td>0</td><td>1</td><td>2</td><td>3</td><td>4</td></tr>
<tr><td>Difficulty projecting voice</td><td>0</td><td>1</td><td>2</td><td>3</td><td>4</td></tr>
<tr><td>Discomfort using voice</td><td>0</td><td>1</td><td>2</td><td>3</td><td>4</td></tr>
</table></td></tr>
<tr><td>Forced Ranking</td><td>A method for prioritizing preferences</td><td>In thinking about health, rank the following from most (1) to least (6) important.
<table>
<tr><td>Physical</td><td>___</td></tr>
<tr><td>Social</td><td>___</td></tr>
<tr><td>Mental</td><td>___</td></tr>
<tr><td>Emotional</td><td>___</td></tr>
<tr><td>Spiritual</td><td>___</td></tr>
<tr><td>Environmental</td><td>___</td></tr>
</table></td></tr>
</table>

(*Continues*)

Table 10.2 Types of Scale Measures *(Continued)*

<table>
<thead>
<tr><th>Scale</th><th>Definition</th><th>Example</th></tr>
</thead>
<tbody>
<tr>
<td>Pick Some</td>
<td>With a long list of choices to rank (e.g., 10 or more), respondents select a fixed subset (e.g., 3, or 5)</td>
<td>Which of the following triggers your cough? Rank your top FIVE (with 1 being the greatest contributor).
<table>
<tr><td>Exercise</td><td>___</td></tr>
<tr><td>Cold weather</td><td>___</td></tr>
<tr><td>Fumes or odors</td><td>___</td></tr>
<tr><td>Stress</td><td>___</td></tr>
<tr><td>Acid reflux</td><td>___</td></tr>
<tr><td>Allergies</td><td>___</td></tr>
<tr><td>Sinus/nasal drainage</td><td>___</td></tr>
<tr><td>Talking</td><td>___</td></tr>
<tr><td>Laughing</td><td>___</td></tr>
<tr><td>Singing</td><td>___</td></tr>
<tr><td>Humidity</td><td>___</td></tr>
<tr><td>Eating dry foods</td><td>___</td></tr>
</table>
</td>
</tr>
<tr>
<td>Paired Comparison</td>
<td>Forces a choice between two alternatives</td>
<td>Of the two pain medications you have used, which do you prefer?
Medication A ___
Medication B ___</td>
</tr>
<tr>
<td>Comparative Scale/ Comparative Intensity</td>
<td>Respondents rate their preference and level of preference</td>
<td>In thinking about the following attributes of CPAP and dental appliance, which do you prefer for treating your obstructive sleep apnea?
<table>
<tr><th></th><th>Strongly Prefer CPAP</th><th>Prefer Neither</th><th>Strongly Prefer Dental Appliance</th></tr>
<tr><td>Cost</td><td>1</td><td>2</td><td>3</td></tr>
<tr><td>Effectiveness</td><td>1</td><td>2</td><td>3</td></tr>
<tr><td>Comfort</td><td>1</td><td>2</td><td>3</td></tr>
</table>
</td>
</tr>
<tr>
<td>Semantic Differential</td>
<td>Used to assess where respondents fall on a continuum of adjectives or attributes (requires polar opposites)</td>
<td>In thinking about your fitness class, how would you rate each of the following attributes?
<table>
<tr><th></th><th>1</th><th>2</th><th>3</th><th>4</th><th>5</th><th></th></tr>
<tr><td>Physically demanding</td><td>o</td><td>o</td><td>o</td><td>o</td><td>o</td><td>Not physically demanding</td></tr>
<tr><td>Socially enjoyable</td><td>o</td><td>o</td><td>o</td><td>o</td><td>o</td><td>Not socially enjoyable</td></tr>
<tr><td>Worth the time</td><td>o</td><td>o</td><td>o</td><td>o</td><td>o</td><td>Not worth the time</td></tr>
</table>
</td>
</tr>
</tbody>
</table>

Table 10.2 Types of Scale Measures ***(Continued)***

<table>
<tr><th>Scale</th><th>Definition</th><th>Example</th></tr>
<tr><td>Adjective Checklist</td><td>Used instead of assigning opposite adjectives</td><td>Which of the following best describes your experience in the fitness class?
<table><tr><td>Demanding</td><td>___</td></tr><tr><td>Worthwhile</td><td>___</td></tr><tr><td>Fun</td><td>___</td></tr><tr><td>Sociable</td><td>___</td></tr><tr><td>Burdensome</td><td>___</td></tr></table></td></tr>
<tr><td>Semantic Distance</td><td>A way to avoid finding polar opposites</td><td>How would you describe the instructions provided with your medication? (1 low and 7 high)
<table><tr><th></th><th>1</th><th>2</th><th>3</th><th>4</th><th>5</th><th>6</th><th>7</th></tr><tr><td>Helpful</td><td>o</td><td>o</td><td>o</td><td>o</td><td>o</td><td>o</td><td>o</td></tr><tr><td>Frustrating</td><td>o</td><td>o</td><td>o</td><td>o</td><td>o</td><td>o</td><td>o</td></tr><tr><td>Complicated</td><td>o</td><td>o</td><td>o</td><td>o</td><td>o</td><td>o</td><td>o</td></tr><tr><td>Understandable</td><td>o</td><td>o</td><td>o</td><td>o</td><td>o</td><td>o</td><td>o</td></tr></table></td></tr>
<tr><td>Pictorial/Graphic</td><td>Instead of selecting a number, respondents select from pictures</td><td><table><tr><td>0</td><td>2</td><td>4</td><td>6</td><td>8</td><td>10</td></tr><tr><td>No hurt</td><td>Hurts little bit</td><td>Hurts little more</td><td>Hurts even more</td><td>Hurts whole lot</td><td>Hurts worst</td></tr></table>Reproduced from Wong-Baker FACES. https://wongbakerfaces.org/</td></tr>
<tr><td>Visual Analog/Slider</td><td>A linear numerical scale without discrete points</td><td>8.7
1 Poor — 10 Excellent
How would you rate your health?</td></tr>
</table>

Data from Sauro J. 15 Common Rating Scales Explained. Measuring U. https://measuringu.com/rating-scales/.

All of us are familiar with rating scales like these. Rating scales may be simple or complex. A simple rating scale may assign people as having excellent health, good health, fair health, or poor health; to different levels of marital status; or as satisfied, neutral, or not satisfied. Sometimes a complex rating scale is needed to understand an issue like voice quality, quality of life, or socio-economic status. For example, quality of life reflects various dimensions (e.g., physical, social, mental). Although each measure explains some of the concept, any one of these indicators alone fails to reflect the complexity of quality of life. However, together the indicators may be combined to produce a single scale measure of quality of life.

One example of a complex scale involves the Medical Outcomes Study Short Form 36 (SF-36) survey, a psychometrically validated questionnaire, developed to assess two overall summary scale components of quality of life (Physical Health and Mental Health), and four subscales for each of these indicators.[14]

Physical health subscales consist of physical function, role-physical, bodily pain, and general health. Mental health subscales consist of vitality, social functioning, role-emotional, and mental health. Each of the quality-of-life measures is converted to a 0 to 100 scale, with 100 representing highest quality of life for that domain measure. For example, a score of 100 on the physical functioning score is obtained by performing all types of physical activity, including the most vigorous without limitations due to health; for the role-physical score by having no problems with work or other daily activities; for the bodily pain scale by having no pain or limitations due to pain; the general health scale by evaluating personal health as excellent; the energy/fatigue scale by feeling full of "pep" and energy all the time; the social functioning scale by performing normal social activities without interference from physical or emotional problems; the role–emotional scale by having no problems with work or other daily activities as a result of emotional problems; and the mental health scale by feeling peaceful, happy, and calm all of the time.

10.6 Cronbach's Alpha

The reliability of a measure can be determined by administering a certain scale two or more times to the same sample respondent to assess response to a score on a variable. Yet, in survey research, administering a scale multiple times is unlikely because of time, cost, and reaction of the respondents. Alternatively, reliability can be measured with respect to internal consistency. A statistic commonly used to evaluate internal consistency is Cronbach's alpha.

Definitions

A **reliability** measure indicates whether a respondent's score on a variable would be the same if the survey were administered again and again.

Internal consistency indicates that all the variables (items) vary according to direction, with a meaningful statistical level of correlation with each other.

Cronbach's alpha is a statistical test that is used to assess how well items in a scale are correlated.[15] Cronbach's alpha is calculated as

$$\alpha = \frac{n\overline{r}}{1+\overline{r}(n-1)}$$

where *n* is the number of items and $\overline{r}$ is the average inter-correlation among the items. Cronbach's alpha ranges from 0 to 1. A value of 1 means that all the items composing the scale are perfectly correlated with each other. As a rule of thumb, the level of internal consistency (reliability) is indicated by **Table 10.3**. For example, a group of individuals were given a survey asking different questions about religious beliefs and practices. High reliability among these questions means that the items are measuring the same underlying construct, which we may choose to call overall religiosity.

Cronbach's alpha is a measure of internal consistency, which shows how closely items among a set of survey items are related. It is an indicator of scale reliability.

Table 10.3 Cronbach's Alpha for Evaluating Internal Consistency

Cronbach's Alpha	Internal Consistency
$\alpha \geq 0.9$	Excellent
$0.9 > \alpha \geq 0.8$	Good
$0.8 > \alpha \geq 0.7$	Acceptable
$0.7 > \alpha \geq 0.6$	Questionable
$0.6 > \alpha \geq 0.5$	Poor
$0.5 > \alpha$	Unacceptable

A large number of items can artificially inflate the estimated alpha, whereas a small number can deflate the estimated alpha. In addition, if the alpha approaches 1, this may indicate redundancy among the items. So, this rating of internal consistency should be viewed as a guide, and the goal is to include items that are internally consistent, but that also provide unique information about what is being measured.

Imagine, for example, that we want to measure how well three questions on the Oxford Happiness Questionnaire correlate.[16] A construct is a belief or characteristic that cannot be used as a variable on its own—only through surrogate variables (other examples might include self-confidence, religiosity, or depression). We select from the survey three questions that we believe will help us to understand who is "happy" and who is not, according to our own definition of happiness. These questions follow:

Rate how strongly you agree or disagree with the following three statements:

1. I am intensely interested in other people.
   a. Strongly Agree
   b. Moderately Agree
   c. Slightly Agree
   d. Slightly Disagree
   e. Moderately Disagree
   f. Strongly Disagree
2. I feel that life is very rewarding.
   a. Strongly Agree
   b. Moderately Agree
   c. Slightly Agree
   d. Slightly Disagree
   e. Moderately Disagree
   f. Strongly Disagree
3. I laugh a lot.
   a. Strongly Agree
   b. Moderately Agree
   c. Slightly Agree
   d. Slightly Disagree
   e. Moderately Disagree
   f. Strongly Disagree

In order to know whether or not these questions are internally consistent—that is, that they all get at the same idea—we can use Cronbach's alpha. Let us imagine that we find that Cronbach's alpha for these three questions is 0.71. This means that respondents who agreed with question 1 generally also agreed with questions 2 and 3, which shows that the questions seem to be "getting at" the same concept. However, if we find that Cronbach's alpha is low, such as 0.35, this would mean that respondents who agreed with one question frequently disagreed with the others, showing that the test questions were not well correlated.

Most major statistical software packages will calculate Cronbach's alpha. If we use SAS procedure code to estimate Cronbach's alpha, we will select the ALPHA option with the CORR procedure. The output provides both the estimated alpha as well as an estimated standardized alpha. If the variances of some of the variables vary widely, we should use the standardized score to estimate reliability. This standardized alpha coefficient tells us how each variable reflects the reliability of the scale with standardized variables.

Example 10.3

For this example we will use the CORR procedure in SAS. Suppose the following responses to the questions in this section were obtained for eight individuals.

Subject	Q1	Q2	Q3
1	2	3	5
2	3	2	3
3	4	4	3
4	1	1	1
5	5	6	4
6	5	4	4
7	3	3	2
8	2	2	1

To compute Cronbach's alpha using SAS, a data set was created and the following procedure code applied to the data:

```
PROC CORR ALPHA DATA=EX_10_3;
VAR Q1 Q2 Q3;
RUN;
```

Partial SAS output is presented here.

Simple Statistics						
Variable	N	Mean	Std Dev	Sum	Minimum	Maximum
Q1	8	3.12500	1.45774	25.00000	1.00000	5.00000
Q2	8	3.12500	1.55265	25.00000	1.00000	6.00000
Q3	8	2.87500	1.45774	23.00000	1.00000	5.00000

Cronbach Coefficient Alpha	
Variables	Alpha
Raw	0.869222
Standardized	0.868162

Cronbach Coefficient Alpha with Deleted Variable				
	Raw Variables		Standardized Variables	
Deleted Variable	Correlation with Total	Alpha	Correlation with Total	Alpha
Q1	0.791029	0.778846	0.785378	0.779792
Q2	0.861411	0.706522	0.861411	0.706522
Q3	0.613445	0.932773	0.611954	0.933763

The standard deviations are similar, so the raw and standardized Cronbach's alpha estimates are similar. The value of 0.869 indicates that there is good internal consistency among the three variables. The last table indicates that if the third question was dropped, Cronbach's alpha would increase to 0.934, for example. Hence, removing this question would make the construct more reliable.

10.7 Factor Analysis

Suppose we want to know if the variables of a survey have similar patterns of responses. Is there a factor that can explain the interrelationship among a set of variables? For example, do a set of items together measure a construct such as intelligence or anxiety. Factor analysis is a process of reducing several variables into a fewer number of dimensions. It can help condense the size of a questionnaire and the number of variables included in the analysis. The process is sometimes referred to as "dimension reduction," in which the dimensions of your data may be reduced into one or more unobserved (latent) variables. In other words, factor analysis helps identify latent factors that drive observable variables. For example, does a set of items actually measure what we call voice-related quality of life (V-RQOL)?

In factor analysis we gain a better understanding of how different underlying factors impact the variance among a select group of variables. Although each factor will have an influence, some will explain more variance than others. Those factors with higher variance will more accurately reflect the variables it comprises. To achieve the goal of factor extraction from a set of data, different methods are available: principal component analysis, common factor analysis, image factoring, maximum likelihood, and others. The most commonly used method, which will be used in this chapter, is principle component analysis. It starts by extracting the maximum variance and putting it into the first factor. Removing the variance explained by the first factor, it then extracts the maximum variance for the second factor. This process continues to the last factor.[17]

The level of variance a factor explains is reflected by an **eigenvalue**. An eigenvalue of at least 1 means the factor explains more variance than any one variable. If the eigenvalue is less than 1, it accounts for less variance than a single variable, so that factor is not retained.

A **factor score** (loading) is the numerical value that indicates how strongly a given variable relates to a factor. Each factor should have three or more variables with high factor loading (typically at least |0.4|) on at least one of the factors. If the variable does not reach this level, it may be deleted. Variables that load on a single factor are related to one another and can be grouped together based on their conceptual knowledge. In addition, each variable should have at least 20 observations to ensure stable results. Principal component analysis can result in correlated components. When two or more correlated components are retained in the analysis, the interpretation can be difficult. To facilitate interpretation a process called rotation can be used. A **rotation** is a linear transformation of the factor result that makes the solution easier to interpret. Varimax rotation will be used in the following example. It is an orthogonal rotation, which means its results are uncorrelated components.

Example 10.4

For this example, we will use the FACTOR procedure in SAS to perform principal components analysis.

The V-RQOL measure is an indicator based on 10 questions about the voice, according to the voice occurrence within the past two weeks. Subjects respond to each of the questions on a 5-point scale (1 = none, 2 = small amount, 3 = moderate amount, 4 = a lot, and 5 = as bad as can be). For a sample of 94 respondents, the following SAS code was applied:

```
PROC FACTOR FUZZ=.4 NFACTORS=2 ROTATE=VARIMAX OUT=DATA;
VAR Q1-Q10;
RUN;
```

Partial output shows the eigenvalues. By convention the number of factors selected equal the number eigenvalues that are at least one.

The FACTOR Procedure
Initial Factor Method: Principal Components

Prior Communality Estimates: ONE

Eigenvalues of the Correlation Matrix: Total = 10 Average = 1				
	Eigenvalue	Difference	Proportion	Cumulative
1	5.68465127	4.49142917	0.5685	0.5685
2	1.19322210	0.23029082	0.1193	0.6878
3	0.96293127	0.27353479	0.0963	0.7841
4	0.68939648	0.32085046	0.0689	0.8530
5	0.36854602	0.02518594	0.0369	0.8899
6	0.34336008	0.08032810	0.0343	0.9242
7	0.26303197	0.07120605	0.0263	0.9505
8	0.19182592	0.02212774	0.0192	0.9697
9	0.16969818	0.03636146	0.0170	0.9867
10	0.13333672		0.0133	1.0000

In this example, two components (factors) appeared, so the program was rewritten with NFACTOR = 2 to produce the results that follow. After the factors are extracted, the aim is to obtain a simple structure that makes interpretability more straightforward. Specifically, the ROTATE = VARIMAX option was used. Again, rotations help minimize the complexity of the factor loadings, making the structure easier to interpret. The FUZZ = .4 option only reports factor loadings whose value is at least |.4|. If both factors were to have had a factor loading less than 0.4 for a given item, this question should be deleted. The following results show loadings for two factors.

Rotated Factor Pattern			
		Factor1	Factor2
Q1	Do you have trouble speaking loudly or being heard in noisy situations?	0.83411	.
Q2	Do you run out of air and need to take frequent breaths when talking?	0.73039	.
Q3	Do you not know what will come out when you begin speaking?	0.67043	.
Q4	Do you get anxious or frustrated?	0.79493	0.42655
Q5	Do you get depressed?	0.47356	0.63845
Q6	Do you have trouble using the telephone?	0.49907	0.58106
Q7	Do you have trouble doing your job or practicing your profession?	0.71178	0.49218
Q8	Do you avoid going out socially?	.	0.88163
Q9	Do you have to repeat yourself to be understood?	0.72976	.
Q10	Have you become less outgoing?	.	0.80521
Values less than 0.4 are not printed.			

We can name the factors based on the variables loading high on each factor. Factor1 represents a construct we could label as "Trouble Speaking," and Factor2 represents a construct we could label as "Social Consequences." Therefore, the 10 variables can be represented by two factors.

Also included in the output are the standardized scoring coefficients. These are used to compute values on each factor that are put back into the data set for each respondent. In the output data set, called "DATA," two factor variables are included. In subsequent analyses, values for these two factors can be used rather than all 10 variables.

Standardized Scoring Coefficients			
		Factor1	Factor2
Q1	Do you have trouble speaking loudly or being heard in noisy situations?	0.40590	-0.33783
Q2	Do you run out of air and need to take frequent breaths when talking?	0.20123	-0.02351
Q3	Do you not know what will come out when you begin speaking?	0.19485	-0.03947
Q4	Do you get anxious or frustrated?	0.21217	-0.01349
Q5	Do you get depressed?	0.00170	0.21218
Q6	Do you have trouble using the telephone?	0.03157	0.17102
Q7	Do you have trouble doing your job or practicing your profession?	0.15421	0.05108
Q8	Do you avoid going out socially?	-0.25527	0.48253
Q9	Do you have to repeat yourself to be understood?	0.19738	-0.01697
Q10	Have you become less outgoing?	-0.15448	0.38283

10.8 Content

The content making up the survey depends on the purpose and corresponding objectives of the survey. Questions should be included if they help address the main objectives of the study. It is good practice to begin constructing a survey by writing a detailed list of information to be collected and the concepts to be measured. The first draft of an instrument should have a broad reach, with more questions than will be ultimately included in the study. The investigator should answer each question as a respondent and imagine how they may be misinterpreted. It is also good practice to have colleagues and experts in questionnaire design review the instrument for face, content, and construct validity. The process of developing a survey should involve revising and shortening the set of items in the questionnaire.

The variables associated with the survey questions will each play a unique role. A variable may be independent or dependent. Variation in the independent variable does not depend on another variable. Variation in the dependent variable depends on another variable. A variable may also be a confounder, mediator, or moderator. Each of these types of variables should be included in the survey. We determine the role of these variables according to experience and theory. A third variable is a confounder if it produces a spurious (distorted) association between two variables. For example, the association between sleep deprivation and reaction time may be explained by cigarette smoking. A third variable is a mediator if it mediates the relationship between the independent variable and the dependent variable. For example, diet influences the risk of polyps, which, in turn, affects the risk of colon cancer. Finally, a moderator is a third variable that moderates the association between an independent and dependent variable. For example, coffee drinking is associated with heart disease among smokers but not among nonsmokers. The direction and nature of associations are theoretical causal concepts.

10.9 Things to Consider When Writing Questions

Writing questions that are clear and get at what you want to measure is imperative. Writing a clear and concise question takes care. This section provides some things to consider when writing your questions.

10.9.1 Ask Questions That Can Be Answered

Survey questions should be answerable. It may be that survey respondents do not have the information to answer a question. For example, most people probably cannot accurately answer how many times they had a drink of water in a day, but they can give a vague response (never, rarely, sometimes, or often).

Many people will forget information about the distant past. For example, although some might remember whether they regularly ate at least five or more servings of fruit and vegetables per day a year ago, many will not. Questions that require long-term memory should be avoided. In addition, associating events in time may be difficult. For example, although I might remember being screened for a certain disease, I may not remember well the exact time I was screened.

10.9.2 Social Desirability Bias

Survey research is sometimes susceptible to the threat of social desirability bias. This occurs if individuals answer questions in a way they think is socially acceptable. Respondents tend to over-report good behavior (e.g., I exercise every day) and under-report negative behavior (e.g., I drink soda whenever I eat at a restaurant). Possible ways to minimize this bias is to include a statement as to why the question is being asked; indicate that the survey is anonymous; put sensitive and demographic questions at the end; and encourage honest answers.

10.9.3 Avoid Ambiguity

Survey questions should be clear and concise in order to avoid a poor response rate and inaccurate answers. Providing instructions, definitions, and examples may help to avoid ambiguity. For example, "A voice disorder is when voice quality, pitch, and loudness differs from what you believe is normal for your age, sex, cultural background, or geographic location.[18] "Have you experienced a voice disorder in the past week?"

10.9.4 Phrasing of Questions

In order to avoid negatively impacting the validity and reproducibility of the responses, the wording of questions should be simple, clear, neutral, free of ambiguity, and encourage accurate and honest responses. When questions are about frequency of behavior, they must include a unit of time, such as on a typical day or during the last 7 days. Diaries can be more accurate, though time consuming. Further, survey questions need to be phrased appropriately. In particular, avoid **loaded questions** in which a respondent may be placed in a situation where they are pushed to confirm an argument to which they may not agree. For example, "Do you think there is less frequent mask wearing during the COVID-19 pandemic because of the community's poor levels of education?" This question is problematic because it requires the respondent to agree that the community has poor education. It also imposes a causal association between mask wearing and education that the respondent may not see.

Double-barreled questions are difficult to answer because a person may agree with part of the question but not the other. For example, "Do you consistently exercise and get adequate sleep?" This question should be separated into two questions.

Questions with **hidden assumptions** should be avoided. Such a question may cause the respondent to answer a question incorrectly or not answer at all. For example, a respondent may be asked to indicate their level of agreement with the statement, "Wearing a mask is wrong because it is unnatural." This is not a valid statement because it contains the hidden assumption that unnatural things are wrong.

Questions should avoid biasing the respondent with your opinion or triggering emotional responses.[19] For example, "Do you agree that mandatory mask wearing is a violation of our inalienable rights?" Such a question has the potential of leading the respondent to a biased answer.

Allow respondents to skip questions that do not apply to them.

Questions should focus on individuals' firsthand knowledge rather than secondhand knowledge, with which they may be unfamiliar.[19] For example, rather than ask, "Does your community have a problem adhering to the mask mandate?" a better question may be, "Do you regularly wear a mask while in public?"

Hypothetical questions should also be avoided because individuals tend to have a hard time predicting future behavior, especially for situations they have not experienced.[18] For example, "If you were moved into an administrative position in the company that requires more meetings, would you spend less time exercising each week?" In addition to having a difficult time predicting future behavior, their response is likely very situational, such as would the new position really result in less time to exercise, does the person need to exercise more, does the time of year and corresponding weather conditions influence exercise, and so on.

10.10 Layout

The format of the survey instrument should reflect several features:

1. A concise and clear title.
2. A place for recording informed consent.
3. Clear and concise survey instructions. In some situations, it may be helpful to provide an example of how to complete a question.
4. Sufficient white space.
5. Emotionally neutral questions near the start and sensitive questions toward the end.
6. Important questions early in order to improve the chance of obtaining that information in the event the respondent does not complete the survey.
7. Questions concerning major subject areas grouped together, one topic at a time, with transitional phrases from one topic to the next.
8. Easy way to complete responses.
9. Avoidance of questions that may influence responses on subsequent questions.
10. Questions ordered from factual to attitudinal to behavioral.

10.11 Pretest

Newly formulated questions require pilot testing. Pilot studies are used to assess an instruments validity and reliability. Pretesting an instrument indicates whether the respondents understand the questions as they were intended to be understood. Pretesting can also identify errors in the questionnaire and whether answer choices produce an adequate range.

A **pilot test** is a smaller preliminary study that evaluates a proposed research study prior to its full-scale administration.

Validity indicates how accurately a method measures something. If a survey measures what it claims to measure, then the instrument is considered valid. To validate a survey instrument, we consider face validity, content validity, construct validity, and criterion validity.

Face validity is whether the measurements are inherently reasonable.

Content validity is how well the measurements represent the phenomena under study.

Construct validity is the degree to which the measurements agree with a theoretical construct, thereby measuring what it claims to measure.

Criterion validity is the extent to which a measure of interest is related to a measure of established validity (a known standard).

An instrument has face validity if it "appears" to be effective at achieving its stated objectives. Suppose a primary objective of a survey is to measure a person's aptitude for a certain type of work. If the survey "looks like" it is going to be effective at accomplishing this aim, it has face validity. Content validity is when an instrument is fully representative of what it is aiming to measure. If a survey is intended to measure the affective dimension of depression, to have content validity it must capture the different dimensions of depression: psychological symptoms (e.g., depressed mood, feelings of worthlessness, guilt), cognitive symptoms (e.g., impaired ability to concentrate or think), and neuro-vegetative symptoms (e.g., sleep problems, fatigue, low energy, changes in appetite).[20] Construct validity assesses whether an instrument measures the concept it claims to measure. A survey intended to measure quality of life has construct validity if high scores on a set of items reflect greater quality of life. Criterion validity is established if the results correspond with a different test measuring the same thing. For example, a new screening test could be statistically analyzed against a standard screening test. If the new screening test produces similar results as the standard, it has criterion validity.

10.12 Conduct the Survey

Once the survey instrument is completed, a sample size determined, and permissions obtained, the survey can be administered through the chosen method (mail, online/email, or interview). High response rates and survey completions are critical to obtain survey results that are representative of the target population

10.12.1 Response Rate

A response rate should accompany the written report of the results of every survey. A **response rate** represents the number of completed surveys divided by the number of people who make up the total sample group (usually expressed as a percentage). For example, a survey was sent online to 1000 employees. The number of respondents who started the survey was 500. The number who completed the survey was 400. The response rate is 50%.

A **completion rate** is the number of completed surveys among respondents who entered the survey. In this example, the completion rate is 80%.

A low response rate means a higher margin of error and poorer reliability. Understanding why people are not responding to the survey is the first step to improving the response rate. It may be that the survey does not appear to be professional, interesting, or from a credible entity. It may also cover a sensitive topic, not be anonymous, or simply be interpreted by the computer as spam. When there is a low response rate, it can indicate a nonresponse bias. Nonresponse bias occurs when statistics estimated from the survey are biased due to the responders being different from the nonresponders in how they answer the questions.

A low completion rate means that respondents are not completing some of the questions in the survey. In this case, questions with a lower number of responses will have lower reliability. A low completion rate means your survey respondents do not like the length, organization, or content of the instrument. Focus groups and pilot testing the instrument should help identify and minimize these problems. Incentives are also an important means for increasing the response and completion rates.

10.12.2 Minimizing Errors

Survey data may be entered into the computer during the process of data collection or after the data are completed. To minimize data entry errors, double-data entry may be used, which means the data are entered twice, by different people. Then, discrepancies are checked and resolved. This process of data entry by hand is less common these days because of the availability of computer programs that are used for both data entry and editing at the same time. For example, programs like Epi Info usually lists the question from the survey on the computer and allows movement to the next question only if the response is acceptable. An acceptable entry may be an entry of 1–5, but if another number is entered, the respondent cannot proceed; a male cannot subsequently say that they have had a diagnosis of cervical cancer; or a person indicating they are a nonsmoker cannot later say they smoke one or more cigarettes per day. The computer program may show where errors are most likely to occur, such that the survey can be revised to minimize these errors.

Some errors may not be caught with a computer program, such as a data entry error within the range of possible choices. These misclassified responses may never be caught. To minimize these errors, instructions should be clear, questions written to minimize bias, and sufficient time, without distractions, provided.

An initial look at the data using frequency distribution tables will identify missing responses and outliers, which may be checked with the completed questionnaires before the main data analysis begins. Even in the analysis stage of the study, it may be useful to return to the original questionnaire to check questionable results. However, destroying cover letters containing personal identifying information should be done once the data entry and edits are complete.

Consistently applied standards in recruitment and training of those who will conduct the survey is an important part of the quality control process. In addition, proper review and evaluation will ensure that the survey is carried out as planned in the study design. Implementing quality control procedures at all stages of the survey can help minimize errors resulting in inaccurate results.

If the survey is conducted carefully, some broad categories of errors can be avoided: coverage error, sampling error, measurement error, nonresponse error, and data processing error.[6,21]

Definitions

Coverage error occurs if the sample is not representative of the target population. An inaccurate sampling frame will contribute to this type of error.

Sampling error occurs when the sample is selected in a way so that some individuals are less likely to be included than others. Sampling error is related to the design and size of the survey.

Measurement error is the difference between the true value and the actual value. Questions that are unclear, sensitive, threatening, or require recalling things from the distant past, and interviewers who are authoritative or inconsistent are a primary source of measurement error.

Nonresponse error refers to responders differing from non-responders in an important way. Ways to minimize nonresponse and loss to follow-up in our sample include choosing a design that avoids invasive and uncomfortable tests, allaying individual concerns, and providing incentives.

Data processing error may occur because of incorrect transcription, coding, data entry, or arithmetic tabulation. The availability of computer programs (e.g., Epi Info) for both data entry and editing greatly lower the risk of data processing error. Coding open-ended questions may require training and supervision from an experienced coder.

10.13 Analysis Plan

Open-ended questions will require coding the answers by assigning labels to the responses and organizing them into categories or themes. Closed-ended questions are more directly assessed using the statistical techniques covered in this book. Survey data are typically described using tables, graphs, and summary statistics. A number of statistical measures of association may also be applied to the data. Statistical analysis is generally performed using Excel, SAS, or other computer software.

10.14 Report of the Results

Once the analysis is complete, the survey results should be described in a written report. The report should consist of the purpose of the survey, methods, results, discussion, and conclusion. The report is then communicated to those who need to know, such as funding sources, policy makers, program managers, and the target population.[5] The methods portion of the report is used to demonstrate the scientific soundness and reliability of the results. Describing the findings must be tailored to the appropriate audience, who may not be researchers or scientists. Basic summary statistics (e.g., percentages and means), tables, and graphs are typically used to help communicate the findings in a concise and effective way.

10.15 Existing Data

In some situations, existing data can be accessed for answering questions on a topic of interest. Much of the survey data collected in the United States and other countries throughout the world are available in large databases. Scientists often access these databases to address important research questions. In the outset of this chapter, some examples were given of existing data. Existing data can be classified as secondary data, ancillary data, or systematic reviews.

10.15.1 Secondary Data

In contrast to primary data, which are collected by the researcher carrying out the study, secondary data are collected by someone other than the actual researcher. These data sources are common, including census, government supported surveys, organizational surveys, research studies, medical records, healthcare billing files, death certificates, national data sets, tumor registries, biological databases, renal registries, diabetes registries, autoimmune registries, Medicare data, and many other sources of data that initially were collected for other purposes, but now are being used to address a new question. They may be available online or in a physical archive.

Use of secondary data can be quick and inexpensive, and the data quality is often very good. On the other hand, secondary data may not represent the ideal population of study, the measurement approach may not be ideal, the data quality poor, or gaining access to the data may be difficult.

If high-quality secondary data that can answer your research question are available, it is always preferred to "reinventing the wheel." Some examples of surveys that provide secondary data are the National Health and Nutrition Examination Survey (NHANES), which is a survey conducted by the National Center for Health Statistics that assesses the health and nutritional status of adults and children in the United States, and assesses changes with time;[22] The National Health Interview Survey (NHIS), which provides national estimates of health status and utilization on a wide range of indicators;[23] the National Hospital Care Survey, which is a source of healthcare statistics on topics such as healthcare resources, quality of health care, disparities in healthcare services according to population subgroups in the United States;[24] the Behavioral Risk Factor Surveillance System, which is a survey conducted in the United States that considers health-related risk behaviors, chronic conditions, and use of screening services;[25] the National Mental Health Services Survey, which provides locations, characteristics, and utilization of mental health facilities in the United States;[26] the European Health Interview Survey, which provides information on health status, health care use, health determinants, and socioeconomic variables in Europe;[27] and the European Health Examination Survey, which combines a health questionnaire and physical measurement data.[28]

Health, United States, is an annual report on the health status of the nation. Its publication is in compliance with Section 308 of the Public Health Service Act.[29] The report contains information on health and health care in the United States. Much of the information is directly obtained from surveys such as NHANES or the NHIS. For example, based on NHANES data, a report indicates that diabetes prevalence (%) among adults aged 20 years and over by age increased between 1999–2000 and 2015–2016 from 4.3% to 5.6% for ages 20–44, from 14.7% to 21.9% for ages 45–64, and 17.9% to 28.2% for ages 65 and over.[29] Diabetes is associated with obesity.[30] During the same time period the age-adjusted prevalence of obesity increased from 33.3% to 41.2% for women and 27.4% to 38.1% for men.[29]

10.15.2 Ancillary Data

Ancillary studies add one or more new measures to a study, often in a subset of the participants, in order to answer a separate research question. For example, in order to evaluate the association between health and religion, researchers added questions about religious preference and activity to the Utah Health Status Survey.[31] This made it possible to compare the health profiles of Latter-day Saints in Utah who are religiously active versus not religiously active. The study also compared these results with those of other religious preferences and church activity levels.

Ancillary studies have the advantages of secondary data by being less costly and more efficient. The addition of a question or questions can involve cross-sectional, case-control, cohort, or experimental studies. Banks of stored sera, DNA images, and the like found in many large cohort studies and clinical trials offer an ideal opportunity to propose new measurements. Adding questions at the start of the study is ideal, but it may be difficult to identify relevant questions in the planning phase. Nevertheless, even when additional variables are not measured at baseline, but during or at the end of the study, useful information can be obtained.[3]

10.15.3 Systematic Reviews and Meta-Analysis

Reviewing the literature allows us to learn what is already known about a topic. We then decide what still needs to be learned. A **systematic review** involves a detailed plan and search strategy determined *a priori*, with the goal of identifying, appraising, and synthesizing relevant studies that address a particular research question.[32] A systematic review involves eight stages: (1) formulate the review question, (2) define inclusion and exclusion criteria, (3) develop search strategy and locate studies, (4) select studies, (5) extract data, (6) access study quality, (7) analyze and interpret results, and (8) disseminate findings. These stages are each nicely developed in a paper by Uman.[32]

Systematic reviews sometimes use statistical techniques to synthesize the results from several studies into a single summary measure. When appropriate, summary estimates of the overall results should be calculated and reported. The statistical aspects of a systematic review (calculated summary effect estimates and variance, statistical tests of heterogeneity, and statistical estimates of publication bias) are called meta-analysis. Meta-analysis is often, but not always, based on randomized, clinical trials.[33]

A **meta-analysis** is a statistical assessment used to systematically evaluate previous research studies addressing the same subject to derive conclusions about a specific body of research.

News File

Moderate alcohol consumption has been negatively associated with coronary disease. However, the association has been controversial. A meta-analysis of 34 prospective studies was conducted to further investigate this association. The study confirmed a J-shaped relationship between alcohol and total mortality: One to two drinks per day for women and one to four drinks per day for men. The greatest protection was associated with one drink of alcohol per day. The analysis also confirmed that higher levels of drinking were associated with increased total mortality. For example, six drinks of alcohol per day (compared with zero) is associated with an increased risk of total mortality of about 40% for women ($n = 16$) and 10% for men ($n = 32$). In men, one drink of alcohol per day (compared with zero) was associated with a decrease in total mortality of 25% in the United States ($n = 9$), 18% in Europe ($n = 14$), and 15% in other countries ($n = 9$).[34]

Data from Castelnuovo AD, Costanzo S, Bagnardi V, Donati MB, Iacoviello L, Gaetano GD. Alcohol dosing and total mortality in men and women: An updated meta-analysis of 34 prospective studies. *Arch Intern Med.* 2006;166:2437–2445.

The statistical analysis phase of the study (meta-analysis) typically involves estimating an overall combined effect. If each study in an analysis has a similar level of precision, we could just compute the mean of the effect sizes. However, because some studies are more precise than others, we want to weight the more precise studies more heavily when obtaining an overall summary measure. Thus, in meta-analysis, rather than compute a simple mean of study effect estimates, we derive a weighted mean, with more weight given to those studies with small variance.

How we assign weights in order to obtain a weighed summary effect estimate depends on whether we choose a fixed-effects model or a random-effects model. The two models have different assumptions, which lead to different definitions of the summary effect estimate and different approaches for assigning weights. Some of the introductory ideas presented in the next two sections come from a meta-analysis book by Borenstein, Hedges, and Rothstein.[35]

10.15.3.1 Fixed Effects Model

The fixed effects model assumes that each of the included studies has a common effect size. Observed effects will be distributed about the common effect size, with a variance that depends largely on the sample size for each study. There is one level of sampling because all the studies considered are sampled from a population with the common effect size.

The aim is to assign studies with larger sample sizes (less variance) more weight. The weight (w) for study i is the inverse of the within-study variance (v):

$$w_i = \frac{1}{v_i}$$

The weighted average of the observed effects T_i is calculated as

$$T = \frac{\sum_i^k w_i T_i}{\sum_i^k w_i}.$$

The variance of the combined effect is the reciprocal of the summed weights:

$$v = \frac{1}{\sum_i^k w_i}$$

The standard error of the combined effect is

$$SE(T) = \sqrt{v}.$$

The 95% confidence interval for the combined effect is calculated as

$$T \pm 1.96 \times SE(T).$$

The Z value is

$$Z = \frac{T}{SE(T)}.$$

Finally, the p-value is as follows:

$$1-\phi(Z) \qquad \text{One tailed}$$

$$2\times\left[1-\phi(|Z|)\right] \qquad \text{Two-tailed}$$

The expression $\phi(Z)$ is the standard normal cumulative distribution function.

Example 10.5

Suppose six similar studies are available in the literature that have independently assessed the ability of the Mediterranean diet to lower cholesterol. In each study, cholesterol scores were compared between individuals on the Mediterranean diet and a control group. The studies used Hedge's g, which is a measure of effect size that uses a sample-size-weighted pooled standard deviation.

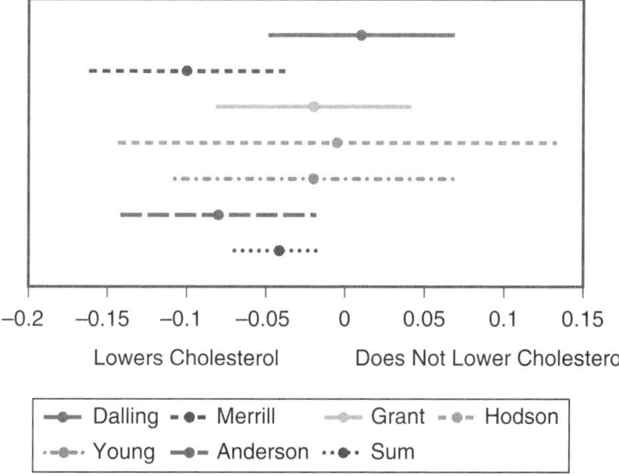

Computations for the fixed effects model are shown in the following spreadsheet.

	A	B	C	D	E	F	G	H	I	J	K	L
1	Data					Fixed Effect			Fixed Effect			
2	Study	ES	Std Error	Variance		Weight	ES x Weight					
3	Dalling	0.01	0.030	0.001		1111.111	11.111		Effect size	-0.042	=G9/F9	
4	Holman	-0.1	0.032	0.001		1000.000	-100.000		Variance	0.000	=1/F9	
5	Grant	-0.02	0.032	0.001		1000.000	-20.000		Standard error	0.014	=SQRT(J4)	
6	Hodson	-0.005	0.071	0.005		200.000	-1.000		95% LCL	-0.070	=J3-1.96*J5	
7	Young	-0.02	0.045	0.002		500.000	-10.000		95% UCL	-0.013	=J3+1.96*J5	
8	Stevens	-0.08	0.032	0.001		1000.000	-80.000		Z value	-2.882	=J3/J5	
9	Sum	-0.042	0.014	0.000		4811.111	-199.889		p-value (1-tailed)	0.002	=NORMDIST(J8,0,1,TRUE)	
10									p-value (2-tailed)	0.004	=2*J9	
11	Column F	=1/D3										
12	Column G	=B3*F3										
13	F9	=SUM(F3:F8)										
14	G9	=SUM(G3:G8)										
15	B9	=G9/F9										
16	C9	=SQRT(1/F9)										

A summary of the studies indicate that the Mediterranean diet significantly lowers cholesterol.

10.15.3.2 Random Effects Model

While the fixed effects model assumes that the true effect is the same in each study, the random effects model does not assume that they are exactly the same. Incorporating studies in a meta-analysis assumes that the studies are similar enough to synthesize the information, although the effect sizes are not necessarily identical across all studies. If we suppose that there is a distribution of true effect sizes, the combined effect should represent an average of the population of true effects.

With the random effects model, two sources of sampling error are considered, within studies and between studies. For each study, within sampling error is the variance for that study. Between sampling error is derived by first computing total variance:

$$Q = \sum_{i=1}^{k} w_i (T_i - T)^2 = \sum_{i=1}^{k} w_i T_i^2 - \frac{\left(\sum_{i=1}^{k} w_i T_i\right)^2}{\sum_{i=1}^{k} w_i}$$

$$df = k - 1$$

We then compute the between-studies variance as

$$\tau^2 = \begin{cases} \dfrac{Q - df}{C} & \text{if } Q > df \\ 0 & \text{if } Q \le df, \end{cases}$$

where

$$C = \sum_{i=1}^{k} w_i - \frac{\sum_{i=1}^{k} w_i^2}{\sum_{i=1}^{k} w_i}.$$

Now we sum the within-study variance and the between study variance for study i as

$$v_i' = v_i + \tau^2.$$

The weight assigned to each study under the random effects model is

$$w_i' = \frac{1}{v_i'}.$$

The weighted average of the observed effects T_i is calculated as

$$T' = \frac{\sum_i^k w_i' T_i}{\sum_i^k w_i'}.$$

The variance of the combined effect is the reciprocal of the summed weights:

$$v' = \frac{1}{\sum_i^k w_i'}$$

The standard error of the combined effect is

$$SE(T') = \sqrt{v'}.$$

The 95% confidence interval for the combined effect is derived as

$$T' \pm 1.96 \times SE(T').$$

The Z value is

$$Z' = \frac{T'}{SE(T')}.$$

Finally, the p-value is as follows:

$$P = 1 - \phi(Z') \qquad \text{One tailed}$$

$$P = 2 \times [1 - \phi(|Z'|)] \qquad \text{Two-tailed}$$

The expression $\phi(Z)$ is the standard normal cumulative distribution function

Example 10.6

This example is based on the same study results that were used for the fixed effects example. The spreadsheet computations for random effects analyses builds on the data for the fixed effects analysis. We now add columns for tau-squared (Columns M–Q) and random effects (Columns S–Z). The definition of the variance differs between the fixed effects analysis and the random effects analysis. The variance for the fixed effects analysis (Column D) is the variance within studies. The variance for the random effects analysis is the sum of the variance within studies and the variance between studies.

M	N	O	P	Q	R	S	T	U	V	W	X	Y	Z	AA	AB	AC
Computed Tau^2			Compute Tau^2			Random Effects						Random Effects				
ES^2xWT	WT^2					Within	Between	Total	WT	ESxWT						
0.111	1234568		Q	8.811	=M9-G9^2/F9	0.001	0.001	0.002	530.602	5.306		Effect size	-0.040	=W9/V9		
10.000	1000000		df	5.000	=COUNT(B3:B8)-1	0.001	0.001	0.002	503.867	-50.387		Variance	0.000	=1/V9		
0.400	1000000		Numerator	3.811	=MAX(Q3-Q4,0)	0.001	0.001	0.002	503.867	-10.077		Standard error	0.020	=SQRT(Z4)		
0.005	40000		C	3870.670	=F9-N9/F9	0.005	0.001	0.006	167.094	-0.835		95% LCL	-0.079	=Z3-1.96*Z5		
0.200	250000		Tau-sq	0.001	=(Q3-Q4)/Q6	0.002	0.001	0.003	335.048	-6.701		95% UCL	-0.002	=Z3+1.96*Z5		
6.400	1000000					0.001	0.001	0.002	503.867	-40.309		Z value	-2.042	=Z3/Z5		
17.116	4524568								2544.345	-103.004		p-value (1-tailed)	0.021	=NORMDIST(Z8,0,1,TRUE)		
												p-value (2-tailed)	0.041	=2*Z9		
Column M	=B3^2*F3				Column S	=D3										
Column N	=F3^2				Column T	=$Q$7										
M9	=SUM(M3:M8)				Column U	=S3+T3										
N9	=SUM(N3:N8)				Column V	=1/U3										
					Column W	=B3*V3										
					V9	=SUM(V3:V8)										
					W9	=SUM(W3:W8)										

10.16 Summary

The focus of this chapter was on survey research. When a problem is identified in the biological and medical sciences, we are interested in answering questions related to that problem: What are the clinical characteristics of the problem? Who is affected? Where are they affected? When are they affected? Why and how is the problem occurring? Answers to such questions can be obtained from health surveys. In general, a health survey is useful for monitoring and assessing health-related information, which may be used to inform individuals and populations on ways to prevent and control health problems. A survey may involve a census of the entire population or a sample of the population. Sometimes existing data from validated instruments are available for investigators to address their research questions. However, often such data are not accessible, and investigators are left to carry out their own survey in order to obtain data to answer their questions. Several steps were presented here for conducting a survey.

A survey proposal contains several elements, one of which is the study plan (protocol), which consists of a statement of purpose, a description of the survey population, the sample size (necessary for sufficient power), and the type of survey (questionnaire or interview, cross-sectional or longitudinal, probability or nonprobability) used. The protocol also includes a description of the content, questions (open- or closed-ended, factual, or attitudinal), and layout of the survey. It should also list steps that will be taken to validate and pretest the survey, the process of conducting the survey and cleaning the data, the analysis plan, and to whom the survey results will be reported.

Rating scales are useful when asking respondents to rate abstract concepts. A number of rating scales were presented. In addition, Cronbach's alpha was presented. This statistic shows how closely items among a set of survey items are related. It is an indicator of scale reliability. Principal component analysis and common factor analysis were also introduced. These are methods used to reduce dimensionality of the dataset to fewer unobserved constructs than variables.

Construction of a survey should begin with a written, detailed list of information to be collected and the concepts to be measured. Variables of interest should be classified accordingly (i.e., independent, dependent, confounder, moderator, and mediator). Corresponding questions to the variables should be answerable, unambiguous, and appropriately phrased. In order to avoid biased results, the investigator should avoid loaded questions, double-barreled questions, and questions with hidden assumptions. New surveys require pilot testing to appraise validity and reliability. Measures of validity to consider include face validity, content validity, construct validity, and criterion validity. In general, these validity measures indicate how accurately a method measures what it is supposed to measure. Factors that influence validity include the response rate, the completion rate, and error related to coverage, sampling, measurement, and data processing.

Once the data analysis is complete, a written report should be prepared, oriented toward those who will benefit from the report. The report may be improved by incorporating tables and graphs, which are often useful for effectively communicating data. The report should include the following elements: purpose, methods, results, discussion, and conclusions.

If data are already available, by utilizing this data rather than creating, validating, and administering your own survey instrument can save time and money and make the results more comparable. Sources of existing data are secondary, ancillary, and systematic reviews. Related to the systematic review is meta-analysis, which is a statistical approach to summarize the results of studies that fit certain eligibility criteria. If the studies to be combined in a meta-analysis each has a similar level of precision, we would simply derive the mean of the effect sizes. Yet, not all studies have the same level of precision, so we should weigh the more precise studies more heavily when obtaining an overall summary measure. Two models were presented for assigning weights in order to compute a weighed summary effect estimate. The fixed effects model assumes that the true effect is the same in each study. Alternatively, the random effects model assumes that the true effect is different across the studies.

Exercises

1. A census survey is most feasible if the target population is large. True/False
2. Advantages of using existing data are that they save time and money and make results comparable. True/False
3. Two primary uses of a written research proposal are to obtain funding and to receive institutional review board approval. True/False
4. A protocol is the study plan. True/False
5. Major elements of the written protocol include the budget, timeline, and the researcher's qualifications. True/False
6. A focus group can not only help focus a survey and formulate relevant questions but assist in interpreting the results of these questions. True/False
7. The accessible population is the target population. True/False
8. Recall bias in a case-control study occurs if cases tend to recall exposure status more/less accurately than do controls. This is an example of systematic error. True/False
9. A low response rate means a lower margin of error. True/False.
10. Another name for serial survey is longitudinal survey. True/False.
11. A completion rate means the same thing as a response rate. True/False.
12. Summary statistics, tables, and graphs are best not included in a final report. True/False.
13. Secondary data have already been collected through primary sources and can be used by researchers for answering their own questions. True/False.
14. Another name for an ancillary study is a meta-analysis. True/False.
15. In survey research, a pilot test evaluates whether the aims of a proposed research study were met after the survey has been administered. True/False.
16. Which of the following is a nonprobability version of stratified sampling?
    a. Convenience sampling
    b. Snowball sampling
    c. Consecutive sampling
    d. Judgmental sampling
    e. Quota sampling
17. An inaccurate sampling frame will contribute to which type of error?
    a. Coverage error
    b. Sampling error
    c. Measurement error
    d. Nonresponse error
    e. Data processing error

18. Avoiding invasive and uncomfortable tests, allaying individual concerns, and providing incentives are ways to help minimize which type of error?
    a. Coverage error
    b. Sampling error
    c. Measurement error
    d. Nonresponse error
    e. Data processing error
19. Probability sampling can help minimize which type of error?
    a. Coverage error
    b. Sampling error
    c. Measurement error
    d. Nonresponse error
    e. Data processing error
20. Which of the following is a coefficient of reliability (internal consistency)?
    a. Factor loading
    b. Eigenvalue
    c. Cronbach's alpha
    d. Tau
21. We are interested in whether the true prevalence of the SARS-CoV-2 in a population is 10%. A random sample of the population is planned to estimate the prevalence. The desired sample size will be able to identify the prevalence of the virus with a 5% margin of error. What is the required sample size using a 95% confidence level if the population size is 20,000?
22. Referring to the previous exercise, if the population size was 1000, then what sample size is required?
23. A survey is conducted with a primary aim to identify mean body mass index among a group of adults aged 50 years and older who have been diagnosed with obstructive sleep apnea (OSA). What is the required size of the survey using a 95% confidence level, a margin of error of 1, and a standard deviation of 5? The population size of patients with OSA is 500.
24. Referring to the previous exercise, if the population size is 50, what is the required sample size of OSA patients?
25. Referring to the previous exercise, the population in stratum 1 is 15. Based on proportionate sampling, what is the required sample size for this stratum?
26. Suppose you evaluated a set of 10 cough-related items (each measured from 0 [never] to 4 [always]). There were 94 respondents who completed the survey. You are interested in measuring the internal consistency of these items and decide to calculate Cronbach's alpha. The following SAS output was obtained:

Cronbach Coefficient Alpha	
Variables	**Alpha**
Raw	0.927390
Standardized	0.931260

Cronbach Coefficient Alpha with Deleted Variable					
	Raw Variables		Standardized Variables		
Deleted Variable	Correlation with Total	Alpha	Correlation with Total	Alpha	Label
x127A	0.549739	0.930400	0.546683	0.933355	My cough is worse when I lie down.
x127B	0.726317	0.920318	0.735143	0.923895	My coughing problem causes me to restrict my personal and social life.
x127C	0.753720	0.919126	0.761511	0.922537	I tend to avoid places because of my cough problem.
x127D	0.774125	0.917605	0.777161	0.921726	I feel embarrassed because of my coughing problem.
x127E	0.776938	0.916975	0.783684	0.921387	People ask, "What's wrong?" because I cough a lot.
x127F	0.800751	0.915360	0.799355	0.920571	I run out of air when I cough.
x127G	0.634771	0.925231	0.627190	0.929368	My coughing problem affects my voice.
x127H	0.786323	0.916413	0.790038	0.921057	my coughing problem limits my physical activity.
x127I	0.701936	0.921045	0.703270	0.925526	My coughing problem upsets me.
x127J	0.776794	0.916767	0.776151	0.921778	People ask me if I am sick because I cough a lot.

How would you rate the internal consistency of these items and can you improve it by eliminating any specific item?

For Questions 27–29. Refer to the following data, which represents responses from 10 individuals to five items related to voice symptoms. Responses ranged from 0 (never) to 5 (daily).

Subject	I1	I2	I3	I4	I5
1	0	0	0	0	0
2	3	2	3	1	2
3	0	3	0	0	5
4	3	3	4	5	5
5	0	0	0	0	0
6	1	0	0	0	1
7	2	2	0	0	0
8	1	1	1	1	1
9	0	0	0	0	0
10	0	0	0	0	0

27. Compute and interpret Cronbach's alpha.
28. Using factor analysis, how many eigenvalues are greater than 1 and what are their values?

29. In your assessment of the data using Cronbach's alpha and factor analysis, are there any items that should be deleted?

30. Suppose six similar studies are available in the literature that have assessed the ability of an intervention to increase steps per day. In each study, total steps were compared between those on the intervention and a control group. The studies used Hedge's g, which is a measure of effect size that uses a sample-size-weighted pooled standard deviation.

Study	Estimate	Standard Error	Variance
James	0.1	0.165	0.027
Phillip	0.3	0.153	0.023
Marty	0.35	0.201	0.040
Martell	0.12	0.101	0.010
Andrew	0.04	0.104	0.011
Dallin	0.15	0.141	0.020

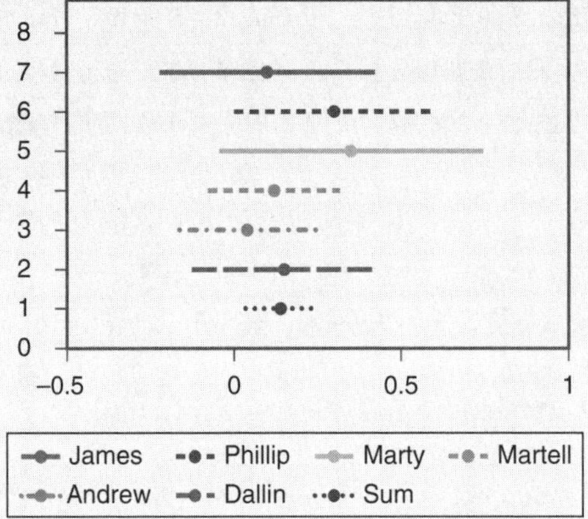

Calculate a one-tailed *p*-value using a fixed effects model, and indicate your conclusion about the intervention on lowering total steps.

31. Do you come to a similar conclusion using the random effects model?

References

1. Terlizzi EP, Villarroel MA. Symptoms of generalized anxiety disorder among adults: United States, 2019. *NCHS Data Brief*, no *378*. Hyattsville, MD: National Center for Health Statistics; 2020.
2. Bureau USC. List of All Surveys & Programs. The United States Census Bureau. https://www.census.gov/content/census/en/programs-surveys/surveys-programs.html/. Accessed April 6, 2021.
3. Health Surveys. RAND Corporation. https://www.rand.org/health-care/surveys_tools.html. Accessed April 6, 2021.
4. Grady, DG, Cummings SR, Hulley SB. Research using existing data. Chapter 13. In: Hulley SB, Cummings SR, Browner WS, Grady DG, Newman TB. *Designing Clinical Research*. 4th ed. Philadelphia, PA: Lippincott Williams & Wilkins; 2013.
5. Cummings SR, Grady DG, Hulley SB. Writing a proposal for funding research. Chapter 19. In: Hulley SB, Cummings SR, Browner WS, Grady DG, Newman TB. *Designing Clinical Research*. 4th ed. Philadelphia, PA: Lippincott Williams & Wilkins; 2013.
6. Herold JM. Survey and sampling. Chapter 6. In: Gregg MB. *Field Epidemiology*, 3rd ed. Oxford, UK: Oxford University Press; 2008.

7. Gupta RS, Warren CM, Smith BM, et al. Prevalence and severity of food allergies among US Adults. *JAMA Netw Open.* 2019;2(1):e185630.
8. International Public Opinion Survey on Cancer. UICC global cancer control. https://www.uicc.org/sites/main/files/atoms/files/WCD20_IntPublicOpinionPoll_Report_FA_Screen_0.pdf. Accessed April 6, 2021.
9. Aiyer A, Surani S, Gill Y, Iyer R, Surani Z. Mental health impact of COVID-19 on healthcare workers in the USA: A cross-sectional web-based Survey. *J Depress Anxiety*. 2020;9(5).
10. Pew Research Center. Religion and public life. https://www.pewforum.org/. Accessed April 6, 2021.
11. Lemeshow S, Hosmer DW, Klar J, Lwanga SK. *Adequacy of Sample Size in Health Studies*. Chichester, UK: Wiley; 1990. https://apps.who.int/iris/handle/10665/41607. Accessed April 6, 2021.
12. Fowler FJ. *Survey Research Methods*. Thousand Oaks, CA: SAGE Publications, Inc.; 2013.
13. Sauro J. 15 Common Rating Scales Explained. Measuring U. https://measuringu.com/rating-scales/. Accessed April 6, 2021.
14. Ware JE Jr, Sherbourne CD. The MOS 36-item short-form health survey (SF-36). I. Conceptual framework and item selection. *Med Care*. 1992;*30*(6):473–483.
15. Cronbach LJ. Coefficient alpha and the internal structure of tests. *Psychometrika.* 1951;*16*(3):297–334.
16. Hills P, Argyle M. The Oxford Happiness Questionnaire: A compact scale for the measurement of psychological well-being. *Pers Individ Differ.* 2002;*33*(7):1073–1082.
17. Principal Components (PCA) and Exploratory Factor Analysis (EFA) with SPSS. IDRE Stats. https://stats.idre.ucla.edu/spss/seminars/efa-spss/. Accessed April 6, 2021.
18. William C. Shiel Jr. MD. Definition of Voice disorder. MedicineNet. https://www.medicinenet.com/voice_disorder/definition.htm. Accessed April 6, 2021.
19. Survey Questions 101: Question Types, Examples, and Tips. Typeform. https://www.typeform.com/surveys/question-types/. Accessed April 6, 2021.
20. Majd M, Saunders EF, Engeland CG. Inflammation and the dimensions of depression: A review. *Front Neuroendocrinol.* 2020;*56*:100800.
21. Kasprzyk D, Shettle C, Giesbrecht L, et al. *Measuring and Reporting Sources of Error in Surveys*. Washington, DC: National Center for Education Statistics; 2001. https://nces.ed.gov/FCSM/pdf/spwp31.pdf. Accessed April 6, 2021.
22. Centers for Disease Control and Prevention. National Health and Nutrition Examination Survey (NHANES) Homepage. https://www.cdc.gov/nchs/nhanes/index.htm. Accessed April 6, 2021.
23. Centers for Disease Control and Prevention. National Health Interview Survey (NHIS). https://www.cdc.gov/nchs/nhis/index.htm. Accessed April 6, 2021.
24. Centers for Disease Control and Prevention. About the National Hospital Care Survey (NHCS). https://www.cdc.gov/nchs/nhcs/index.htm. Accessed April 6, 2021.
25. Centers for Disease Control and Prevention. CDC BRFSS. https://www.cdc.gov/brfss/index.html. Published August 31, 2020. Accessed December 14, 2020.
26. Substance Abuse & Mental Health Services Administration. National Mental Health Services Survey (NMHSS). DASIS: Drug & Alcohol Services Information System. https://wwwdasis.samhsa.gov/dasis2/nmhss.htm. Accessed April 6, 2021.
27. Eurostat. European Health Interview Survey; Access to microdata. https://ec.europa.eu/eurostat/web/microdata/european-health-interview-survey. Accessed April 6, 2021.
28. European Health Examination Survey (EHES). http://www.ehes.info/. Accessed April 6, 2021.
29. National Center for Health Statistics. *Health, United States, 2018*. Hyattsville, MD; 2019.
30. Leitner DR, Frühbeck G, Yumuk V, et al. Obesity and type 2 diabetes: Two diseases with a need for combined treatment strategies—EASO can lead the way. *Obes Facts.* 2017;*10*(5):483–492.
31. Daniels M, White GL, Standord JB, Lyon JL, Merrill RM. Associations between breast cancer risk factors and religious practices in Utah. *Prev Med.* 2004;*38*(1):28–38.
32. Uman LS. Systematic reviews and meta-analyses. *J Can Acad Child Adolesc Psychiatry.* 2011;*20*(1):57–59.
33. Haidich AB. Meta-analysis in medical research. *Hippokratia.* 2010;*14*(Suppl 1):29–37.
34. Castelnuovo AD, Costanzo S, Bagnardi V, Donati MB, Iacoviello L, Gaetano GD. Alcohol dosing and total mortality in men and women: An updated meta-analysis of 34 prospective studies. *Arch Intern Med.* 2006;*166*:2437–2445.
35. Borenstein M, Hedges L, Rothstein H. *Meta-analysis: Fixed effect vs. random effects*. Englewood, NJ: Biostat Inc.; 2007. https://www.meta-analysis.com/downloads/M-a_f_e_v_r_e_sv.pdf. Accessed April 6, 2021.

Appendix A

Answers to Odd-Numbered Exercises

Chapter 1

1. Descriptive statistics, probability, inference, and statistical techniques. Descriptive statistics are measures of frequency, tendency, dispersion (variation), and position that represent either a sample or a population. Probability is used when discussing the chance or likelihood that a given event will occur. It is the foundation of statistical inference. Statistical inference is when conclusions are drawn about a population based on sample information taken from the population. Statistical techniques are analytic approaches that utilize various statistical methods to investigate research questions.
3. A, B, A, B, A
5. Frequency (count, percent rate); central tendency (mean, median, mode); dispersion (standard deviation, range, interquartile range); position (percentile, rank)
7. Inferential statistics involves probability by drawing conclusions about the population based on sample data beyond what would be expected by random chance.
9. 8, 5.75, 5.34, 1, 16.

Chapter 2

1. A – Ratio
3. C – Rate
5. 34/63 × 100 = 54.0 per 100
7. A, B, A, B, C
9. The age distribution is younger in Utah; older in Florida.

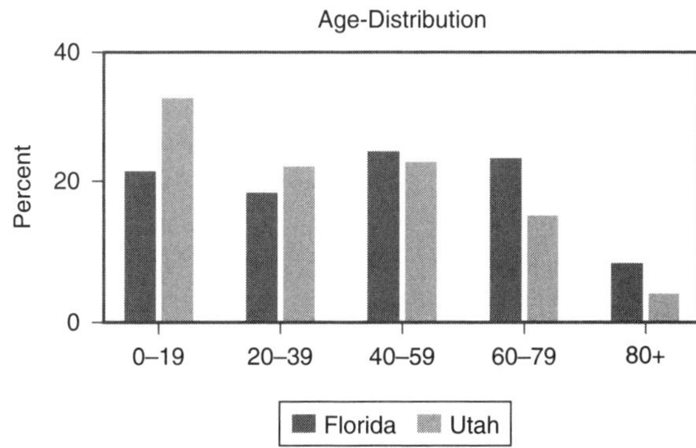

11. The age-adjusted rate in Utah using the Florida population as the standard is 1011.1 per 100,000.
13. Seven for ages 45–54, 12 for ages 55–64, 19 for ages 65–74, 31 for ages 75–84, and 52 for ages 85 and older.
15. Yes, if the age-distribution between groups are similar or if the rate is not dependent on age.
17. The crude rate represents the actual risk of the event in the population. If the age-distribution differs between populations being compared or in a given population over time, then to make comparisons in rates that are not confounded by age, age-adjustment is necessary.
19. Arizona has a greater relative variability, as indicated by the coefficient of variation.

Analysis Variable : Utah						
Mean	Median	Variance	Std Dev	Range	Quartile Range	Coeff of Variation
424.7	429.5	3892.2	62.4	164.0	122.0	14.7

Analysis Variable : Arizona						
Mean	Median	Variance	Std Dev	Range	Quartile Range	Coeff of Variation
2319.6	2223.0	680442.7	824.9	2710.0	1179.0	35.6

21. No outliers were seen this week because no observations are < Q1 – (1.5 × IQR) = 350 or > Q3 + (1.5 × IQR) = 6126.
23. A
25. Yes, $\sqrt{.75 \times 8} = 2.4$ and $\sqrt{.8 \times 5} = 2.0$.
27. Degrees of freedom of an estimate is the number of independent pieces of information used to obtain the estimate.
29. 68%, 95%, 99.7%

Chapter 3

1. If an experiment is repeated *n* times under the same conditions, and if the event A occurs *m* times, then as *n* grows larger, the ratio *m*/*n* approaches a fixed limit that is the probability of A. $P(A) = m/n$.
3. Subjective probability involves using one's own experience, judgment, or opinion to find probabilities.
5. Mutually exclusive events involve two or more events for which the occurrence of one event precludes the occurrence of the other(s). Independent events are events whose occurrence or outcome has no effect on the probability of the other. There is a link between mutually exclusive events in that they cannot both happen at once. However, there is no link between independent events.
7. $P(A \text{ or } B) = P(A) + P(B) - P(A \text{ and } B)$
9. When the events are independent: $P(A \text{ and } B) = P(A)P(B)$
11. 0.966, 0.033, 0.001
13. No, like the situation with twins, the proportion of women having triplets or higher increases exponentially with age. Beware if you get pregnant at age 45 or older!

15. 3.93%
17. 0.009
19. Bayes' Theorem relates the probability of the occurrence of an event to the presence or nonpresence of an associated event; that is, it shows that if we know the conditional probability of B given A and $P(B)$ and $P(A)$, we can identify the conditional probability of A given B.
21. $PV^+ = 0.227$; of those with a positive physical exam for abuse, 22.7% have been abused. $PV^- = 0.998$; of those with a negative physical exam for abuse, 99.8% have not been abused.
23. Cluster sampling.
25. Do not use systematic sampling if the data exhibits patterns. On the other hand, if it does not exhibit patterns and the risk of data manipulation by a researcher is low, it may be a less expensive, straightforward approach.
27. Use "=RANDBETWEEN(1,500)" in a given cell and copy and paste it into the number of cells of your desired sample size.

Chapter 4

1. A random variable is usually written as X, with possible values that are numerical outcomes of a random phenomenon of interest.
3. A probability distribution is a statistical function that describes the values and corresponding likelihoods that a random variable can assume within a specified range.
5. i. The experiment consists of a countable number of events occurring during a given time interval or area or volume.
   ii. The probability that an event occurs remains constant throughout the experiment.
   iii. The occurrence of an event is independent of the occurrence of all other events.
   iv. The mean (expected) number of events in each interval is denoted by the Greek letter lambda, λ.
7. Mean, median, and mode are the same value; the normal curve is bell-shaped and symmetric about the mean; it is known as a normal random variable with its probability distribution called a normal distribution.
9. It allows us to determine the probability of a score that occurs in a normal distribution, as well as to compare two scores originating from different normal distributions.
11. B
13. Drug B because the mean tolerability score is higher with a smaller variance and standard deviation. Apply the formulas for the expected value of a discrete random variable and the variance of a discrete random variable.

	μ_X	σ_X^2	σ_X
Drug A	3.05	1.65	1.28
Drug B	3.65	1.43	1.19

15.

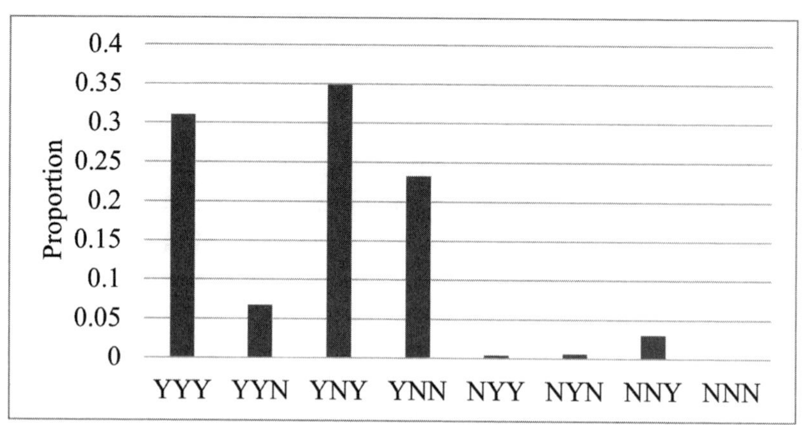

17. 0.349
19. $P(X = 0 \mid n = 10,\ p = 0.3) =$ 0.0282. In Excel use =BINOMDIST(0,10,0.3, FALSE)

    $P(X < 5 \mid n = 10,\ p = 0.3) =$ 0.8497. In Excel use =BINOMDIST(4,10,0.3, TRUE)
21. Binomial = 0.4698. In Excel use =BINOMDIST(5,100,0.01596,TRUE)–BINOMDIST(1,100,0.01596,TRUE). Poisson = 0.4678. The expected number is .01596 × 100 = 1.596. In Excel use =POISSON(5,1.596,TRUE)–POISSON (1,1.596,TRUE)
23. $\mu, \sigma / \sqrt{n}$
25. $(\bar{X} < 15) = P\left(Z < \frac{15-20}{20}\right) =$ 0.1318. In Excel use =NORMDIST(15,20, SQRT(20),TRUE)
27. $P(\bar{X} \geq 3) = P\left(Z > \frac{3-1.9}{1.1}\right) =$ 0.1587. In Excel use = 1–NORMDIST(3,1.9, 1.1,TRUE)
29. We can use the standard normal distribution to evaluate this problem because the sample size is large. $P(22 < \bar{X} < 24) =$ $P\left(\frac{22-23}{8/\sqrt{50}} < Z < \frac{24-20}{8/\sqrt{50}}\right) =$ 0.6232. In Excel use =NORMDIST(24,23,8/ SQRT(50),TRUE)–NORMDIST(22,23,8/SQRT(50),TRUE)
31. 0.176; use standard error $= \frac{8}{\sqrt{50}}\sqrt{\frac{500-50}{500-1}} = 1.074$. In Excel use =NORMDIST(22,23,1.074,TRUE)
33. First, the z value that corresponds with the area less than 0.6 is 0.2533. Now, solve for x: $\frac{x-2.5}{2.8} = 0.2533$, so $x = 2.8 \times 0.2533 + 2.5 = 3.2$.
35. D

Chapter 5

1. a. 4.0, 31.1, 5.6, 1.8; b. 1.8, 10.5, 3.2, 0.7; c. 10.0, 62.5, 7.9, 3.5
3. If X_i is a normally distributed random variable with mean μ and variance σ^2, then $E(X_i) = \mu$.
5. To obtain the z value for a confidence level of 90%, 95%, and 99%, use the Excel formula =NORM.S.INV(1–0.1/2) = 1.645, =NORM.S.INV(1–0.05/2) = 1.96, and =NORM.S.INV(1–0.01/2) = 2.576, respectively. a. 90% CI = 18.9 – 21.1; b. 95% CI = 19.8 – 22.2; c. 99% CI = 94.7 – 105.3

7. To obtain the t value for a confidence level of 95%, use the Excel formula =T.INV.2T(.05,9) = 2.262, =T.INV.2T(.05,19) = 2.093, and =T.INV.2T(.05,4) = 2.776, respectively. a. 95% CI = 0.01–7.99; b. 95% CI = 0.23–3.27; c. 95% CI = 0.18–19.82
9. 95% CI = −5.57, −2.33
11. a. 0.333, 0.096; b. 0.462, 0.062; c. 0.400, 0.022
13. 95% CI = 0.618–0.678
15. The process of selecting between the null and alternative hypothesis.
17. Negative (inverse).
19. $z = 0.745$; because p-value = 0.456 > 0.05, we fail to reject the null hypothesis. To calculate the p-value in Excel use =2*(1–NORM.S.DIST (0.745,TRUE)) or =T.DIST.2T(0.745,500)
21. a. Type 1: reject that the product is contaminated when it is; Type 2: accept that the product is contaminated when it is not; b. small α.
23. The sample of pigs should be a simple random sample, and there should be no outliers in the change scores in weight in the sample.
25. Six steps of hypothesis testing: 1. $H_0: \mu \leq 65$; 2. $H_a: \mu > 65$; 3. $\alpha = 0.05$, $n = 200$; 4. t test, with a critical value of 1.97; 5. $t = \dfrac{69.7 - 65}{32.5 / \sqrt{200}} = 2.045$;

   6. Because $t = 2.045 > 1.97$ (and the corresponding p-value = 0.0211 < 0.05), reject H_0 and conclude that the mean percentage of adults in the United States seeing a dentist in the past year is greater than 65%. The critical value was obtained using the Excel formula =T.INV(0.975,199). The p-value was obtained using the Excel formula =T.DIST.RT(2.045,199).
27. Six steps of hypothesis testing: 1. H_0: $\mu_d = 0$; 2. H_a: $\mu_d < 0$; 3. $n = 348$, $\alpha = 0.05$; 4. t test; 5. $t = \dfrac{-1.53 - 0}{3.38 / \sqrt{348}} = -8.44$; 6. The p-value < 0.0001

   (obtained by typing the Excel formula =T.DIST(–8.44,347,TRUE)). Because p-value < 0.05, reject H_0 and conclude the 6-week coronary heart disease prevention program significantly lowered depression.
29. Six steps of hypothesis testing: 1. H_0: $\mu_d = 0$; 2. H_a: $\mu_d \neq 0$; 3. $\alpha = 0.05$, $n = 10$; 4. t test with $10 - 1 = 9$ degrees of freedom. The critical value is |2.26|; 5. t value = −2.32; 6. Because $t = -2.32 < -2.26$ (and the corresponding p-value = 0.0451 < 0.05), reject H_0 and conclude that percentage of restless sleep after 6 weeks is lower for those in the intervention group compared with the control group. The critical value was obtained in Excel using the formula =T.INV.2T(0.05,9). The p-value was obtained in Excel using the formula =T.DIST.2T(2.32,9).
31. Six steps of hypothesis testing: 1. H_0: $\mu_I \geq \mu_C$; 2. H_a: $\mu_I < \mu_C$; 3. α = 0.05, $n_1 = 174$, $n_2 = 174$; 4. t test with 174 + 174 − 2 = 342 degrees of freedom. The critical t value is −1.97; 5. t = −7.06; 6. Because $t = -7.06 < -1.97$ (and the corresponding p-value < 0.0001), reject the null hypothesis and conclude that those in the intervention group experienced significantly greater decrease in depression than those in the control group over the six-month period.
33. Six steps of hypothesis testing: 1. H_0: $p_I = p_C$; 2. H_a: $p_I < p_C$; 3. $\alpha = 0.05$, $n_1 = 100$, $n_2 = 100$; 4. Z test, with critical value −1.645; 5. $z = -1.99$; 6. Because $z = -1.99 < -1.645$ (and the corresponding p-value = 0.0233 < 0.05), reject H_0 and conclude that percentage of restless sleep after six weeks is lower for those in the intervention group compared with the control group. The p-value was obtained using the Excel formula =NORM.S.DIST(–1.99,TRUE).

35. Six steps of hypothesis testing: 1. H_0: $p \geq 0.8$; 2. H_a: $p < 0.8$; 3. $\alpha = 0.05$, $n = 100$; 4. $np_0 > 10$, $np_0(1 - p_0) > 10$, so is it appropriate to use the Z test. The critical value is -1.645; 5. $z = -1.25$; 6. Because $z = -1.25 > -1.645$ (and the corresponding p-value $= 0.1057 > 0.05$), we fail to reject the null hypothesis. There is insufficient evidence to say that the proportion of women in the United States ages 40 years and older who received a mammogram within the past 2 years is less than 0.80. The p-value was obtained in Excel using the formula =NORM.S.DIST (–1.25,TRUE).
37. The kappa coefficient is 0.6333, with 95% CI = 0.4403 – 0.8264. This score represents "good agreement" between the raters.
39. $z = -2.88$, p-value $= 2 \times 0.0020 = 0.0040$; the difference is –0.13 and 95% CI = –0.218, –0.042. The $\chi^2 = 8.30$, p-value $= 0.0040$. Attrition is significantly greater for men than women.
41. Six steps of hypothesis testing: 1. H_0: $\sigma^2 = 25$; 2. H_a: $\sigma^2 \neq 25$; 3. $\alpha = 0.05$, $n = 10$; 4. χ^2 with $10 - 1 = 9$ degree of freedom; 5. $\chi^2 = 17.53$; 6. With Excel, =CHISQ.INV(0.975,9) returns 19.02 and =CHISQ.INV(0.025,9) returns 2.70. Because the calculated value does not lie in the rejection region, we fail to reject the null hypothesis that the standard deviation equals 5.
43. Six steps of hypothesis testing: 1. H_0: $p \leq 0.25$; 2. H_a: $p > 0.25$; 3. $\alpha = 0.05$, $n = 94$; 4. Z statistic with a critical value of $z_{0.05} = 1.645$; 5. $z = \dfrac{f - p_0}{\sqrt{\dfrac{p_0(1 - p_0)}{n}}} = \dfrac{0.3936 - 0.25}{\sqrt{\dfrac{0.25(1 - 0.25)}{94}}} = 3.22$; 6. Because $z = 3.22 > 1.645$, reject the null hypothesis and conclude that the prevalence of a voice problem is greater among adult patients with obstructive sleep apnea. The p-value can be obtained in Excel by the formula: =T.DIST.RT(3.22,1000)
45. The mean component quality of life is 69.09 for patients with no voice problem versus 49.31 for patients with a voice problem. We are 95% confident that the mean difference (for no voice problem versus voice problem) in component quality of life for all adults with obstructive sleep apnea is 10.60 – 28.96. Statistical significance exists at the 0.05 level because the confidence interval does not overlap 0.
47. Six steps of hypothesis testing: 1. H_0: Tobacco smoking is independent of marijuana use; 2. H_a: Tobacco smoking is NOT independent of marijuana use. 3. $\alpha = 0.05$, $n = 94$; 4. Fisher's Exact Test; 5. Calculating the row percentages show that 17.24% of tobacco smokers use marijuana compared with 3.08% of non-tobacco smokers who use marijuana. Hence, tobacco smokers are 5.6 times more likely to use marijuana than non-tobacco smokers; 6. The two-sided p-value is $0.0273 < 0.05$, so reject the null hypothesis and conclude that tobacco smoking and marijuana use are not independent. Calculating the row percentages show that 17.24% of tobacco smokers use marijuana is compared with 3.08% of non-tobacco smokers who use marijuana.
49. The mean death rate (per 100,000) in the North East Region is 83.92 compared with 27.80 in other regions of the United States. We are 95% confident that the true mean difference in rates is 19.52 – 92.71 (obtained using SAS). The difference in means is statistically significant at the 0.05 level because the confidence interval does not overlap 0.

Chapter 6

1. $J = 3$ and $N = 348$. The degrees of freedom for the model and the error are 2 and 345, respectively.
3. 3.021, obtained from the Excel formula =F.INV.RT(0.05,2,345). Thus, reject the null hypothesis because $F = 8.91 > 3.021$.
5. One-way because there was a single independent variable (weight classification).
7. a. 4.12; 2.72 (NM), 5.00 (M), 3.00 (D), 5.71 (W); b. 45.82; c. 3; d. 15.27, e. 40.86; f. 24; g. 1.70; h. $F = 8.97$. The critical value is 3.01, obtained from the Excel formula =F.INV.RT(0.05,3,24). Because $F = 8.97 > 3.01$, reject the null hypothesis of equality of means and conclude that at least one mean differs from the others. We can look at the p-value, which also indicates significance;

i.

Source	DF	Sum of Squares	Mean Square	F Value	Pr > F
Model	3	45.82142857	15.27380952	8.97	0.0004
Error	24	40.85714286	1.70238095		
Corrected Total	27	86.67857143			

j.

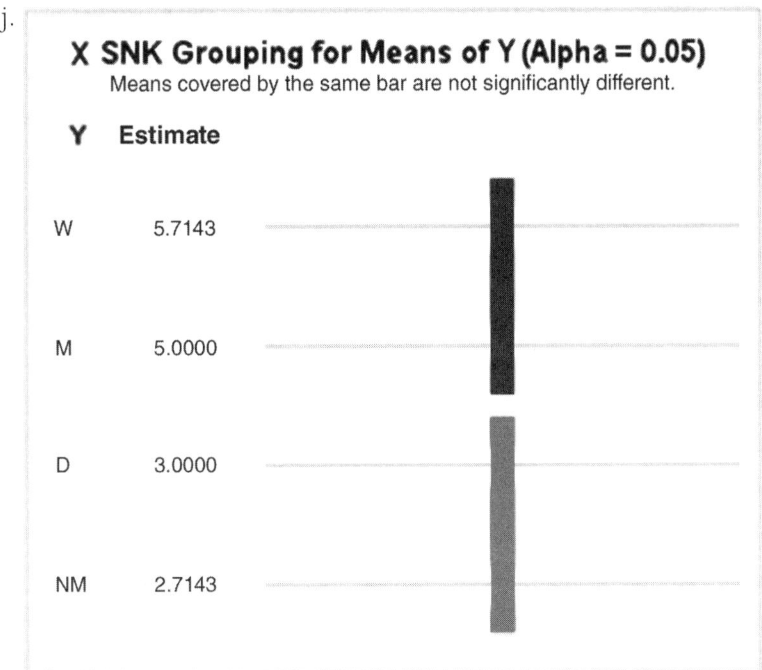

k. $\alpha' = \dfrac{0.05}{3} = 0.0167$

9. The SAS program is as follow:

```
DATA Study;
Do Group='GD','Normal';
Do Drug='Drug','Placebo';
Do Subj=1 to 4;
Input Score @;
```

```
Output;
End;
End;
End;
DATALINES;
10 10 11 9 6 9 6 7 7 4 5 7 11 10 12 11
;

PROC ANOVA DATA=Study;
TITLE 'Depression Treatment Study';
Class Group Drug;
Model Score=Group|Drug;
MEANS Group|Drug;RUN;
```

We do not need to request a multiple-comparison test because each variable has two levels. A portion of the output is shown here:

Source	DF	Anova SS	Mean Square	F Value	Pr > F
Group	1	0.06250000	0.06250000	0.04	0.8360
Drug	1	5.06250000	5.06250000	3.63	0.0811
Group*Drug	1	68.06250000	68.06250000	48.76	<.0001

There is a strong Group*Drug interaction term (p-value < .0001). This means that the effect of the drug on depression depends on the status of genetic deficiency. Additional output shows that the drug decreases the depression score for those with no genetic deficiency but increases it for those with a genetic deficiency.

Level of Group	Level of Drug	N	Score	
			Mean	Std Dev
GD	Drug	4	10.0000000	0.81649658
GD	Plac	4	7.0000000	1.41421356
No	Drug	4	5.7500000	1.50000000
No	Plac	4	11.0000000	0.81649658

11. a. 6.25 for drug A, 9.50 for drug B, 7.62 for drug C, 10.0 for drug D.
    b. Here is the SAS program:

```
DATA Pain;
INPUT SUBJ PAIN1 PAIN2 PAIN3 PAIN4;
Datalines;
1   5   8   6   9
2   3   12  8   8
3   7   12  10  11
4   11  9   5   14
5   5   10  7   9
6   5   7   8   10
7   6   10  10  11
8   8   8   7   8
;
```

```
PROC ANOVA DATA=Pain;
TITLE "One-way Repeated Measures ANOVA";
MODEL PAIN1-PAIN4=/NOUNI;
REPEATED DRUG 4 (1 2 3 4);
RUN;
```

c. A portion of the output is here, with Wilks' lambda statistic rejecting the hypothesis of no drug effect.

MANOVA Test Criteria and Exact F Statistics for the Hypothesis of no DRUG Effect H = Anova SSCP Matrix for DRUG E = Error SSCP Matrix S=1 M=0.5 N=1.5					
Statistic	**Value**	**F Value**	**Num DF**	**Den DF**	**Pr > F**
Wilks' Lambda	0.10935431	13.57	3	5	0.0077
Pillai's Trace	0.89064569	13.57	3	5	0.0077
Hotelling-Lawley Trace	8.14458704	13.57	3	5	0.0077
Roy's Greatest Root	8.14458704	13.57	3	5	0.0077

d. Drug A is preferred because it corresponds with the lowest average pain score.

13. Six steps of hypothesis testing: 1. H_0: $p_1 = p_2 = p_3$; 2. H_a: At least one p_i differs from the others; 3. $\alpha = 0.05$, $n = 94$; 4. χ^2 test of independence. Degrees of freedom = (Row − 1)(Columns − 1) = (2 − 1)(3 − 1) = 2. The critical value is $\chi^2_{0.05,2} = 5.99$; 5. The F value = 5.44. 6. Because $F = 5.44 < 5.99$ (and the corresponding p-value = 0.0659 > 0.05), we fail to reject the null hypothesis. There is insufficient evidence to conclude that CPAP use is associated with obstructive sleep apnea severity.
15. Based on the Cochran-Mantel-Haenszel statistic (10.9287, p-value = 0.0042), there is a significant linear trend between general health and daytime sleepiness.

Cochran-Mantel-Haenszel Statistics (Based on Table Scores)				
Statistic	**Alternative Hypothesis**	**DF**	**Value**	**Prob**
1	Nonzero Correlation	1	10.3933	0.0013
2	Row Mean Scores Differ	2	10.9287	0.0042
3	General Association	6	13.1276	0.0411

Conditional column percentages show that general health shifts from more excellent to more poor as daytime sleepiness becomes more severe.

Frequency Percent Row Pct Col Pct	Table of GH by DS					
		DS				
	GH	1	2	3	4	Total
	1	13 13.83 40.63 59.09	12 12.77 37.50 36.36	4 4.26 12.50 20.00	3 3.19 9.38 15.79	32 34.04
	2	6 6.38 15.00 27.27	15 15.96 37.50 45.45	11 11.70 27.50 55.00	8 8.51 20.00 42.11	40 42.55
	3	3 3.19 13.64 13.64	6 6.38 27.27 18.18	5 5.32 22.73 25.00	8 8.51 36.36 42.11	22 23.40
	Total	22 23.40	33 35.11	20 21.28	19 20.21	94 100.00

Chapter 7

1. D, B, C, E, A
3. 95% CI = 1.37 – 5.43
5. Rate Ratio = 2.17
7. 12.65 per 1000
9. Odds Ratio = 4.00
11. $AF_e = 75.0\%$
13. a. Risk ratio = 0.77; Fifth grade school children who were bullied were 23% less likely to be happy three years later.
    b. We are 95% confident that being happy among those who were bullied compared with those who were not for the whole fifth grade population of children is in the interval 0.66 – 0.91. Given that the confidence interval does not include 1, the risk ratio is significant at the 0.05 level.
    c. Being happy among those who were bullied in fifth grade is 13.0 per 100 lower than among those who were not bullied.
15. The odds ratio is a good estimate of the risk ratio for rare outcomes where less than 10% of the population is affected.
17. a. PR (Men) = 1.17, 95% CI = 0.98 – 1.40; PR (Women) = 1.24, 95% CI = 0.86 – 1.78
    b. Yes. We fail to reject the hypothesis of homogeneity according to the Breslow-Day test.

Breslow-Day Test for Homogeneity of the Odds Ratios	
Chi-Square	0.0163
DF	1
Pr > ChiSq	0.8986

    c. Yes
    d. $PR_{MH} = 1.19$, 95% CI = 1.01 – 1.40. Perceived health is greater for those whose religious faith is very important to them, after adjusting for sex.
19. a. Six steps of hypothesis testing: 1. H_0: Odds Ratio = 1; 2. H_a: Odds Ratio ≠ 1; 3. $\alpha = 0.05$, $n = 4{,}156$; 4. χ^2 test of independence with 1 degree of freedom, $\chi^2_{0.05,1} = 3.84$; 5. Odds Ratio = 0.99. 6. Because

$\chi^2_{0.05,1} = 3.84 > 0.037$ (or because the p-value > 0.05), we fail to reject the null hypothesis.

b. We are 95% confident that the true odds ratio for oral contraceptive use and breast cancer for all women is in the interval 0.85 – 1.15. Because the interval contains 1, the association is not significant at the 0.05 level.

21. C, A, B

23. a. $r = 0.79$; $t = 4.03$, p-value $= 0.0024$ (obtained from the Excel formula =T.DIST.2T(4.03,10)). Reject the null hypothesis.

b. $r = 0.60$; $t = 3.25$, p-value $= 0.0042$ (obtained from the Excel formula =T.DIST.2T(3.25,19)). Reject the null hypothesis.

25. a

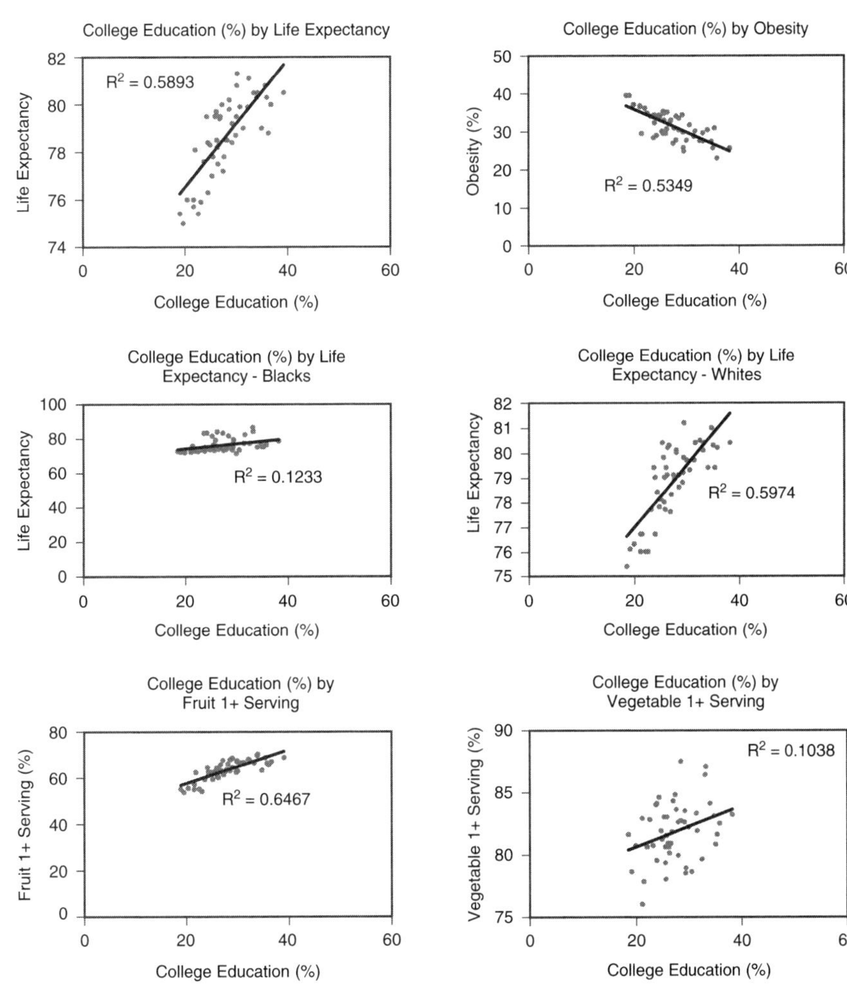

b. 0.77 (LE), 0.35 (LE-B), 0.77 (LE-W), 0.80 (F), 0.32 (V), –0.73 (O)

d. Whites

e. Fruit

f. There is a strong negative (inverse) association between the college education (%) and obesity (%) among the states in the United States.

g. 0.78 (LE), 0.48 (LE-B), 0.75 (LE-W), 0.82 (F), 0.28 (V), –0.68 (O)

h. This variable is more skewed and so less normally distributed.

i. The correlation coefficients between life expectancy and fruit, vegetable, obesity, and college graduate are 0.90, 0.16, –0.80, and 0.77, respectively. Corresponding estimates based on Spearman's correlation coefficient are 0.85, 0.08, –0.76, and 0.78, respectively. The association is greatest for fruit, based on the absolute value of the correlation coefficient.

j. The strength of the linear association between life expectancy and fruit, life expectancy and obesity, and life expectancy and college education is stronger for whites. The strength of the linear association between life expectancy and vegetables is stronger for blacks. Note that the four correlation coefficients are 0.50, 0.48, –0.49, and 0.35 for blacks and 0.86, 0.17, –0.76, and 0.77 for whites. Corresponding estimates based on Spearman's correlation coefficient are 0.57, 0.33, –0.65, and 0.48 for blacks and 0.80, 0.08, –0.72, and 0.75 for whites.

27. We are 95% confident that the true value of the correlation in the population is bounded in the interval 0.626 – 0.863.

Chapter 8

1. No. The simple linear regression model is: $Y_i = \beta_0 + \beta_1 X_i + \varepsilon_i$; $E(Y_i) = \beta_0 + \beta_1 X_i$.
3. There is a positive association (i.e., for a serving increase in fruit and vegetables per day, HDL increases by 0.5, on average). However, information is insufficient to conclude that the association is statistically significant (i.e., standard error of the slope is not provided).
5. a. MM = 157.47 – 1.16 × Age; b. 87.87; c. $r^2 = 0.73$. Approximately 73% of the variation in muscle mass is explained by age; d. The residual plot shows a scattering about the 0, indicating a linear relationship with constant variance.

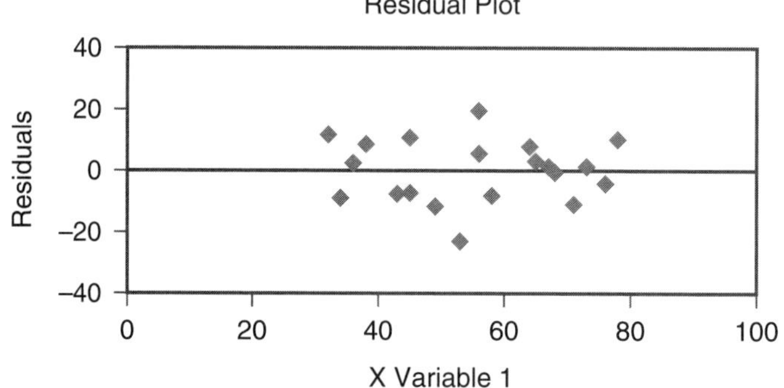

7. a. HDL2 = 10.56 + 0.94 × HDL1. b. Satisfied.

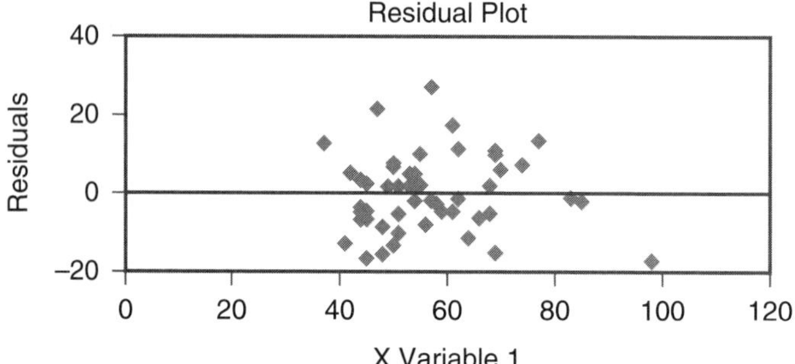

c. This graph is produced by SAS using PROC REG.

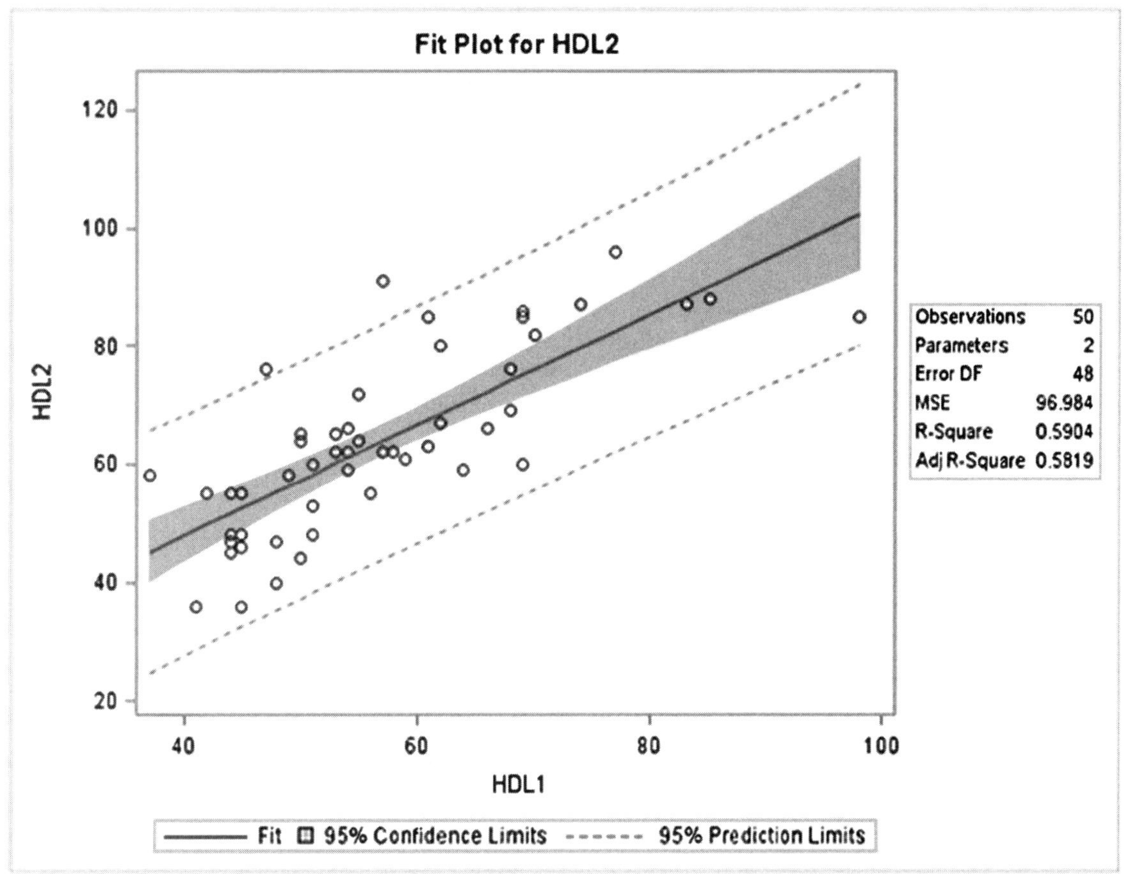

d. Yes = 38 and No = 12.
e. HDL2 = 6.41 + 0.91 × HDL1 + 7.72 × Diet
f. Yes, t value = 2.47, p-value = 0.0170.
g. Adjusted $R^2 = 0.6222$, which indicates the model is better than with just HDL1, where $R^2 = 0.5819$.
h. No, t value = 0.88, p-value = 0.3848.
i. No. Drop it in order to provide more power for evaluating the remaining estimates in the model.
j. No. The main effects that make up a significant interaction should always be retained, regardless of statistical significance.
k. Change = 1.25 + 7.41 × Diet
l. We are 95% confident that the true slope coefficient measuring the association between diet and the change in HDL is bounded by the interval 1.19 – 13.63.
m. Those in the dietary intervention have significantly greater change in HDL, 7.41 on average.

9. a. Awareness is positively associated with age ($r = 0.70$, p-value < 0.0001). Mean awareness is significantly lower for males (M = 48.3, SD = 10.7) than for females (M = 61.6, SD = 11.1) (p-value = 0.0024). Mean age is significantly younger for males (M = 33.9, SD = 9.3) than for females (M = 51.1, SD = 15.4) (p-value = 0.0011).
   b. Flu Shot = −13.76 – 0.25 × Awareness; OR = 1.28, 95% CI = 1.05 – 1.55.
   Flu Shot = −8.54 + 0.20 × Age; OR = 1.22, 95% CI = 1.02 – 1.46.
   Flu Shot = −1.39 – 2.77 × Sex; OR = 0.63, 95% CI = 0.007 – 0.559.

c. No, because they cannot independently predict the value of the dependent variable.
d. The dependent variable is binary, the observations are independent of each other and the sample size is sufficiently large (a general rule is 10 observations per independent variable). However, there is multicollinearity among the independent variables, so it is not appropriate to include all the independent variables in the model simultaneously.

11. Hazard ratios and 95% confidence intervals.

Local stage	Referent	95% LCL	95% UCL
Regional stage	3.52	3.10	3.99
Distant stage	21.93	18.42	26.11
Unknown Stage	5.15	3.95	6.71
Grade I	Referent		
Grade II	2.25	1.57	3.23
Grade III	4.35	3.05	6.21
Unknown grade	3.18	2.24	4.53
Age (1 yr)	1.01	1.00	1.01

13.

```
PROC LOGISTIC DATA=a;
CLASS H (REF='0') Y (REF='0') SEX;  MODEL Y=H SEX;RUN;
```

Odds Ratio Estimates			
Effect	Point Estimate	95% Wald Confidence Limits	
H 1 vs 0	5.253	1.070	25.796
SEX F vs M	0.477	0.097	2.354

15.

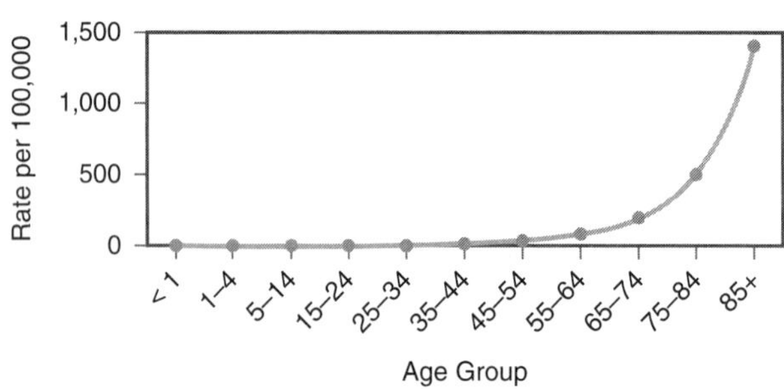

Chapter 9

1. D, F, C, E, C, B, A
3. p-value = 0.1250 > 0.05 = α, so according to the sign test there is not sufficient evidence to conclude that the depression scores significantly decrease.

5. p-value = 0.0245 < 0.05 = α, so reject the null hypothesis and conclude that the median difference is not equal to zero. Because most of the differences are positive, the reduction in FVC is greater during treatment with the placebo than during treatment with the drug. So treatment with the drug does reduce the loss of pulmonary function.
7. a. Using Excel, a histogram of the data show a left-skewed distribution.

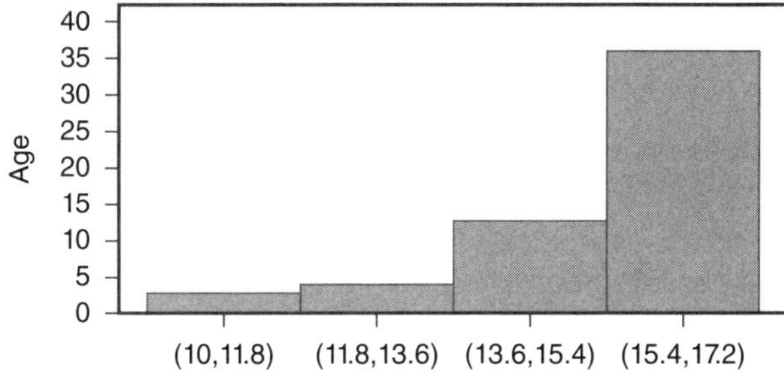

The normality tests executed in SAS:

Tests for Normality				
Test	Statistic		p Value	
Shapiro-Wilk	W	0.779215	Pr < W	<0.0001
Kolmogorov-Smirnov	D	0.251912	Pr > D	<0.0100
Cramer-von Mises	W-Sq	0.722649	Pr > W-Sq	<0.0050
Anderson-Darling	A-Sq	4.273521	Pr > A-Sq	<0.0050

Therefore, the age variable is not normally distributed.

b. The Mann-Whitney U test is shown in the following SAS output.

Wilcoxon Two-Sample Test	
Statistic	323.5000
Normal Approximation	
Z	-2.0108
One-Sided Pr < Z	0.0222
Two-Sided Pr > |Z|	0.0444
t Approximation	
One-Sided Pr < Z	0.0246
Two-Sided Pr > |Z|	0.0493
Z includes a continuity correction of 0.5.	

Because p-value = 0.0444 < 0.05 = α, we reject the null hypothesis. Therefore, median age of first marijuana smoking among those who indicated that they have previously smoked marijuana is significantly different for Hispanics than non-Hispanics.

9. Six steps of hypothesis testing: 1. H_0: Mandatory requirements had no effect on the positive test rate; 2. H_a: Mandatory requirements affected the positive test rate; 3. α = 0.05, n = 12 counties; 4. Friedman's test. Using

the chi-square table with $k - 1$ degrees of freedom gives a critical value of 5.99; 5. The Q statistic = 18.5; 6. Because Q = 18.5 > 5.99 (and the corresponding p-value < 0.0001), reject the null hypothesis. Mandatory requirements significantly change the positive test rate for SARS-CoV-2.

Chapter 10

1. False
3. True
5. False
7. False
9. False
11. False
13. True
15. False
17. A
19. B
21. 138; here is a website that may be helpful: http://www.raosoft.com/samplesize.html.
23. 81
25. 10
27. 0.90, which indicates excellent internal consistency.
29. No — deleting any one item does not increase Cronbach's alpha and all the factor loadings on the single factor are high.
31. Yes

M	N	O	P	Q	R	S	T	U	V	W	X	Y	Z
Computed Tau^2			Compute Tau^2			Random Effects						Random Effects	
ES^2xWT	WT^2					Within	Between	Total	WT	ESxWT			
0.367	1349.162		Q	3.213		0.027	-0.007	0.021	48.302	4.830		Effect size	0.120
3.845	1824.880		df	5.000		0.023	-0.007	0.017	59.218	17.765		Variance	0.001
3.032	612.655		Numerator	0.000		0.040	-0.007	0.034	29.517	10.331		Standard error	0.037
1.412	9609.803		C	274.042		0.010	-0.007	0.004	271.822	32.619		95% LCL	0.047
0.148	8548.042		Tau-sq	-0.007		0.011	-0.007	0.004	232.889	9.316		95% UCL	0.193
1.132	2530.018					0.020	-0.007	0.013	74.857	11.228		Z value	3.216
9.935	24474.560								716.604	86.089		p-value (1-tailed)	0.001
												p-value (2-tailed)	0.001

Appendix B

Tables

Table 1. Cumulative Binomial Probabilities

n	*r*	0.01	0.05	0.1	0.15	0.2	0.25	0.3	0.35	0.4	0.45	0.5
2	0	0.9801	0.9025	0.8100	0.7225	0.6400	0.5625	0.4900	0.4225	0.3600	0.3025	0.2500
	1	0.9999	0.9975	0.9900	0.9775	0.9600	0.9375	0.9100	0.8775	0.8400	0.7975	0.7500
	2	1.0000	1.0000	1.0000	1.0000	1.0000	1.0000	1.0000	1.0000	1.0000	1.0000	1.0000
3	0	0.9703	0.8574	0.7290	0.6141	0.5120	0.4219	0.3430	0.2746	0.2160	0.1664	0.1250
	1	0.9997	0.9928	0.9720	0.9393	0.8960	0.8438	0.7840	0.7183	0.6480	0.5748	0.5000
	2	1.0000	0.9999	0.9990	0.9966	0.9920	0.9844	0.9730	0.9571	0.9360	0.9089	0.8750
	3	1.0000	1.0000	1.0000	1.0000	1.0000	1.0000	1.0000	1.0000	1.0000	1.0000	1.0000
4	0	0.9606	0.8145	0.6561	0.5220	0.4096	0.3164	0.2401	0.1785	0.1296	0.0915	0.0625
	1	0.9994	0.9860	0.9477	0.8905	0.8192	0.7383	0.6517	0.5630	0.4752	0.3910	0.3125
	2	1.0000	0.9995	0.9963	0.9880	0.9728	0.9492	0.9163	0.8735	0.8208	0.7585	0.6875
	3	1.0000	1.0000	0.9999	0.9995	0.9984	0.9961	0.9919	0.9850	0.9744	0.9590	0.9375
	4	1.0000	1.0000	1.0000	1.0000	1.0000	1.0000	1.0000	1.0000	1.0000	1.0000	1.0000
5	0	0.9510	0.7738	0.5905	0.4437	0.3277	0.2373	0.1681	0.1160	0.0778	0.0503	0.0313
	1	0.9990	0.9774	0.9185	0.8352	0.7373	0.6328	0.5282	0.4284	0.3370	0.2562	0.1875
	2	1.0000	0.9988	0.9914	0.9734	0.9421	0.8965	0.8369	0.7648	0.6826	0.5931	0.5000
	3	1.0000	1.0000	0.9995	0.9978	0.9933	0.9844	0.9692	0.9460	0.9130	0.8688	0.8125
	4	1.0000	1.0000	1.0000	0.9999	0.9997	0.9990	0.9976	0.9948	0.9898	0.9816	0.9688
	5	1.0000	1.0000	1.0000	1.0000	1.0000	1.0000	1.0000	1.0000	1.0000	1.0000	1.0000
6	0	0.9415	0.7351	0.5314	0.3772	0.2621	0.1780	0.1177	0.0754	0.0467	0.0277	0.0156
	1	0.9985	0.9672	0.8857	0.7765	0.6554	0.5339	0.4202	0.3191	0.2333	0.1636	0.1094
	2	1.0000	0.9978	0.9842	0.9527	0.9011	0.8306	0.7443	0.6471	0.5443	0.4415	0.3438
	3	1.0000	0.9999	0.9987	0.9941	0.9830	0.9624	0.9295	0.8826	0.8208	0.7447	0.6563
	4	1.0000	1.0000	0.9999	0.9996	0.9984	0.9954	0.9891	0.9777	0.9590	0.9308	0.8906
	5	1.0000	1.0000	1.0000	1.0000	0.9999	0.9998	0.9993	0.9982	0.9959	0.9917	0.9844
	6	1.0000	1.0000	1.0000	1.0000	1.0000	1.0000	1.0000	1.0000	1.0000	1.0000	1.0000
7	0	0.9321	0.6983	0.4783	0.3206	0.2097	0.1335	0.0824	0.0490	0.0280	0.0152	0.0078
	1	0.9980	0.9556	0.8503	0.7166	0.5767	0.4450	0.3294	0.2338	0.1586	0.1024	0.0625
	2	1.0000	0.9962	0.9743	0.9262	0.8520	0.7564	0.6471	0.5323	0.4199	0.3164	0.2266
	3	1.0000	0.9998	0.9973	0.9879	0.9667	0.9294	0.8740	0.8002	0.7102	0.6083	0.5000
	4	1.0000	1.0000	0.9998	0.9988	0.9953	0.9871	0.9712	0.9444	0.9037	0.8471	0.7734
	5	1.0000	1.0000	1.0000	0.9999	0.9996	0.9987	0.9962	0.9910	0.9812	0.9643	0.9375
	6	1.0000	1.0000	1.0000	1.0000	1.0000	0.9999	0.9998	0.9994	0.9984	0.9963	0.9922
	7	1.0000	1.0000	1.0000	1.0000	1.0000	1.0000	1.0000	1.0000	1.0000	1.0000	1.0000

n	r	0.01	0.05	0.1	0.15	0.2	0.25	0.3	0.35	0.4	0.45	0.5
8	0	0.9227	0.6634	0.4305	0.2725	0.1678	0.1001	0.0577	0.0319	0.0168	0.0084	0.0039
	1	0.9973	0.9428	0.8131	0.6572	0.5033	0.3671	0.2553	0.1691	0.1064	0.0632	0.0352
	2	1.0000	0.9942	0.9619	0.8948	0.7969	0.6785	0.5518	0.4278	0.3154	0.2201	0.1445
	3	1.0000	0.9996	0.9950	0.9787	0.9437	0.8862	0.8059	0.7064	0.5941	0.4770	0.3633
	4	1.0000	1.0000	0.9996	0.9972	0.9896	0.9727	0.9420	0.8939	0.8263	0.7396	0.6367
	5	1.0000	1.0000	1.0000	0.9998	0.9988	0.9958	0.9887	0.9747	0.9502	0.9115	0.8555
	6	1.0000	1.0000	1.0000	1.0000	0.9999	0.9996	0.9987	0.9964	0.9915	0.9819	0.9648
	7	1.0000	1.0000	1.0000	1.0000	1.0000	1.0000	0.9999	0.9998	0.9993	0.9983	0.9961
	8	1.0000	1.0000	1.0000	1.0000	1.0000	1.0000	1.0000	1.0000	1.0000	1.0000	1.0000
9	0	0.9135	0.6303	0.3874	0.2316	0.1342	0.0751	0.0404	0.0207	0.0101	0.0046	0.0020
	1	0.9966	0.9288	0.7748	0.5995	0.4362	0.3003	0.1960	0.1211	0.0705	0.0385	0.0195
	2	0.9999	0.9916	0.9470	0.8592	0.7382	0.6007	0.4628	0.3373	0.2318	0.1495	0.0898
	3	1.0000	0.9994	0.9917	0.9661	0.9144	0.8343	0.7297	0.6089	0.4826	0.3614	0.2539
	4	1.0000	1.0000	0.9991	0.9944	0.9804	0.9511	0.9012	0.8283	0.7334	0.6214	0.5000
	5	1.0000	1.0000	0.9999	0.9994	0.9969	0.9900	0.9747	0.9464	0.9007	0.8342	0.7461
	6	1.0000	1.0000	1.0000	1.0000	0.9997	0.9987	0.9957	0.9888	0.9750	0.9502	0.9102
	7	1.0000	1.0000	1.0000	1.0000	1.0000	0.9999	0.9996	0.9986	0.9962	0.9909	0.9805
	8	1.0000	1.0000	1.0000	1.0000	1.0000	1.0000	1.0000	0.9999	0.9997	0.9992	0.9981
	9	1.0000	1.0000	1.0000	1.0000	1.0000	1.0000	1.0000	1.0000	1.0000	1.0000	1.0000
10	0	0.9044	0.5987	0.3487	0.1969	0.1074	0.0563	0.0283	0.0135	0.0061	0.0025	0.0010
	1	0.9957	0.9139	0.7361	0.5443	0.3758	0.2440	0.1493	0.0860	0.0464	0.0233	0.0107
	2	0.9999	0.9885	0.9298	0.8202	0.6778	0.5256	0.3828	0.2616	0.1673	0.0996	0.0547
	3	1.0000	0.9990	0.9872	0.9500	0.8791	0.7759	0.6496	0.5138	0.3823	0.2660	0.1719
	4	1.0000	0.9999	0.9984	0.9901	0.9672	0.9219	0.8497	0.7515	0.6331	0.5044	0.3770
	5	1.0000	1.0000	0.9999	0.9986	0.9936	0.9803	0.9527	0.9051	0.8338	0.7384	0.6231
	6	1.0000	1.0000	1.0000	0.9999	0.9991	0.9965	0.9894	0.9740	0.9452	0.8980	0.8281
	7	1.0000	1.0000	1.0000	1.0000	0.9999	0.9996	0.9984	0.9952	0.9877	0.9726	0.9453
	8	1.0000	1.0000	1.0000	1.0000	1.0000	1.0000	0.9999	0.9995	0.9983	0.9955	0.9893
	9	1.0000	1.0000	1.0000	1.0000	1.0000	1.0000	1.0000	1.0000	0.9999	0.9997	0.9990
	10	1.0000	1.0000	1.0000	1.0000	1.0000	1.0000	1.0000	1.0000	1.0000	1.0000	1.0000
11	0	0.8953	0.5688	0.3138	0.1673	0.0859	0.0422	0.0198	0.0088	0.0036	0.0014	0.0005
	1	0.9948	0.8981	0.6974	0.4922	0.3221	0.1971	0.1130	0.0606	0.0302	0.0139	0.0059
	2	0.9998	0.9848	0.9104	0.7788	0.6174	0.4552	0.3127	0.2001	0.1189	0.0652	0.0327
	3	1.0000	0.9985	0.9815	0.9306	0.8389	0.7133	0.5696	0.4256	0.2963	0.1911	0.1133
	4	1.0000	0.9999	0.9973	0.9841	0.9496	0.8854	0.7897	0.6683	0.5328	0.3971	0.2744
	5	1.0000	1.0000	0.9997	0.9973	0.9884	0.9657	0.9218	0.8513	0.7535	0.6331	0.5000
	6	1.0000	1.0000	1.0000	0.9997	0.9980	0.9924	0.9784	0.9499	0.9007	0.8262	0.7256
	7	1.0000	1.0000	1.0000	1.0000	0.9998	0.9988	0.9957	0.9878	0.9707	0.9390	0.8867
	8	1.0000	1.0000	1.0000	1.0000	1.0000	0.9999	0.9994	0.9980	0.9941	0.9852	0.9673
	9	1.0000	1.0000	1.0000	1.0000	1.0000	1.0000	1.0000	0.9998	0.9993	0.9978	0.9941
	10	1.0000	1.0000	1.0000	1.0000	1.0000	1.0000	1.0000	1.0000	1.0000	0.9999	0.9995
	11	1.0000	1.0000	1.0000	1.0000	1.0000	1.0000	1.0000	1.0000	1.0000	1.0000	1.0000
12	0	0.8864	0.5404	0.2824	0.1422	0.0687	0.0317	0.0138	0.0057	0.0022	0.0008	0.0002
	1	0.9938	0.8816	0.6590	0.4435	0.2749	0.1584	0.0850	0.0424	0.0196	0.0083	0.0032
	2	0.9998	0.9804	0.8891	0.7358	0.5584	0.3907	0.2528	0.1513	0.0834	0.0421	0.0193
	3	1.0000	0.9978	0.9744	0.9078	0.7946	0.6488	0.4925	0.3467	0.2253	0.1345	0.0730
	4	1.0000	0.9998	0.9957	0.9761	0.9274	0.8424	0.7237	0.5834	0.4382	0.3044	0.1939
	5	1.0000	1.0000	0.9995	0.9954	0.9806	0.9456	0.8822	0.7873	0.6652	0.5269	0.3872
	6	1.0000	1.0000	1.0000	0.9993	0.9961	0.9858	0.9614	0.9154	0.8418	0.7393	0.6128
	7	1.0000	1.0000	1.0000	0.9999	0.9994	0.9972	0.9905	0.9745	0.9427	0.8883	0.8062

n	r	0.01	0.05	0.1	0.15	0.2	0.25	0.3	0.35	0.4	0.45	0.5
	8	1.0000	1.0000	1.0000	1.0000	0.9999	0.9996	0.9983	0.9944	0.9847	0.9644	0.9270
	9	1.0000	1.0000	1.0000	1.0000	1.0000	1.0000	0.9998	0.9992	0.9972	0.9921	0.9807
	10	1.0000	1.0000	1.0000	1.0000	1.0000	1.0000	1.0000	0.9999	0.9997	0.9989	0.9968
	11	1.0000	1.0000	1.0000	1.0000	1.0000	1.0000	1.0000	1.0000	1.0000	0.9999	0.9998
	12	1.0000	1.0000	1.0000	1.0000	1.0000	1.0000	1.0000	1.0000	1.0000	1.0000	1.0000
13	0	0.8775	0.5133	0.2542	0.1209	0.0550	0.0238	0.0097	0.0037	0.0013	0.0004	0.0001
	1	0.9928	0.8646	0.6213	0.3983	0.2337	0.1267	0.0637	0.0296	0.0126	0.0049	0.0017
	2	0.9997	0.9755	0.8661	0.6920	0.5017	0.3326	0.2025	0.1132	0.0579	0.0269	0.0112
	3	1.0000	0.9969	0.9658	0.8820	0.7473	0.5843	0.4206	0.2783	0.1686	0.0929	0.0461
	4	1.0000	0.9997	0.9935	0.9658	0.9009	0.7940	0.6543	0.5005	0.3530	0.2280	0.1334
	5	1.0000	1.0000	0.9991	0.9925	0.9700	0.9198	0.8346	0.7159	0.5744	0.4268	0.2905
	6	1.0000	1.0000	0.9999	0.9987	0.9930	0.9757	0.9376	0.8705	0.7712	0.6437	0.5000
	7	1.0000	1.0000	1.0000	0.9998	0.9988	0.9944	0.9818	0.9538	0.9023	0.8212	0.7095
	8	1.0000	1.0000	1.0000	1.0000	0.9998	0.9990	0.9960	0.9874	0.9679	0.9302	0.8666
	9	1.0000	1.0000	1.0000	1.0000	1.0000	0.9999	0.9994	0.9975	0.9922	0.9797	0.9539
	10	1.0000	1.0000	1.0000	1.0000	1.0000	1.0000	0.9999	0.9997	0.9987	0.9959	0.9888
	11	1.0000	1.0000	1.0000	1.0000	1.0000	1.0000	1.0000	1.0000	0.9999	0.9995	0.9983
	12	1.0000	1.0000	1.0000	1.0000	1.0000	1.0000	1.0000	1.0000	1.0000	1.0000	0.9999
	13	1.0000	1.0000	1.0000	1.0000	1.0000	1.0000	1.0000	1.0000	1.0000	1.0000	1.0000
14	0	0.8688	0.4877	0.2288	0.1028	0.0440	0.0178	0.0068	0.0024	0.0008	0.0002	0.0001
	1	0.9916	0.8470	0.5846	0.3567	0.1979	0.1010	0.0475	0.0205	0.0081	0.0029	0.0009
	2	0.9997	0.9700	0.8416	0.6479	0.4481	0.2811	0.1608	0.0839	0.0398	0.0170	0.0065
	3	1.0000	0.9958	0.9559	0.8535	0.6982	0.5213	0.3552	0.2205	0.1243	0.0632	0.0287
	4	1.0000	0.9996	0.9908	0.9533	0.8702	0.7415	0.5842	0.4227	0.2793	0.1672	0.0898
	5	1.0000	1.0000	0.9985	0.9885	0.9562	0.8883	0.7805	0.6405	0.4859	0.3373	0.2120
	6	1.0000	1.0000	0.9998	0.9978	0.9884	0.9617	0.9067	0.8164	0.6925	0.5461	0.3953
	7	1.0000	1.0000	1.0000	0.9997	0.9976	0.9897	0.9685	0.9247	0.8499	0.7414	0.6047
	8	1.0000	1.0000	1.0000	1.0000	0.9996	0.9979	0.9917	0.9757	0.9417	0.8811	0.7880
	9	1.0000	1.0000	1.0000	1.0000	1.0000	0.9997	0.9983	0.9940	0.9825	0.9574	0.9102
	10	1.0000	1.0000	1.0000	1.0000	1.0000	1.0000	0.9998	0.9989	0.9961	0.9886	0.9713
	11	1.0000	1.0000	1.0000	1.0000	1.0000	1.0000	1.0000	0.9999	0.9994	0.9979	0.9935
	12	1.0000	1.0000	1.0000	1.0000	1.0000	1.0000	1.0000	1.0000	0.9999	0.9998	0.9991
	13	1.0000	1.0000	1.0000	1.0000	1.0000	1.0000	1.0000	1.0000	1.0000	1.0000	0.9999
	14	1.0000	1.0000	1.0000	1.0000	1.0000	1.0000	1.0000	1.0000	1.0000	1.0000	1.0000
15	0	0.8601	0.4633	0.2059	0.0874	0.0352	0.0134	0.0048	0.0016	0.0005	0.0001	0.0000
	1	0.9904	0.8291	0.5490	0.3186	0.1671	0.0802	0.0353	0.0142	0.0052	0.0017	0.0005
	2	0.9996	0.9638	0.8159	0.6042	0.3980	0.2361	0.1268	0.0617	0.0271	0.0107	0.0037
	3	1.0000	0.9945	0.9444	0.8227	0.6482	0.4613	0.2969	0.1727	0.0905	0.0424	0.0176
	4	1.0000	0.9994	0.9873	0.9383	0.8358	0.6865	0.5155	0.3519	0.2173	0.1204	0.0592
	5	1.0000	1.0000	0.9978	0.9832	0.9390	0.8516	0.7216	0.5643	0.4032	0.2608	0.1509
	6	1.0000	1.0000	0.9997	0.9964	0.9819	0.9434	0.8689	0.7548	0.6098	0.4522	0.3036
	7	1.0000	1.0000	1.0000	0.9994	0.9958	0.9827	0.9500	0.8868	0.7869	0.6535	0.5000
	8	1.0000	1.0000	1.0000	0.9999	0.9992	0.9958	0.9848	0.9578	0.9050	0.8182	0.6964
	9	1.0000	1.0000	1.0000	1.0000	0.9999	0.9992	0.9964	0.9876	0.9662	0.9231	0.8491
	10	1.0000	1.0000	1.0000	1.0000	1.0000	0.9999	0.9993	0.9972	0.9907	0.9745	0.9408
	11	1.0000	1.0000	1.0000	1.0000	1.0000	1.0000	0.9999	0.9995	0.9981	0.9937	0.9824
	12	1.0000	1.0000	1.0000	1.0000	1.0000	1.0000	1.0000	0.9999	0.9997	0.9989	0.9963
	13	1.0000	1.0000	1.0000	1.0000	1.0000	1.0000	1.0000	1.0000	1.0000	0.9999	0.9995
	14	1.0000	1.0000	1.0000	1.0000	1.0000	1.0000	1.0000	1.0000	1.0000	1.0000	1.0000
	15	1.0000	1.0000	1.0000	1.0000	1.0000	1.0000	1.0000	1.0000	1.0000	1.0000	1.0000

n	r	0.01	0.05	0.1	0.15	0.2	0.25	0.3	0.35	0.4	0.45	0.5
20	0	0.8179	0.3585	0.1216	0.0388	0.0115	0.0032	0.0008	0.0002	0.0000	0.0000	0.0000
	1	0.9831	0.7358	0.3918	0.1756	0.0692	0.0243	0.0076	0.0021	0.0005	0.0001	0.0000
	2	0.9990	0.9245	0.6769	0.4049	0.2061	0.0913	0.0355	0.0121	0.0036	0.0009	0.0002
	3	1.0000	0.9841	0.8671	0.6477	0.4115	0.2252	0.1071	0.0444	0.0160	0.0049	0.0013
	4	1.0000	0.9974	0.9568	0.8299	0.6297	0.4148	0.2375	0.1182	0.0510	0.0189	0.0059
	5	1.0000	0.9997	0.9888	0.9327	0.8042	0.6172	0.4164	0.2454	0.1256	0.0553	0.0207
	6	1.0000	1.0000	0.9976	0.9781	0.9133	0.7858	0.6080	0.4166	0.2500	0.1299	0.0577
	7	1.0000	1.0000	0.9996	0.9941	0.9679	0.8982	0.7723	0.6010	0.4159	0.2520	0.1316
	8	1.0000	1.0000	0.9999	0.9987	0.9900	0.9591	0.8867	0.7624	0.5956	0.4143	0.2517
	9	1.0000	1.0000	1.0000	0.9998	0.9974	0.9861	0.9520	0.8782	0.7553	0.5914	0.4119
	10	1.0000	1.0000	1.0000	1.0000	0.9994	0.9961	0.9829	0.9468	0.8725	0.7507	0.5881
	11	1.0000	1.0000	1.0000	1.0000	0.9999	0.9991	0.9949	0.9804	0.9435	0.8692	0.7483
	12	1.0000	1.0000	1.0000	1.0000	1.0000	0.9998	0.9987	0.9940	0.9790	0.9420	0.8684
	13	1.0000	1.0000	1.0000	1.0000	1.0000	1.0000	0.9997	0.9985	0.9935	0.9786	0.9423
	14	1.0000	1.0000	1.0000	1.0000	1.0000	1.0000	1.0000	0.9997	0.9984	0.9936	0.9793
	15	1.0000	1.0000	1.0000	1.0000	1.0000	1.0000	1.0000	1.0000	0.9997	0.9985	0.9941
	16	1.0000	1.0000	1.0000	1.0000	1.0000	1.0000	1.0000	1.0000	1.0000	0.9997	0.9987
	17	1.0000	1.0000	1.0000	1.0000	1.0000	1.0000	1.0000	1.0000	1.0000	1.0000	0.9998
	18	1.0000	1.0000	1.0000	1.0000	1.0000	1.0000	1.0000	1.0000	1.0000	1.0000	1.0000
	19	1.0000	1.0000	1.0000	1.0000	1.0000	1.0000	1.0000	1.0000	1.0000	1.0000	1.0000
	20	1.0000	1.0000	1.0000	1.0000	1.0000	1.0000	1.0000	1.0000	1.0000	1.0000	1.0000

Table 2. Cumulative Poisson Probabilities

	λ									
r	0.005	0.01	0.02	0.03	0.04	0.05	0.06	0.07	0.08	0.09
0	0.9950	0.9900	0.9802	0.9704	0.9608	0.9512	0.9418	0.9324	0.9231	0.9139
1	1.0000	1.0000	0.9998	0.9996	0.9992	0.9988	0.9983	0.9977	0.9970	0.9962
2	1.0000	1.0000	1.0000	1.0000	1.0000	1.0000	1.0000	0.9999	0.9999	0.9999
3	1.0000	1.0000	1.0000	1.0000	1.0000	1.0000	1.0000	1.0000	1.0000	1.0000

	λ									
r	0.1	0.2	0.3	0.4	0.5	0.6	0.7	0.8	0.9	1
0	0.9048	0.8187	0.7408	0.6703	0.6065	0.5488	0.4966	0.4493	0.4066	0.3679
1	0.9953	0.9825	0.9631	0.9384	0.9098	0.8781	0.8442	0.8088	0.7725	0.7358
2	0.9998	0.9989	0.9964	0.9921	0.9856	0.9769	0.9659	0.9526	0.9371	0.9197
3	1.0000	0.9999	0.9997	0.9992	0.9982	0.9966	0.9942	0.9909	0.9865	0.9810
4	1.0000	1.0000	1.0000	0.9999	0.9998	0.9996	0.9992	0.9986	0.9977	0.9963
5	1.0000	1.0000	1.0000	1.0000	1.0000	1.0000	0.9999	0.9998	0.9997	0.9994
6	1.0000	1.0000	1.0000	1.0000	1.0000	1.0000	1.0000	1.0000	1.0000	0.9999
7	1.0000	1.0000	1.0000	1.0000	1.0000	1.0000	1.0000	1.0000	1.0000	1.0000

	λ									
r	1.1	1.2	1.3	1.4	1.5	1.6	1.7	1.8	1.9	2
0	0.3329	0.3012	0.2725	0.2466	0.2231	0.2019	0.1827	0.1653	0.1496	0.1353
1	0.6990	0.6626	0.6268	0.5918	0.5578	0.5249	0.4932	0.4628	0.4337	0.4060
2	0.9004	0.8795	0.8571	0.8335	0.8088	0.7834	0.7572	0.7306	0.7037	0.6767
3	0.9743	0.9662	0.9569	0.9463	0.9344	0.9212	0.9068	0.8913	0.8747	0.8571
4	0.9946	0.9923	0.9893	0.9857	0.9814	0.9763	0.9704	0.9636	0.9559	0.9473
5	0.9990	0.9985	0.9978	0.9968	0.9955	0.9940	0.9920	0.9896	0.9868	0.9834

	λ									
r	**1.1**	**1.2**	**1.3**	**1.4**	**1.5**	**1.6**	**1.7**	**1.8**	**1.9**	**2**
6	0.9999	0.9997	0.9996	0.9994	0.9991	0.9987	0.9981	0.9974	0.9966	0.9955
7	1.0000	1.0000	0.9999	0.9999	0.9998	0.9997	0.9996	0.9994	0.9992	0.9989
8	1.0000	1.0000	1.0000	1.0000	1.0000	1.0000	0.9999	0.9999	0.9998	0.9998
9	1.0000	1.0000	1.0000	1.0000	1.0000	1.0000	1.0000	1.0000	1.0000	1.0000

	λ									
r	**2.1**	**2.2**	**2.3**	**2.4**	**2.5**	**2.6**	**2.7**	**2.8**	**2.9**	**3**
0	0.1225	0.1108	0.1003	0.0907	0.0821	0.0743	0.0672	0.0608	0.0550	0.0498
1	0.3796	0.3546	0.3309	0.3084	0.2873	0.2674	0.2487	0.2311	0.2146	0.1991
2	0.6496	0.6227	0.5960	0.5697	0.5438	0.5184	0.4936	0.4695	0.4460	0.4232
3	0.8386	0.8194	0.7993	0.7787	0.7576	0.7360	0.7141	0.6919	0.6696	0.6472
4	0.9379	0.9275	0.9162	0.9041	0.8912	0.8774	0.8629	0.8477	0.8318	0.8153
5	0.9796	0.9751	0.9700	0.9643	0.9580	0.9510	0.9433	0.9349	0.9258	0.9161
6	0.9941	0.9925	0.9906	0.9884	0.9858	0.9828	0.9794	0.9756	0.9713	0.9665
7	0.9985	0.9980	0.9974	0.9967	0.9958	0.9947	0.9934	0.9919	0.9901	0.9881
8	0.9997	0.9995	0.9994	0.9991	0.9989	0.9985	0.9981	0.9976	0.9969	0.9962
9	0.9999	0.9999	0.9999	0.9998	0.9997	0.9996	0.9995	0.9993	0.9991	0.9989
10	1.0000	1.0000	1.0000	1.0000	0.9999	0.9999	0.9999	0.9998	0.9998	0.9997
11	1.0000	1.0000	1.0000	1.0000	1.0000	1.0000	1.0000	1.0000	0.9999	0.9999
12	1.0000	1.0000	1.0000	1.0000	1.0000	1.0000	1.0000	1.0000	1.0000	1.0000

	λ									
r	**3.1**	**3.2**	**3.3**	**3.4**	**3.5**	**3.6**	**3.7**	**3.8**	**3.9**	**4**
0	0.0450	0.0408	0.0369	0.0334	0.0302	0.0273	0.0247	0.0224	0.0202	0.0183
1	0.1847	0.1712	0.1586	0.1468	0.1359	0.1257	0.1162	0.1074	0.0992	0.0916
2	0.4012	0.3799	0.3594	0.3397	0.3208	0.3027	0.2854	0.2689	0.2531	0.2381
3	0.6248	0.6025	0.5803	0.5584	0.5366	0.5152	0.4942	0.4735	0.4532	0.4335
4	0.7982	0.7806	0.7626	0.7442	0.7254	0.7064	0.6872	0.6678	0.6484	0.6288
5	0.9057	0.8946	0.8829	0.8705	0.8576	0.8441	0.8301	0.8156	0.8006	0.7851
6	0.9612	0.9554	0.9490	0.9421	0.9347	0.9267	0.9182	0.9091	0.8995	0.8893
7	0.9858	0.9832	0.9802	0.9769	0.9733	0.9692	0.9648	0.9599	0.9546	0.9489
8	0.9953	0.9943	0.9931	0.9917	0.9901	0.9883	0.9863	0.9840	0.9815	0.9786
9	0.9986	0.9982	0.9978	0.9973	0.9967	0.9960	0.9952	0.9942	0.9931	0.9919
10	0.9996	0.9995	0.9994	0.9992	0.9990	0.9987	0.9984	0.9981	0.9977	0.9972
11	0.9999	0.9999	0.9998	0.9998	0.9997	0.9996	0.9995	0.9994	0.9993	0.9991
12	1.0000	1.0000	1.0000	0.9999	0.9999	0.9999	0.9999	0.9998	0.9998	0.9997
13	1.0000	1.0000	1.0000	1.0000	1.0000	1.0000	1.0000	1.0000	0.9999	0.9999
14	1.0000	1.0000	1.0000	1.0000	1.0000	1.0000	1.0000	1.0000	1.0000	1.0000

	λ									
r	**4.1**	**4.2**	**4.3**	**4.4**	**4.5**	**4.6**	**4.7**	**4.8**	**4.9**	**5**
0	0.0166	0.0150	0.0136	0.0123	0.0111	0.0101	0.0091	0.0082	0.0074	0.0067
1	0.0845	0.0780	0.0719	0.0663	0.0611	0.0563	0.0518	0.0477	0.0439	0.0404
2	0.2238	0.2102	0.1974	0.1851	0.1736	0.1626	0.1523	0.1425	0.1333	0.1247
3	0.4142	0.3954	0.3772	0.3594	0.3423	0.3257	0.3097	0.2942	0.2793	0.2650
4	0.6093	0.5898	0.5704	0.5512	0.5321	0.5132	0.4946	0.4763	0.4582	0.4405
5	0.7693	0.7531	0.7367	0.7199	0.7029	0.6858	0.6684	0.6510	0.6335	0.6160
6	0.8786	0.8675	0.8558	0.8436	0.8311	0.8180	0.8046	0.7908	0.7767	0.7622
7	0.9427	0.9361	0.9290	0.9214	0.9134	0.9049	0.8960	0.8867	0.8769	0.8666
8	0.9755	0.9721	0.9683	0.9642	0.9597	0.9549	0.9497	0.9442	0.9382	0.9319
9	0.9905	0.9889	0.9871	0.9851	0.9829	0.9805	0.9778	0.9749	0.9717	0.9682

	λ									
r	4.1	4.2	4.3	4.4	4.5	4.6	4.7	4.8	4.9	5
10	0.9966	0.9959	0.9952	0.9943	0.9933	0.9922	0.9910	0.9896	0.9880	0.9863
11	0.9989	0.9986	0.9983	0.9980	0.9976	0.9971	0.9966	0.9960	0.9953	0.9945
12	0.9997	0.9996	0.9995	0.9993	0.9992	0.9990	0.9988	0.9986	0.9983	0.9980
13	0.9999	0.9999	0.9998	0.9998	0.9997	0.9997	0.9996	0.9995	0.9994	0.9993
14	1.0000	1.0000	1.0000	0.9999	0.9999	0.9999	0.9999	0.9999	0.9998	0.9998
15	1.0000	1.0000	1.0000	1.0000	1.0000	1.0000	1.0000	1.0000	0.9999	0.9999
16	1.0000	1.0000	1.0000	1.0000	1.0000	1.0000	1.0000	1.0000	1.0000	1.0000

	λ									
r	5.1	5.2	5.3	5.4	5.5	5.6	5.7	5.8	5.9	6
0	0.0061	0.0055	0.0050	0.0045	0.0041	0.0037	0.0033	0.0030	0.0027	0.0025
1	0.0372	0.0342	0.0314	0.0289	0.0266	0.0244	0.0224	0.0206	0.0189	0.0174
2	0.1165	0.1088	0.1016	0.0948	0.0884	0.0824	0.0768	0.0715	0.0666	0.0620
3	0.2513	0.2381	0.2254	0.2133	0.2017	0.1906	0.1800	0.1700	0.1604	0.1512
4	0.4231	0.4061	0.3895	0.3733	0.3575	0.3422	0.3272	0.3127	0.2987	0.2851
5	0.5984	0.5809	0.5635	0.5461	0.5289	0.5119	0.4950	0.4783	0.4619	0.4457
6	0.7474	0.7324	0.7171	0.7017	0.6860	0.6703	0.6544	0.6384	0.6224	0.6063
7	0.8560	0.8449	0.8335	0.8217	0.8095	0.7970	0.7841	0.7710	0.7576	0.7440
8	0.9252	0.9181	0.9106	0.9027	0.8944	0.8857	0.8766	0.8672	0.8574	0.8472
9	0.9644	0.9603	0.9559	0.9512	0.9462	0.9409	0.9352	0.9292	0.9228	0.9161
10	0.9844	0.9823	0.9800	0.9775	0.9747	0.9718	0.9686	0.9651	0.9614	0.9574
11	0.9937	0.9927	0.9916	0.9904	0.9890	0.9875	0.9859	0.9841	0.9821	0.9799
12	0.9976	0.9972	0.9967	0.9962	0.9955	0.9949	0.9941	0.9932	0.9922	0.9912
13	0.9992	0.9990	0.9988	0.9986	0.9983	0.9980	0.9977	0.9973	0.9969	0.9964
14	0.9997	0.9997	0.9996	0.9995	0.9994	0.9993	0.9991	0.9990	0.9988	0.9986
15	0.9999	0.9999	0.9999	0.9998	0.9998	0.9998	0.9997	0.9996	0.9996	0.9995
16	1.0000	1.0000	1.0000	0.9999	0.9999	0.9999	0.9999	0.9999	0.9999	0.9998
17	1.0000	1.0000	1.0000	1.0000	1.0000	1.0000	1.0000	1.0000	1.0000	0.9999
18	1.0000	1.0000	1.0000	1.0000	1.0000	1.0000	1.0000	1.0000	1.0000	1.0000

	λ									
r	6.1	6.2	6.3	6.4	6.5	6.6	6.7	6.8	6.9	7
0	0.0022	0.0020	0.0018	0.0017	0.0015	0.0014	0.0012	0.0011	0.0010	0.0009
1	0.0159	0.0146	0.0134	0.0123	0.0113	0.0103	0.0095	0.0087	0.0080	0.0073
2	0.0577	0.0536	0.0498	0.0463	0.0430	0.0400	0.0371	0.0344	0.0320	0.0296
3	0.1425	0.1342	0.1264	0.1189	0.1118	0.1052	0.0988	0.0928	0.0871	0.0818
4	0.2719	0.2592	0.2469	0.2351	0.2237	0.2127	0.2022	0.1920	0.1823	0.1730
5	0.4298	0.4141	0.3988	0.3837	0.3690	0.3547	0.3406	0.3270	0.3137	0.3007
6	0.5902	0.5742	0.5582	0.5423	0.5265	0.5108	0.4953	0.4799	0.4647	0.4497
7	0.7301	0.7160	0.7017	0.6873	0.6728	0.6581	0.6433	0.6285	0.6136	0.5987
8	0.8367	0.8259	0.8148	0.8033	0.7916	0.7796	0.7673	0.7548	0.7420	0.7291
9	0.9090	0.9016	0.8939	0.8858	0.8774	0.8686	0.8596	0.8502	0.8405	0.8305
10	0.9531	0.9486	0.9437	0.9386	0.9332	0.9274	0.9214	0.9151	0.9084	0.9015
11	0.9776	0.9750	0.9723	0.9693	0.9661	0.9627	0.9591	0.9552	0.9510	0.9467
12	0.9900	0.9887	0.9873	0.9857	0.9840	0.9821	0.9801	0.9779	0.9755	0.9730
13	0.9958	0.9952	0.9945	0.9937	0.9929	0.9920	0.9909	0.9898	0.9885	0.9872
14	0.9984	0.9981	0.9978	0.9974	0.9970	0.9966	0.9961	0.9956	0.9950	0.9943
15	0.9994	0.9993	0.9992	0.9990	0.9988	0.9986	0.9984	0.9982	0.9979	0.9976
16	0.9998	0.9997	0.9997	0.9996	0.9996	0.9995	0.9994	0.9993	0.9992	0.9990
17	0.9999	0.9999	0.9999	0.9999	0.9998	0.9998	0.9998	0.9997	0.9997	0.9996
18	1.0000	1.0000	1.0000	1.0000	0.9999	0.9999	0.9999	0.9999	0.9999	0.9999

r	λ 6.1	6.2	6.3	6.4	6.5	6.6	6.7	6.8	6.9	7
19	1.0000	1.0000	1.0000	1.0000	1.0000	1.0000	1.0000	1.0000	1.0000	1.0000
20	1.0000	1.0000	1.0000	1.0000	1.0000	1.0000	1.0000	1.0000	1.0000	1.0000

r	λ 7.1	7.2	7.3	7.4	7.5	7.6	7.7	7.8	7.9	8
0	0.0008	0.0007	0.0007	0.0006	0.0006	0.0005	0.0005	0.0004	0.0004	0.0003
1	0.0067	0.0061	0.0056	0.0051	0.0047	0.0043	0.0039	0.0036	0.0033	0.0030
2	0.0275	0.0255	0.0236	0.0219	0.0203	0.0188	0.0174	0.0161	0.0149	0.0138
3	0.0767	0.0719	0.0674	0.0632	0.0591	0.0554	0.0518	0.0485	0.0453	0.0424
4	0.1641	0.1555	0.1473	0.1395	0.1321	0.1249	0.1181	0.1117	0.1055	0.0996
5	0.2881	0.2759	0.2640	0.2526	0.2414	0.2307	0.2203	0.2103	0.2006	0.1912
6	0.4349	0.4204	0.4060	0.3920	0.3782	0.3646	0.3514	0.3384	0.3257	0.3134
7	0.5838	0.5689	0.5541	0.5393	0.5246	0.5100	0.4956	0.4812	0.4670	0.4530
8	0.7160	0.7027	0.6892	0.6757	0.6620	0.6482	0.6343	0.6204	0.6065	0.5925
9	0.8202	0.8096	0.7988	0.7877	0.7764	0.7649	0.7531	0.7411	0.7290	0.7166
10	0.8942	0.8867	0.8788	0.8707	0.8622	0.8535	0.8445	0.8352	0.8257	0.8159
11	0.9420	0.9371	0.9319	0.9265	0.9208	0.9148	0.9085	0.9020	0.8952	0.8881
12	0.9703	0.9673	0.9642	0.9609	0.9573	0.9536	0.9496	0.9454	0.9409	0.9362
13	0.9857	0.9841	0.9824	0.9805	0.9784	0.9762	0.9739	0.9714	0.9687	0.9658
14	0.9935	0.9927	0.9918	0.9908	0.9897	0.9886	0.9873	0.9859	0.9844	0.9827
15	0.9972	0.9969	0.9964	0.9959	0.9954	0.9948	0.9941	0.9934	0.9926	0.9918
16	0.9989	0.9987	0.9985	0.9983	0.9980	0.9978	0.9974	0.9971	0.9967	0.9963
17	0.9996	0.9995	0.9994	0.9993	0.9992	0.9991	0.9989	0.9988	0.9986	0.9984
18	0.9998	0.9998	0.9998	0.9997	0.9997	0.9996	0.9996	0.9995	0.9994	0.9993
19	0.9999	0.9999	0.9999	0.9999	0.9999	0.9999	0.9998	0.9998	0.9998	0.9997
20	1.0000	1.0000	1.0000	1.0000	1.0000	1.0000	0.9999	0.9999	0.9999	0.9999
21	1.0000	1.0000	1.0000	1.0000	1.0000	1.0000	1.0000	1.0000	1.0000	1.0000

r	λ 8.1	8.2	8.3	8.4	8.5	8.6	8.7	8.8	8.9	9
0	0.0003	0.0003	0.0002	0.0002	0.0002	0.0002	0.0002	0.0002	0.0001	0.0001
1	0.0028	0.0025	0.0023	0.0021	0.0019	0.0018	0.0016	0.0015	0.0014	0.0012
2	0.0127	0.0118	0.0109	0.0100	0.0093	0.0086	0.0079	0.0073	0.0068	0.0062
3	0.0396	0.0370	0.0346	0.0323	0.0301	0.0281	0.0262	0.0244	0.0228	0.0212
4	0.0940	0.0887	0.0837	0.0789	0.0744	0.0701	0.0660	0.0621	0.0584	0.0550
5	0.1822	0.1736	0.1653	0.1573	0.1496	0.1422	0.1352	0.1284	0.1219	0.1157
6	0.3013	0.2896	0.2781	0.2670	0.2562	0.2457	0.2355	0.2256	0.2160	0.2068
7	0.4391	0.4254	0.4119	0.3987	0.3856	0.3728	0.3602	0.3478	0.3357	0.3239
8	0.5786	0.5647	0.5507	0.5369	0.5231	0.5094	0.4958	0.4823	0.4689	0.4557
9	0.7041	0.6915	0.6788	0.6659	0.6530	0.6400	0.6269	0.6137	0.6006	0.5874
10	0.8058	0.7955	0.7850	0.7743	0.7634	0.7522	0.7409	0.7294	0.7178	0.7060
11	0.8807	0.8731	0.8652	0.8571	0.8487	0.8400	0.8311	0.8220	0.8126	0.8030
12	0.9313	0.9261	0.9207	0.9150	0.9091	0.9029	0.8965	0.8898	0.8829	0.8758
13	0.9628	0.9595	0.9561	0.9524	0.9486	0.9445	0.9403	0.9358	0.9311	0.9261
14	0.9810	0.9791	0.9771	0.9749	0.9726	0.9701	0.9675	0.9647	0.9617	0.9585
15	0.9908	0.9898	0.9887	0.9875	0.9862	0.9848	0.9832	0.9816	0.9798	0.9780
16	0.9958	0.9953	0.9947	0.9941	0.9934	0.9926	0.9918	0.9909	0.9899	0.9889
17	0.9982	0.9979	0.9977	0.9973	0.9970	0.9966	0.9962	0.9957	0.9952	0.9947
18	0.9992	0.9991	0.9990	0.9989	0.9987	0.9985	0.9983	0.9981	0.9978	0.9976
19	0.9997	0.9997	0.9996	0.9995	0.9995	0.9994	0.9993	0.9992	0.9991	0.9989

	λ									
r	**8.1**	**8.2**	**8.3**	**8.4**	**8.5**	**8.6**	**8.7**	**8.8**	**8.9**	**9**
20	0.9999	0.9999	0.9998	0.9998	0.9998	0.9998	0.9997	0.9997	0.9996	0.9996
21	1.0000	1.0000	0.9999	0.9999	0.9999	0.9999	0.9999	0.9999	0.9998	0.9998
22	1.0000	1.0000	1.0000	1.0000	1.0000	1.0000	1.0000	1.0000	0.9999	0.9999
23	1.0000	1.0000	1.0000	1.0000	1.0000	1.0000	1.0000	1.0000	1.0000	1.0000

	λ									
r	**9.1**	**9.2**	**9.3**	**9.4**	**9.5**	**9.6**	**9.7**	**9.8**	**9.9**	**10**
0	0.0001	0.0001	0.0001	0.0001	0.0001	0.0001	0.0001	0.0001	0.0001	0.0000
1	0.0011	0.0010	0.0009	0.0009	0.0008	0.0007	0.0007	0.0006	0.0005	0.0005
2	0.0058	0.0053	0.0049	0.0045	0.0042	0.0038	0.0035	0.0033	0.0030	0.0028
3	0.0198	0.0184	0.0172	0.0160	0.0149	0.0138	0.0129	0.0120	0.0111	0.0103
4	0.0517	0.0486	0.0456	0.0429	0.0403	0.0378	0.0355	0.0333	0.0312	0.0293
5	0.1098	0.1041	0.0986	0.0935	0.0885	0.0838	0.0793	0.0750	0.0710	0.0671
6	0.1978	0.1892	0.1808	0.1727	0.1649	0.1574	0.1502	0.1433	0.1366	0.1301
7	0.3123	0.3010	0.2900	0.2792	0.2687	0.2584	0.2485	0.2388	0.2294	0.2202
8	0.4426	0.4296	0.4168	0.4042	0.3918	0.3796	0.3676	0.3558	0.3442	0.3328
9	0.5742	0.5611	0.5479	0.5349	0.5218	0.5089	0.4960	0.4832	0.4705	0.4579
10	0.6941	0.6820	0.6699	0.6576	0.6453	0.6329	0.6205	0.6080	0.5955	0.5830
11	0.7932	0.7832	0.7730	0.7626	0.7520	0.7412	0.7303	0.7193	0.7081	0.6968
12	0.8684	0.8607	0.8529	0.8448	0.8364	0.8279	0.8191	0.8101	0.8009	0.7916
13	0.9210	0.9156	0.9100	0.9042	0.8981	0.8919	0.8853	0.8786	0.8716	0.8645
14	0.9552	0.9517	0.9480	0.9441	0.9400	0.9357	0.9312	0.9265	0.9216	0.9165
15	0.9760	0.9738	0.9715	0.9691	0.9665	0.9638	0.9609	0.9579	0.9546	0.9513
16	0.9878	0.9865	0.9852	0.9838	0.9823	0.9806	0.9789	0.9770	0.9751	0.9730
17	0.9941	0.9934	0.9927	0.9919	0.9911	0.9902	0.9892	0.9881	0.9870	0.9857
18	0.9973	0.9969	0.9966	0.9962	0.9957	0.9952	0.9947	0.9941	0.9935	0.9928
19	0.9988	0.9986	0.9985	0.9983	0.9980	0.9978	0.9975	0.9972	0.9969	0.9965
20	0.9995	0.9994	0.9993	0.9992	0.9991	0.9990	0.9989	0.9987	0.9986	0.9984
21	0.9998	0.9998	0.9997	0.9997	0.9996	0.9996	0.9995	0.9995	0.9994	0.9993
22	0.9999	0.9999	0.9999	0.9999	0.9999	0.9998	0.9998	0.9998	0.9997	0.9997
23	1.0000	1.0000	1.0000	1.0000	0.9999	0.9999	0.9999	0.9999	0.9999	0.9999
24	1.0000	1.0000	1.0000	1.0000	1.0000	1.0000	1.0000	1.0000	1.0000	1.0000

	λ									
r	**11**	**12**	**13**	**14**	**15**	**16**	**17**	**18**	**19**	**20**
0	0.0000	0.0000	0.0000	0.0000	0.0000	0.0000	0.0000	0.0000	0.0000	0.0000
1	0.0002	0.0001	0.0000	0.0000	0.0000	0.0000	0.0000	0.0000	0.0000	0.0000
2	0.0012	0.0005	0.0002	0.0001	0.0000	0.0000	0.0000	0.0000	0.0000	0.0000
3	0.0049	0.0023	0.0011	0.0005	0.0002	0.0001	0.0000	0.0000	0.0000	0.0000
4	0.0151	0.0076	0.0037	0.0018	0.0009	0.0004	0.0002	0.0001	0.0000	0.0000
5	0.0375	0.0203	0.0107	0.0055	0.0028	0.0014	0.0007	0.0003	0.0002	0.0001
6	0.0786	0.0458	0.0259	0.0142	0.0076	0.0040	0.0021	0.0010	0.0005	0.0003
7	0.1432	0.0895	0.0540	0.0316	0.0180	0.0100	0.0054	0.0029	0.0015	0.0008
8	0.2320	0.1550	0.0998	0.0621	0.0374	0.0220	0.0126	0.0071	0.0039	0.0021
9	0.3405	0.2424	0.1658	0.1094	0.0699	0.0433	0.0261	0.0154	0.0089	0.0050
10	0.4599	0.3472	0.2517	0.1757	0.1185	0.0774	0.0491	0.0304	0.0183	0.0108
11	0.5793	0.4616	0.3532	0.2600	0.1848	0.1270	0.0847	0.0549	0.0347	0.0214
12	0.6887	0.5760	0.4631	0.3585	0.2676	0.1931	0.1350	0.0917	0.0606	0.0390
13	0.7813	0.6815	0.5730	0.4644	0.3632	0.2745	0.2009	0.1426	0.0984	0.0661
14	0.8540	0.7720	0.6751	0.5704	0.4657	0.3675	0.2808	0.2081	0.1497	0.1049

r	λ 11	12	13	14	15	16	17	18	19	20
15	0.9074	0.8444	0.7636	0.6694	0.5681	0.4667	0.3715	0.2867	0.2148	0.1565
16	0.9441	0.8987	0.8355	0.7559	0.6641	0.5660	0.4677	0.3751	0.2920	0.2211
17	0.9678	0.9370	0.8905	0.8272	0.7489	0.6593	0.5640	0.4686	0.3784	0.2970
18	0.9823	0.9626	0.9302	0.8826	0.8195	0.7423	0.6550	0.5622	0.4695	0.3814
19	0.9907	0.9787	0.9573	0.9235	0.8752	0.8122	0.7363	0.6509	0.5606	0.4703
20	0.9953	0.9884	0.9750	0.9521	0.9170	0.8682	0.8055	0.7307	0.6472	0.5591
21	0.9977	0.9939	0.9859	0.9712	0.9469	0.9108	0.8615	0.7991	0.7255	0.6437
22	0.9990	0.9970	0.9924	0.9833	0.9673	0.9418	0.9047	0.8551	0.7931	0.7206
23	0.9995	0.9985	0.9960	0.9907	0.9805	0.9633	0.9367	0.8989	0.8490	0.7875
24	0.9998	0.9993	0.9980	0.9950	0.9888	0.9777	0.9594	0.9317	0.8933	0.8432
25	0.9999	0.9997	0.9990	0.9974	0.9938	0.9869	0.9748	0.9554	0.9269	0.8878
26	1.0000	0.9999	0.9995	0.9987	0.9967	0.9925	0.9848	0.9718	0.9514	0.9221
27	1.0000	0.9999	0.9998	0.9994	0.9983	0.9959	0.9912	0.9827	0.9687	0.9475
28	1.0000	1.0000	0.9999	0.9997	0.9991	0.9978	0.9950	0.9897	0.9805	0.9657
29	1.0000	1.0000	1.0000	0.9999	0.9996	0.9989	0.9973	0.9941	0.9882	0.9782
30	1.0000	1.0000	1.0000	0.9999	0.9998	0.9994	0.9986	0.9967	0.9930	0.9865
31	1.0000	1.0000	1.0000	1.0000	0.9999	0.9997	0.9993	0.9982	0.9960	0.9919
32	1.0000	1.0000	1.0000	1.0000	1.0000	0.9999	0.9996	0.9990	0.9978	0.9953
33	1.0000	1.0000	1.0000	1.0000	1.0000	0.9999	0.9998	0.9995	0.9988	0.9973
34	1.0000	1.0000	1.0000	1.0000	1.0000	1.0000	0.9999	0.9998	0.9994	0.9985
35	1.0000	1.0000	1.0000	1.0000	1.0000	1.0000	1.0000	0.9999	0.9997	0.9992
36	1.0000	1.0000	1.0000	1.0000	1.0000	1.0000	1.0000	0.9999	0.9998	0.9996
37	1.0000	1.0000	1.0000	1.0000	1.0000	1.0000	1.0000	1.0000	0.9999	0.9998
38	1.0000	1.0000	1.0000	1.0000	1.0000	1.0000	1.0000	1.0000	1.0000	0.9999
39	1.0000	1.0000	1.0000	1.0000	1.0000	1.0000	1.0000	1.0000	1.0000	0.9999
40	1.0000	1.0000	1.0000	1.0000	1.0000	1.0000	1.0000	1.0000	1.0000	1.0000

Table 3. Normal Probabilities

Z	.00	.01	.02	.03	.04	.05	.06	.07	.08	.09
−3.9	0.0000	0.0000	0.0000	0.0000	0.0000	0.0000	0.0000	0.0000	0.0000	0.0000
−3.8	0.0001	0.0001	0.0001	0.0001	0.0001	0.0001	0.0001	0.0001	0.0001	0.0001
−3.7	0.0001	0.0001	0.0001	0.0001	0.0001	0.0001	0.0001	0.0001	0.0001	0.0001
−3.6	0.0002	0.0002	0.0001	0.0001	0.0001	0.0001	0.0001	0.0001	0.0001	0.0001
−3.5	0.0002	0.0002	0.0002	0.0002	0.0002	0.0002	0.0002	0.0002	0.0002	0.0002
−3.4	0.0003	0.0003	0.0003	0.0003	0.0003	0.0003	0.0003	0.0003	0.0003	0.0002
−3.3	0.0005	0.0005	0.0005	0.0004	0.0004	0.0004	0.0004	0.0004	0.0004	0.0003
−3.2	0.0007	0.0007	0.0006	0.0006	0.0006	0.0006	0.0006	0.0005	0.0005	0.0005
−3.1	0.0010	0.0009	0.0009	0.0009	0.0008	0.0008	0.0008	0.0008	0.0007	0.0007
−3.0	0.0013	0.0013	0.0013	0.0012	0.0012	0.0011	0.0011	0.0011	0.0010	0.0010
−2.9	0.0019	0.0018	0.0018	0.0017	0.0016	0.0016	0.0015	0.0015	0.0014	0.0014
−2.8	0.0026	0.0025	0.0024	0.0023	0.0023	0.0022	0.0021	0.0021	0.0020	0.0019
−2.7	0.0035	0.0034	0.0033	0.0032	0.0031	0.0030	0.0029	0.0028	0.0027	0.0026
−2.6	0.0047	0.0045	0.0044	0.0043	0.0041	0.0040	0.0039	0.0038	0.0037	0.0036
−2.5	0.0062	0.0060	0.0059	0.0057	0.0055	0.0054	0.0052	0.0051	0.0049	0.0048
−2.4	0.0082	0.0080	0.0078	0.0075	0.0073	0.0071	0.0069	0.0068	0.0066	0.0064
−2.3	0.0107	0.0104	0.0102	0.0099	0.0096	0.0094	0.0091	0.0089	0.0087	0.0084
−2.2	0.0139	0.0136	0.0132	0.0129	0.0125	0.0122	0.0119	0.0116	0.0113	0.0110
−2.1	0.0179	0.0174	0.0170	0.0166	0.0162	0.0158	0.0154	0.0150	0.0146	0.0143
−2.0	0.0228	0.0222	0.0217	0.0212	0.0207	0.0202	0.0197	0.0192	0.0188	0.0183
−1.9	0.0287	0.0281	0.0274	0.0268	0.0262	0.0256	0.0250	0.0244	0.0239	0.0233

Z	.00	.01	.02	.03	.04	.05	.06	.07	.08	.09
−1.8	0.0359	0.0351	0.0344	0.0336	0.0329	0.0322	0.0314	0.0307	0.0301	0.0294
−1.7	0.0446	0.0436	0.0427	0.0418	0.0409	0.0401	0.0392	0.0384	0.0375	0.0367
−1.6	0.0548	0.0537	0.0526	0.0516	0.0505	0.0495	0.0485	0.0475	0.0465	0.0455
−1.5	0.0668	0.0655	0.0643	0.0630	0.0618	0.0606	0.0594	0.0582	0.0571	0.0559
−1.4	0.0808	0.0793	0.0778	0.0764	0.0749	0.0735	0.0721	0.0708	0.0694	0.0681
−1.3	0.0968	0.0951	0.0934	0.0918	0.0901	0.0885	0.0869	0.0853	0.0838	0.0823
−1.2	0.1151	0.1131	0.1112	0.1093	0.1075	0.1056	0.1038	0.1020	0.1003	0.0985
−1.1	0.1357	0.1335	0.1314	0.1292	0.1271	0.1251	0.1230	0.1210	0.1190	0.1170
−1.0	0.1587	0.1562	0.1539	0.1515	0.1492	0.1469	0.1446	0.1423	0.1401	0.1379
−0.9	0.1841	0.1814	0.1788	0.1762	0.1736	0.1711	0.1685	0.1660	0.1635	0.1611
−0.8	0.2119	0.2090	0.2061	0.2033	0.2005	0.1977	0.1949	0.1922	0.1894	0.1867
−0.7	0.2420	0.2389	0.2358	0.2327	0.2296	0.2266	0.2236	0.2206	0.2177	0.2148
−0.6	0.2743	0.2709	0.2676	0.2643	0.2611	0.2578	0.2546	0.2514	0.2483	0.2451
−0.5	0.3085	0.3050	0.3015	0.2981	0.2946	0.2912	0.2877	0.2843	0.2810	0.2776
−0.4	0.3446	0.3409	0.3372	0.3336	0.3300	0.3264	0.3228	0.3192	0.3156	0.3121
−0.3	0.3821	0.3783	0.3745	0.3707	0.3669	0.3632	0.3594	0.3557	0.3520	0.3483
−0.2	0.4207	0.4168	0.4129	0.4090	0.4052	0.4013	0.3974	0.3936	0.3897	0.3859
−0.1	0.4602	0.4562	0.4522	0.4483	0.4443	0.4404	0.4364	0.4325	0.4286	0.4247
−0.0	0.5000	0.4960	0.4920	0.4880	0.4840	0.4801	0.4761	0.4721	0.4681	0.4641
0.0	0.5000	0.5040	0.5080	0.5120	0.5160	0.5199	0.5239	0.5279	0.5319	0.5359
0.1	0.5398	0.5438	0.5478	0.5517	0.5557	0.5596	0.5636	0.5675	0.5714	0.5753
0.2	0.5793	0.5832	0.5871	0.5910	0.5948	0.5987	0.6026	0.6064	0.6103	0.6141
0.3	0.6179	0.6217	0.6255	0.6293	0.6331	0.6368	0.6406	0.6443	0.6480	0.6517
0.4	0.6554	0.6591	0.6628	0.6664	0.6700	0.6736	0.6772	0.6808	0.6844	0.6879
0.5	0.6915	0.6950	0.6985	0.7019	0.7054	0.7088	0.7123	0.7157	0.7190	0.7224
0.6	0.7257	0.7291	0.7324	0.7357	0.7389	0.7422	0.7454	0.7486	0.7517	0.7549
0.7	0.7580	0.7611	0.7642	0.7673	0.7704	0.7734	0.7764	0.7794	0.7823	0.7852
0.8	0.7881	0.7910	0.7939	0.7967	0.7995	0.8023	0.8051	0.8078	0.8106	0.8133
0.9	0.8159	0.8186	0.8212	0.8238	0.8264	0.8289	0.8315	0.8340	0.8365	0.8389
1.0	0.8413	0.8438	0.8461	0.8485	0.8508	0.8531	0.8554	0.8577	0.8599	0.8621
1.1	0.8643	0.8665	0.8686	0.8708	0.8729	0.8749	0.8770	0.8790	0.8810	0.8830
1.2	0.8849	0.8869	0.8888	0.8907	0.8925	0.8944	0.8962	0.8980	0.8997	0.9015
1.3	0.9032	0.9049	0.9066	0.9082	0.9099	0.9115	0.9131	0.9147	0.9162	0.9177
1.4	0.9192	0.9207	0.9222	0.9236	0.9251	0.9265	0.9279	0.9292	0.9306	0.9319
1.5	0.9332	0.9345	0.9357	0.9370	0.9382	0.9394	0.9406	0.9418	0.9429	0.9441
1.6	0.9452	0.9463	0.9474	0.9484	0.9495	0.9505	0.9515	0.9525	0.9535	0.9545
1.7	0.9554	0.9564	0.9573	0.9582	0.9591	0.9599	0.9608	0.9616	0.9625	0.9633
1.8	0.9641	0.9649	0.9656	0.9664	0.9671	0.9678	0.9686	0.9693	0.9699	0.9706
1.9	0.9713	0.9719	0.9726	0.9732	0.9738	0.9744	0.9750	0.9756	0.9761	0.9767
2.0	0.9772	0.9778	0.9783	0.9788	0.9793	0.9798	0.9803	0.9808	0.9812	0.9817
2.1	0.9821	0.9826	0.9830	0.9834	0.9838	0.9842	0.9846	0.9850	0.9854	0.9857
2.2	0.9861	0.9864	0.9868	0.9871	0.9875	0.9878	0.9881	0.9884	0.9887	0.9890
2.3	0.9893	0.9896	0.9898	0.9901	0.9904	0.9906	0.9909	0.9911	0.9913	0.9916
2.4	0.9918	0.9920	0.9922	0.9925	0.9927	0.9929	0.9931	0.9932	0.9934	0.9936
2.5	0.9938	0.9940	0.9941	0.9943	0.9945	0.9946	0.9948	0.9949	0.9951	0.9952
2.6	0.9953	0.9955	0.9956	0.9957	0.9959	0.9960	0.9961	0.9962	0.9963	0.9964
2.7	0.9965	0.9966	0.9967	0.9968	0.9969	0.9970	0.9971	0.9972	0.9973	0.9974
2.8	0.9974	0.9975	0.9976	0.9977	0.9977	0.9978	0.9979	0.9979	0.9980	0.9981
2.9	0.9981	0.9982	0.9982	0.9983	0.9984	0.9984	0.9985	0.9985	0.9986	0.9986
3.0	0.9987	0.9987	0.9987	0.9988	0.9988	0.9989	0.9989	0.9989	0.9990	0.9990
3.1	0.9990	0.9991	0.9991	0.9991	0.9992	0.9992	0.9992	0.9992	0.9993	0.9993
3.2	0.9993	0.9993	0.9994	0.9994	0.9994	0.9994	0.9994	0.9995	0.9995	0.9995

Z	.00	.01	.02	.03	.04	.05	.06	.07	.08	.09
3.3	0.9995	0.9995	0.9995	0.9996	0.9996	0.9996	0.9996	0.9996	0.9996	0.9997
3.4	0.9997	0.9997	0.9997	0.9997	0.9997	0.9997	0.9997	0.9997	0.9997	0.9998
3.5	0.9998	0.9998	0.9998	0.9998	0.9998	0.9998	0.9998	0.9998	0.9998	0.9998
3.6	0.9998	0.9998	0.9999	0.9999	0.9999	0.9999	0.9999	0.9999	0.9999	0.9999
3.7	0.9999	0.9999	0.9999	0.9999	0.9999	0.9999	0.9999	0.9999	0.9999	0.9999
3.8	0.9999	0.9999	0.9999	0.9999	0.9999	0.9999	0.9999	0.9999	0.9999	0.9999
3.9	1.0000	1.0000	1.0000	1.0000	1.0000	1.0000	1.0000	1.0000	1.0000	1.0000

Table 4. Percentiles of the *t* Distribution

One Sided	75%	80%	85%	90%	95%	97.50%	99%	99.50%	99.75%	99.90%	99.95%
Two Sided	**50%**	**60%**	**70%**	**80%**	**90%**	**95%**	**98%**	**99%**	**99.50%**	**99.80%**	**99.90%**
df											
1	1	1.376	1.963	3.078	6.314	12.71	31.82	63.66	127.3	318.3	636.6
2	0.816	1.061	1.386	1.886	2.92	4.303	6.965	9.925	14.09	22.33	31.6
3	0.765	0.978	1.25	1.638	2.353	3.182	4.541	5.841	7.453	10.21	12.92
4	0.741	0.941	1.19	1.533	2.132	2.776	3.747	4.604	5.598	7.173	8.61
5	0.727	0.92	1.156	1.476	2.015	2.571	3.365	4.032	4.773	5.893	6.869
6	0.718	0.906	1.134	1.44	1.943	2.447	3.143	3.707	4.317	5.208	5.959
7	0.711	0.896	1.119	1.415	1.895	2.365	2.998	3.499	4.029	4.785	5.408
8	0.706	0.889	1.108	1.397	1.86	2.306	2.896	3.355	3.833	4.501	5.041
9	0.703	0.883	1.1	1.383	1.833	2.262	2.821	3.25	3.69	4.297	4.781
10	0.7	0.879	1.093	1.372	1.812	2.228	2.764	3.169	3.581	4.144	4.587
11	0.697	0.876	1.088	1.363	1.796	2.201	2.718	3.106	3.497	4.025	4.437
12	0.695	0.873	1.083	1.356	1.782	2.179	2.681	3.055	3.428	3.93	4.318
13	0.694	0.87	1.079	1.35	1.771	2.16	2.65	3.012	3.372	3.852	4.221
14	0.692	0.868	1.076	1.345	1.761	2.145	2.624	2.977	3.326	3.787	4.14
15	0.691	0.866	1.074	1.341	1.753	2.131	2.602	2.947	3.286	3.733	4.073
16	0.69	0.865	1.071	1.337	1.746	2.12	2.583	2.921	3.252	3.686	4.015
17	0.689	0.863	1.069	1.333	1.74	2.11	2.567	2.898	3.222	3.646	3.965
18	0.688	0.862	1.067	1.33	1.734	2.101	2.552	2.878	3.197	3.61	3.922
19	0.688	0.861	1.066	1.328	1.729	2.093	2.539	2.861	3.174	3.579	3.883
20	0.687	0.86	1.064	1.325	1.725	2.086	2.528	2.845	3.153	3.552	3.85
21	0.686	0.859	1.063	1.323	1.721	2.08	2.518	2.831	3.135	3.527	3.819
22	0.686	0.858	1.061	1.321	1.717	2.074	2.508	2.819	3.119	3.505	3.792
23	0.685	0.858	1.06	1.319	1.714	2.069	2.5	2.807	3.104	3.485	3.767
24	0.685	0.857	1.059	1.318	1.711	2.064	2.492	2.797	3.091	3.467	3.745
25	0.684	0.856	1.058	1.316	1.708	2.06	2.485	2.787	3.078	3.45	3.725
26	0.684	0.856	1.058	1.315	1.706	2.056	2.479	2.779	3.067	3.435	3.707
27	0.684	0.855	1.057	1.314	1.703	2.052	2.473	2.771	3.057	3.421	3.69
28	0.683	0.855	1.056	1.313	1.701	2.048	2.467	2.763	3.047	3.408	3.674
29	0.683	0.854	1.055	1.311	1.699	2.045	2.462	2.756	3.038	3.396	3.659
30	0.683	0.854	1.055	1.31	1.697	2.042	2.457	2.75	3.03	3.385	3.646
40	0.681	0.851	1.05	1.303	1.684	2.021	2.423	2.704	2.971	3.307	3.551
50	0.679	0.849	1.047	1.299	1.676	2.009	2.403	2.678	2.937	3.261	3.496
60	0.679	0.848	1.045	1.296	1.671	2	2.39	2.66	2.915	3.232	3.46
80	0.678	0.846	1.043	1.292	1.664	1.99	2.374	2.639	2.887	3.195	3.416
100	0.677	0.845	1.042	1.29	1.66	1.984	2.364	2.626	2.871	3.174	3.39
120	0.677	0.845	1.041	1.289	1.658	1.98	2.358	2.617	2.86	3.16	3.373
∞	0.674	0.842	1.036	1.282	1.645	1.96	2.326	2.576	2.807	3.090	3.291

Table 5. χ^2 Distribution Values

df	0.995	0.99	0.975	0.95	0.9	0.1	0.05	0.025	0.01	0.005
1	---	---	0.001	0.004	0.016	2.706	3.841	5.024	6.635	7.879
2	0.01	0.02	0.051	0.103	0.211	4.605	5.991	7.378	9.21	10.597
3	0.072	0.115	0.216	0.352	0.584	6.251	7.815	9.348	11.345	12.838
4	0.207	0.297	0.484	0.711	1.064	7.779	9.488	11.143	13.277	14.86
5	0.412	0.554	0.831	1.145	1.61	9.236	11.07	12.833	15.086	16.75
6	0.676	0.872	1.237	1.635	2.204	10.645	12.592	14.449	16.812	18.548
7	0.989	1.239	1.69	2.167	2.833	12.017	14.067	16.013	18.475	20.278
8	1.344	1.646	2.18	2.733	3.49	13.362	15.507	17.535	20.09	21.955
9	1.735	2.088	2.7	3.325	4.168	14.684	16.919	19.023	21.666	23.589
10	2.156	2.558	3.247	3.94	4.865	15.987	18.307	20.483	23.209	25.188
11	2.603	3.053	3.816	4.575	5.578	17.275	19.675	21.92	24.725	26.757
12	3.074	3.571	4.404	5.226	6.304	18.549	21.026	23.337	26.217	28.3
13	3.565	4.107	5.009	5.892	7.042	19.812	22.362	24.736	27.688	29.819
14	4.075	4.66	5.629	6.571	7.79	21.064	23.685	26.119	29.141	31.319
15	4.601	5.229	6.262	7.261	8.547	22.307	24.996	27.488	30.578	32.801
16	5.142	5.812	6.908	7.962	9.312	23.542	26.296	28.845	32	34.267
17	5.697	6.408	7.564	8.672	10.085	24.769	27.587	30.191	33.409	35.718
18	6.265	7.015	8.231	9.39	10.865	25.989	28.869	31.526	34.805	37.156
19	6.844	7.633	8.907	10.117	11.651	27.204	30.144	32.852	36.191	38.582
20	7.434	8.26	9.591	10.851	12.443	28.412	31.41	34.17	37.566	39.997
21	8.034	8.897	10.283	11.591	13.24	29.615	32.671	35.479	38.932	41.401
22	8.643	9.542	10.982	12.338	14.041	30.813	33.924	36.781	40.289	42.796
23	9.26	10.196	11.689	13.091	14.848	32.007	35.172	38.076	41.638	44.181
24	9.886	10.856	12.401	13.848	15.659	33.196	36.415	39.364	42.98	45.559
25	10.52	11.524	13.12	14.611	16.473	34.382	37.652	40.646	44.314	46.928
26	11.16	12.198	13.844	15.379	17.292	35.563	38.885	41.923	45.642	48.29
27	11.808	12.879	14.573	16.151	18.114	36.741	40.113	43.195	46.963	49.645
28	12.461	13.565	15.308	16.928	18.939	37.916	41.337	44.461	48.278	50.993
29	13.121	14.256	16.047	17.708	19.768	39.087	42.557	45.722	49.588	52.336
30	13.787	14.953	16.791	18.493	20.599	40.256	43.773	46.979	50.892	53.672
40	20.707	22.164	24.433	26.509	29.051	51.805	55.758	59.342	63.691	66.766
50	27.991	29.707	32.357	34.764	37.689	63.167	67.505	71.42	76.154	79.49
60	35.534	37.485	40.482	43.188	46.459	74.397	79.082	83.298	88.379	91.952
70	43.275	45.442	48.758	51.739	55.329	85.527	90.531	95.023	100.425	104.215
80	51.172	53.54	57.153	60.391	64.278	96.578	101.879	106.629	112.329	116.321
90	59.196	61.754	65.647	69.126	73.291	107.565	113.145	118.136	124.116	128.299
100	67.328	70.065	74.222	77.929	82.358	118.498	124.342	129.561	135.807	140.169

Table 6. *F* Distribution Values

F Table for $\alpha = 0.05$

/	$df_1 = 1$	2	3	4	5	6	7	8	12	24	∞
$df_2 = 1$	161.4476	199.5	215.7073	224.5832	230.1619	233.986	236.7684	238.8827	243.906	249.0518	254.3144
2	18.5128	19	19.1643	19.2468	19.2964	19.3295	19.3532	19.371	19.4125	19.4541	19.4957
3	10.128	9.5521	9.2766	9.1172	9.0135	8.9406	8.8867	8.8452	8.7446	8.6385	8.5264
4	7.7086	6.9443	6.5914	6.3882	6.2561	6.1631	6.0942	6.041	5.9117	5.7744	5.6281
5	6.6079	5.7861	5.4095	5.1922	5.0503	4.9503	4.8759	4.8183	4.6777	4.5272	4.365
6	5.9874	5.1433	4.7571	4.5337	4.3874	4.2839	4.2067	4.1468	3.9999	3.8415	3.6689
7	5.5914	4.7374	4.3468	4.1203	3.9715	3.866	3.787	3.7257	3.5747	3.4105	3.2298
8	5.3177	4.459	4.0662	3.8379	3.6875	3.5806	3.5005	3.4381	3.2839	3.1152	2.9276
9	5.1174	4.2565	3.8625	3.6331	3.4817	3.3738	3.2927	3.2296	3.0729	2.9005	2.7067
10	4.9646	4.1028	3.7083	3.478	3.3258	3.2172	3.1355	3.0717	2.913	2.7372	2.5379
11	4.8443	3.9823	3.5874	3.3567	3.2039	3.0946	3.0123	2.948	2.7876	2.609	2.4045
12	4.7472	3.8853	3.4903	3.2592	3.1059	2.9961	2.9134	2.8486	2.6866	2.5055	2.2962
13	4.6672	3.8056	3.4105	3.1791	3.0254	2.9153	2.8321	2.7669	2.6037	2.4202	2.2064
14	4.6001	3.7389	3.3439	3.1122	2.9582	2.8477	2.7642	2.6987	2.5342	2.3487	2.1307
15	4.5431	3.6823	3.2874	3.0556	2.9013	2.7905	2.7066	2.6408	2.4753	2.2878	2.0658
16	4.494	3.6337	3.2389	3.0069	2.8524	2.7413	2.6572	2.5911	2.4247	2.2354	2.0096
17	4.4513	3.5915	3.1968	2.9647	2.81	2.6987	2.6143	2.548	2.3807	2.1898	1.9604
18	4.4139	3.5546	3.1599	2.9277	2.7729	2.6613	2.5767	2.5102	2.3421	2.1497	1.9168
19	4.3807	3.5219	3.1274	2.8951	2.7401	2.6283	2.5435	2.4768	2.308	2.1141	1.878
20	4.3512	3.4928	3.0984	2.8661	2.7109	2.599	2.514	2.4471	2.2776	2.0825	1.8432
21	4.3248	3.4668	3.0725	2.8401	2.6848	2.5727	2.4876	2.4205	2.2504	2.054	1.8117
22	4.3009	3.4434	3.0491	2.8167	2.6613	2.5491	2.4638	2.3965	2.2258	2.0283	1.7831
23	4.2793	3.4221	3.028	2.7955	2.64	2.5277	2.4422	2.3748	2.2036	2.005	1.757
24	4.2597	3.4028	3.0088	2.7763	2.6207	2.5082	2.4226	2.3551	2.1834	1.9838	1.733
25	4.2417	3.3852	2.9912	2.7587	2.603	2.4904	2.4047	2.3371	2.1649	1.9643	1.711
26	4.2252	3.369	2.9752	2.7426	2.5868	2.4741	2.3883	2.3205	2.1479	1.9464	1.6906
27	4.21	3.3541	2.9604	2.7278	2.5719	2.4591	2.3732	2.3053	2.1323	1.9299	1.6717
28	4.196	3.3404	2.9467	2.7141	2.5581	2.4453	2.3593	2.2913	2.1179	1.9147	1.6541
29	4.183	3.3277	2.934	2.7014	2.5454	2.4324	2.3463	2.2783	2.1045	1.9005	1.6376
30	4.1709	3.3158	2.9223	2.6896	2.5336	2.4205	2.3343	2.2662	2.0921	1.8874	1.6223
40	4.0847	3.2317	2.8387	2.606	2.4495	2.3359	2.249	2.1802	2.0035	1.7929	1.5089
60	4.0012	3.1504	2.7581	2.5252	2.3683	2.2541	2.1665	2.097	1.9174	1.7001	1.3893
120	3.9201	3.0718	2.6802	2.4472	2.2899	2.175	2.0868	2.0164	1.8337	1.6084	1.2539
∞	3.8415	2.9957	2.6049	2.3719	2.2141	2.0986	2.0096	1.9384	1.7522	1.5173	1

Appendix C

Formula Sheet

$$\bar{x} = \frac{1}{n}\sum x_i, \quad s = \sqrt{\frac{1}{n-1}\sum (x_i - \bar{x})^2}$$

Outliers lie outside the range $\bar{x} \pm 3s$, or are < Q1 − (1.5 × IQR) or > Q3 + (1.5 × IQR)

$$z = \frac{x - \mu}{\sigma} \qquad x = \mu + z\sigma \qquad \sigma = \sqrt{\frac{1}{N}\sum (x_i - \bar{x})^2}$$

Means Inference

$$z = \frac{\bar{x} - \mu}{\sigma / \sqrt{n}} \qquad \bar{x} \pm z_{1-\alpha/2}\frac{\sigma}{\sqrt{n}} \qquad n = \frac{z_{1-\alpha/2}^2 \sigma^2}{d^2}$$

d = desired margin of error

Means Inference—One-Sample t Test

$$t = \frac{\bar{x} - \mu_0}{s / \sqrt{n}} \qquad \bar{x} \pm t_{1-\alpha/2, n-1}\frac{s}{\sqrt{n}}$$

Means Inference—Two-Sample t Test

$$t = \frac{\bar{x}_1 - \bar{x}_2}{SE_{(\bar{x}_1 - \bar{x}_2)}} \qquad (\bar{x}_1 - \bar{x}_2) \pm t_{1-\alpha/2, n_1+n_2-2} SE_{(\bar{x}_1 - \bar{x}_2)}$$

Proportions Inference—One Sample z Test for Proportions

$$z = \frac{f - p_0}{\sqrt{p_0(1-p_0)/n}} \qquad f \pm z_{1-\alpha/2}\sqrt{\frac{f(1-f)}{n}} \qquad n = \frac{z_{1-\frac{\alpha}{2}}^2 p(1-p)}{d^2}$$

Proportions Inference—Two Sample z Test for Proportions

$$z = \frac{f_1 - f_2}{\sqrt{f_{\text{pooled}}(1 - f_{\text{pooled}})\left[\frac{1}{n_1} + \frac{1}{n_2}\right]}} \qquad (f_1 - f_2) \pm z_{1-\alpha/2}\sqrt{\frac{f_1(1-f_1)}{n_1} + \frac{f_2(1-f_2)}{n_2}}$$

Pooled sample proportion: $f_{\text{pooled}} = \dfrac{x_1 + x_2}{n_1 + n_2}$

Simple Regression Inference—Slope

$$t = \frac{b_1 - \beta_1}{SE_{b_1}} \text{ with } df = n - 2 \qquad b_1 \pm t_{1-\alpha/2, n-2} SE_{b_1}$$

Chi-Square

$$\chi^2 = \sum \frac{(\text{Observed Count} - \text{Expected Count})^2}{\text{Expected Count}}$$

$$\text{Expected Count} = \frac{\text{Row Total} \times \text{Column Total}}{\text{Table Total}}$$

with $df = (\text{Rows} - 1)(\text{Columns} - 1)$

IQR: Interquartile range

Appendix D

Detailed Formula Sheet

Procedure	Role-Type Classification	Hypotheses	Conditions	Test Statistic	Confidence Interval
1-sample t for means	Q	$H_0: \mu = \mu_0$ $H_a: \begin{cases} \mu > \mu_0 \\ \mu < \mu_0 \\ \mu \neq \mu_0 \end{cases}$	**Random** data collection **Normal** population (with no outliers) or large sample size	$t = \dfrac{\overline{x} - \mu_0}{s / \sqrt{n}}$ $df = n - 1$	$\overline{x} \pm t_{1-\alpha/2, n-1} \dfrac{s}{\sqrt{n}}$
Matched pairs t for mean of differences	$C \rightarrow Q$	$H_0: \mu_d = 0$ $H_a: \begin{cases} \mu_d > 0 \\ \mu_d < 0 \\ \mu_d \neq 0 \end{cases}$	**Random** data collection **Normal** population (with no outliers) or large sample size	$t = \dfrac{\overline{d} - 0}{s_d / \sqrt{n}}$ $df = n - 1$	$\overline{d} \pm t_{1-\alpha/2, n-1} \dfrac{s_d}{\sqrt{n}}$
2-sample t for difference of means (pooled variance)	$C \rightarrow Q$	$H_0: \mu_1 = \mu_2$ $H_a: \begin{cases} \mu_1 > \mu_2 \\ \mu_1 < \mu_2 \\ \mu_1 \neq \mu_2 \end{cases}$	**Random** data collection **Normal** population (with no outliers) or large sample size **Equal** population standard deviations (largest s/smallest $s < 2$)	$t = \dfrac{\overline{x}_1 - \overline{x}_2}{SE_{(\overline{x}_1 - \overline{x}_2)}}$ $df = n_1 + n_2 - 2$	$(\overline{x}_1 - \overline{x}_2) \pm t_{1-\alpha/2, n_1+n_2-2} SE_{(\overline{x}_1 - \overline{x}_2)}$
ANOVA (Analysis of Variance)	$C \rightarrow Q$	$H_0: \mu_1 = \mu_2 = \cdots = \mu_n$ H_a: At least one mean is different	**Random** data collection **Normal** populations (with no outliers) or large n **Equal** population standard deviations (Largest s/smallest $s < 2$)	F (obtained from computer output) $df = J - 1,\ N - J$	Obtained from computer output

Procedure	Role-Type Classification	Hypotheses	Conditions	Test Statistic	Confidence Interval
Correlation	Q → Q	$H_0: \rho = 0$ $H_a: \begin{cases} \rho > 0 \\ \rho < 0 \\ \rho \neq 0 \end{cases}$	**Random** data collection **Linearity** – linear association in scatter plot **Normal** populations (no outliers)	$t = r\sqrt{\frac{n-2}{1-r^2}}$	z transform of $r \pm z_{\alpha/2}\sqrt{(1/(n-3))}$ Confidence Interval $= \left[\frac{e^{2L}-1}{e^{2L}+1}, \frac{e^{2U}-1}{e^{2U}+1}\right]$
Linear Regression	Q → Q	$H_0: \beta_1 = 0$ $H_a: \begin{cases} \beta_1 > 0 \\ \beta_1 < 0 \\ \beta_1 \neq 0 \end{cases}$	**Linearity** – linear pattern in scatter plot **Independence** – random data collection **Normality** – histogram of residuals is normal **Equal** population standard deviation – scatterplot has no megaphone pattern	$t = \frac{b_1}{SE_{b_1}}$ $df = n - 2$	$b_1 \pm t_{1-\alpha/2} SE_{b_1}$
Logistic Regression	C, Q → C	$H_0: \beta_1 = 0$ $H_a: \begin{cases} \beta_1 > 0 \\ \beta_1 < 0 \\ \beta_1 \neq 0 \end{cases}$	**Linearity** – linear between log-odds and independent variables **Independence** – random data collection **Binary/ordinal** outcome	Wald Chi-Square (obtained from computer output) Odds Ratio for $x_1 = e^{b_1}$	Obtained from computer output $95\%\ CI(OR) = e^{b_1 \pm 1.96 SE_{b_1}}$
Poisson Regression	C, Q → C	$H_0: \beta_1 = 0$ $H_a: \begin{cases} \beta_1 > 0 \\ \beta_1 < 0 \\ \beta_1 \neq 0 \end{cases}$	**Linearity** – linear between log-rates and independent variables **Independence** – random data collection **Count** or **rate** outcome	Chi-Square (obtained from computer output) Rate Ratio for $x_1 = e^{b_1}$	Obtained from computer output $95\%\ CI(RR) = e^{b_1 \pm 1.96 SE_{b_1}}$
Log-Binomial	C, Q → C	$H_0: \beta_1 = 0$ $H_a: \begin{cases} \beta_1 > 0 \\ \beta_1 < 0 \\ \beta_1 \neq 0 \end{cases}$	**Linearity** – linear between log-risks and independent variables **Independence** – random data collection **Binary** outcome	Chi-Square (obtained from computer output) Risk Ratio for $x_1 = e^{b_1}$	Obtained from computer output $95\%\ CI(RR) = e^{b_1 \pm 1.96 SE_{b_1}}$

Procedure	Role-Type Classification	Hypotheses	Conditions	Test Statistic	Confidence Interval
Cox Regression	Q, Q → Q	$H_0: \beta_1 = 0$ $H_a: \begin{cases} \beta_1 > 0 \\ \beta_1 < 0 \\ \beta_1 \neq 0 \end{cases}$	**Linearity** – linear between log-hazards and independent variables **Independence** – random data collection **Count** outcome	Chi-Square (obtained from computer output) Hazard Ratio for $x_1 = e^{b_1}$	Obtained from computer output $95\%\ CI(HR) = e^{b_1 \pm 1.96 SE_{b_1}}$
1-sample z for proportions	C	$H_0: p = p_0$ $H_a: \begin{cases} p > p_0 \\ p < p_0 \\ p \neq p_0 \end{cases}$	**Random** data collection **Normality** of the sampling distribution of f "Checks" →	$z = \frac{f - p_0}{\sqrt{p_0(1-p_0)/n}}$ $np_0 > 10$ $n(1-p_0) > 10$	$f \pm z_{1-\alpha/2}\sqrt{\frac{f(1-f)}{n}}$ $nf > 10$ $n(1-f) > 10$
2-sample z for proportions	C → C	$H_0: p_1 = p_2$ $H_a: \begin{cases} p_1 > p_2 \\ p_1 < p_2 \\ p_1 \neq p_2 \end{cases}$	**Random** data collection **Normality** of the sampling distribution of $f_1 - f_2$ "Checks" →	$z = \frac{f_1 - f_2}{\sqrt{f_{\text{pooled}}(1-f_{\text{pooled}})\left[\frac{1}{n_1} + \frac{1}{n_2}\right]}}$ Pooled sample proportion: $f_{\text{pooled}} = \frac{x_1 + x_2}{n_1 + n_2}$ $n_1 f_{\text{pooled}} > 5$; $n_1(1-f_{\text{pooled}}) > 5$ $n_2 f_{\text{pooled}} > 5$; $n_2(1-f_{\text{pooled}}) > 5$	$f_1 - f_2 \pm z_{1-\alpha/2}\text{SE}_{f_1 - f_2}$ $n_1 f_1 > 5$; $n_1(1-f_1) > 5$ $n_2 f_2 > 5$; $n_2(1-f_1) > 5$
Chi-Square Goodness of Fit	C → C	H_0: Distribution as hypothesized H_a: Distribution not as hypothesized	**Random** data collection	$\chi^2 = \sum \frac{(O-E)^2}{E}$; $E = \frac{\text{Row Total} \times \text{Column Total}}{\text{Table Total}}$ $df = k - 1$	
Chi-Square Independence	C → C	H_0: No Association H_a: Association	**Random** data collection **Large** sample size (all expected counts > 5)	$\chi^2 = \sum \frac{(O-E)^2}{E}$; $E = \frac{\text{Row Total} \times \text{Column Total}}{\text{Table Total}}$ $df = (\text{Rows} - 1)(\text{Columns} - 1)$	

Q: Quantitative; C: Categorical. For Role-Type Classification, the letter on the left indicates the type of independent variable involved and the letter on the right represents the type of dependent variable involved. For example, with ANOVA the independent variable has 3 or more levels and the dependent variable is quantitative.

Glossary

A

Accessible population A geographically and temporally defined subset of the target population.

Age-adjusted rate A weighted average of the age-group specific rates, where the weights are the proportions of persons in the corresponding age group of a standard population.

Alpha The probability of committing a Type I error, denoted by α. Typically set at 0.05.

Alternative hypothesis This hypothesis (sometimes called the research hypothesis) gives the opposing opinion or conclusion to that of the null hypothesis. The goal is usually to provide sufficient evidence to support this hypothesis.

Analysis of covariance A blend of analysis of variance (ANOVA) and regression that evaluates whether the means of a dependent variable are equal over the levels of a categorical independent variable while adjusting for a covariate.

Analysis of variance A procedure that uses the computation of the variation between groups and the variation within groups to test the hypothesis that *J* populations have the same means.

Arithmetic mean The typical (or average) value of a set of numbers obtained by taking their sum divided by *n*.

Attack rate The number of new cases of a health-related state or event reported during a given time interval divided by the population at risk of becoming a case at the start of the interval. Usually expressed per 100.

Attributable fraction in the population (AF_P) A measure that reflects the expected proportional reduction in risk that would occur if the exposure were removed from the population.

Attributable fraction in the exposed cases (AF_e) A measure that reflects the expected proportional reduction in cases who were exposed had the exposure not occurred.

B

Bayes' Theorem An approach that relates the probability of the occurrence of an event to the presence or nonpresence of an associated event; that is, it shows that if we know the conditional probability of B given A and the probabilities of A and B, we can identify the conditional probability of A given B.

Beta The probability of committing a Type II error, denoted by β. Typically set at 0.20.

Bias The deviation of results from the truth; can result in an observed association between variables that is not real.

Binomial probability distribution A discrete probability distribution that expresses the probability that an outcome will take on one of two values ("success" or "failure") in a finite number of trials.

Binomial logistic regression Application of logistic regression where the dependent variable is binary (two levels).

Biostatistics The branch of statistics concerned with the development and application of methods for collecting, analyzing, and interpreting biological data to assist in decision-making.

Breslow-Day statistic A value used to test the hypothesis of homogeneity of odds ratios.

C

Case-control study design A process by which cases and controls are identified and we investigate whether the cases are more or less likely than the controls to have been exposed.

Censoring A situation where the value of a measurement or observation is not completely known.

Central limit theorem This theorem says that for a population with mean μ and standard deviation σ, if you take sufficiently large random samples from the population with replacement, the distribution of means will have a normal distribution with mean μ and a standard deviation of $\sigma / \sqrt{n}$.

Chance The likelihood of something occurring.

Chi-square distribution A continuous distribution typically derived as the sampling distribution of a sum of squares of independent standard normal variables. It is a skewed distribution, has only positive values, and depends on a single parameter (the degrees of freedom). Many test statistics are approximately distributed as a chi-square.

Chi-square test Any statistical hypothesis test in which the test statistic's sampling distribution is a chi-square distribution assuming that the null hypothesis is true.

Classical probability A measure of the likelihood of something happening, with each outcome being equally likely to occur and the outcomes being mutually exclusive.

Close-ended question In response to a question, the subject selects from a list of predefined choices.

Cluster sample A form of probability sample where respondents are drawn from a random sample of mutually exclusive groups (clusters) within a total population.

Cochran-Mantel-Haenszel test A family of tests for detecting relationships between categorical observations in k strata.

Coefficient of determination The proportion of the total observed variability in the dependent variables that is explained by the independent nominal variable.

Coefficient of variation The ratio of the standard deviation to the mean multiplied by 100; a measure of relative variability.

Cohen's kappa (*k*) A statistic that is commonly used to measure the level of agreement between two observers on a binary (two-level) nominal variable.

Cohort study design A group of subjects banded together in some way is classified according to exposure status and followed over time to evaluate whether the exposure is associated with some outcome measure. Cohorts may be evaluated prospectively or retrospectively.

Completely randomized design A design that involves subjects being randomly assigned to treatments; the same number of subjects are assigned to each treatment.

Completion rate The number of completed surveys among respondents who entered the survey.

Conditional probability The probability of one event given another event has occurred.

Confidence interval A range of values wherein there is a level of probability that the true parameter value lies. It is bounded by a lower and upper limit.

Confidence level $100 \times (1-\alpha)$, which is expressed as a percent.

Confidence limits The numbers at the upper and lower end of a confidence interval.

Confounder A variable that is associated with both the independent variable and dependent variable, resulting in a spurious association; a confounder is a third variable that distorts the association between two other variables.

Consecutive sampling Each subject that meets the criteria for inclusion is selected into the study until the required sample size is met.

Construct validity The degree to which the measurements agree with a theoretical construct, thereby measuring what it claims to measure.

Content validity Indicates how well the measurements represent the phenomena under study.

Contingency table A table showing the distribution of one categorical variable in rows and another categorical variable in columns. It is used to study the association between the two variables.

Continuous random variable A variable able to take on any value in an interval.

Convenience sampling A type of nonprobability sampling in which a sample population is selected because it is readily available.

Coverage error The sample is not representative of the target population. An inaccurate sampling frame will contribute to this type of error.

Cox proportional hazards model A model used to analyze time-to-event (survival) data using the hazard (force of mortality or morbidity) scale.

Criterion validity The extent to which a measure of interest is related to a measure of established validity (a known standard).

Cronbach's alpha A measure of internal consistency that shows how closely items among a set of survey items are related; an indicator of scale reliability.

Cross-sectional study design A collection of data at a single point in time for each subject being studied. This is a useful design for obtaining prevalence data.

Data Information obtained through observation, experiment, or measurement of a phenomenon of interest.

Data processing error Errors due to incorrect transcription, coding, data entry, or arithmetic tabulation.

Degrees of freedom The number of independent pieces of information used to obtain an estimate; the number of independent observations in a sample minus the number of parameters that are estimated from the sample.

Dependent variable The outcome or event studied and expected to change as the independent variable changes.

Descriptive biostatistics Measures of frequency (e.g., count, percent, rate), central tendency (e.g., mean, median, mode), dispersion or variation (e.g., standard deviation, range, interquartile range), and position (e.g., percentile, rank) representing either a sample or a population applied to data relating to living organisms.

Discrete random variable Integers or counts that differ by fixed amounts, with no intermediate values possible.

Distribution A function that shows the possible values of a variable and how often those values occur.

Double-barreled question A question that consists of two separate topics or issues but requires one answer.

Dunn-Šidàk correction An *a priori* multiple comparisons test for assessing which of three or more means significantly differs from one another. It is used to control the family-wise error rate.

Ecologic study design Individual level data are not studied, but rather aggregated population level data are correlated and assessed.

Effect modification Statistical interaction where the association between two variables depends on the level of a third variable.

Eigenvalue The level of variance a factor explains. An eigenvalue of at least 1 means the factor explains more variance than any one variable.

Empirical rule A statistical rule in which for a normal distribution almost all the data lie within three standard deviations of the mean. It is also called the three-sigma rule: 68-95-99.7.

Equation A statement indicating that the values of two mathematical expressions are equal.

Estimate (or point estimate) The actual numerical value of an estimator.

Estimator A random variable or a sample statistic that is used to estimate an unknown population parameter.

Event One or more outcomes of an experiment.

Exponent A quantity that reflects the power to which a number or expression is raised.

Exposure Data that reflect an environmental contaminant (e.g., toxic chemical), a behavior (e.g., tobacco smoking), or an individual attribute (e.g., age).

F

Face validity The extent to which a procedure (i.e., test or assessment) is inherently reasonable based on its stated aims.

Factor analysis A process of reducing several variables into a fewer number of dimensions. It can help condense the size of a questionnaire and the number of variables included in the analysis. The process is sometimes referred to as "dimension reduction," in which the dimensions of a data set are reduced into one or more unobserved (latent) variables.

Factor extraction Can involve one of two approaches, principal components analysis or common factor analysis; its aim is to reduce dimensionality of the dataset to fewer unobserved constructs than variables.

Factor score A numerical value that indicates how strongly a given variable relates to a factor.

Finite population correction factor A value $\sqrt{((N-n)/(N-1))}$ multiplied by the standard error if the sample size is large compared to the population.

Fisher's exact test A statistical test used to assess contingency tables; gives the exact probability of the occurrence of the observed frequencies, according to the assumption of independence and size of the row and column totals (marginal frequencies).

Five-number summary The minimum, the first quartile (25th percentile), the median (50th percentile), the third quartile (75th percentile), and the maximum.

Focus group A group interview, generally conducted with a homogeneous collection of 6–10 individuals whose responses can provide insights.

Formula A special type of equation used to show the relationship between different variables.

Frequency distribution A display, either tabular or graphical, of the number of occurrences at each possible level of a variable.

Frequentist probability The proportion of times an event occurs as the limit of its relative frequency in a large number of trials.

***F* distribution** An asymmetric probability distribution that ranges from 0 to infinity. It has v_1 degrees of freedom for the numerator and v_2 degrees of freedom for the denominator. The distribution has the greatest spread when the degrees of freedom are small.

***F* statistic** The ratio of two variances. It is named after Sir Ronald Fisher.

***F* test** Used to evaluate the hypothesis of equal variances for two independent groups for the *t* test, or to compare the mean-squares among groups to the mean-squares within groups for ANOVA.

Geometric mean An average that indicates the typical value of a set of numbers by taking the *n*th root of the product of their values.

Graph A diagram that shows the relationship between variables, typically a two-dimensional drawing showing a relationship between two sets of information or numbers.

Hazard function A mathematical expression that gives the instantaneous potential for an event to occur given survival up to time *t*.

Heteroscedasticity From the Greek "hetero," which refers to different, and "skedasis," which refers to dispersion; having different variances.

Hidden assumption A question in a questionnaire that requires the respondent to take something for granted or suppose something to be true that the respondent does not believe is true.

Homogeneity Of the same or similar distribution function or values; having the same variances.

Hypothesis testing The process of selecting between the null hypothesis and alternative hypothesis.

Independent variable A variable that does not depend on or change with another variable.

Incidence rate A measure of the number of cases that occur during a given time period divided by the population at risk of becoming a case. This measure reflects risk and is sometimes called an attack rate. When the cases are divided by the cumulative time they are at risk, it is referred to as a person-time rate.

Inferential statistics The process of drawing conclusions about a population based on sample information taken from that population.

Internal consistency Indicates that all the variables (items) vary according to direction, with a meaningful statistical level of correlation with each other.

Interquartile range The middle 50% of the data; the data from the first to the third quartile.

Interval data Numerical values measured along a scale in which there is an order and the difference between two values is meaningful.

J

Judgmental sampling Occurs when the researcher chooses a sample from which the most can be learned (analogous to calling in the experts for their advice).

L

Least squares A statistical method in which we obtain the parameter estimates of the model that yield the minimum sum of squared distances between the data and the model. In regression, it provides the best fitting line to the data.

Level of confidence The probability that a parameter value will fall within a given, specified range of values.

Level of significance The probability of a Type I error, denoted by the Greet letter α.

Likert scale Rating scale (usually 1–5 or 1–7, ranging from least to most) used to measure attitudes, opinions, or perceptions.

Loaded question A question that pushes a respondent to confirm an argument with which he or she may not agree.

Log-binomial regression A regression technique that is used when the dependent variable is binary. The parameter estimate is a relative risk rather than an odds ratio, as obtained using logistic regression.

Logistic regression A regression technique that is appropriate if the dependent variable is categorical. It describes the relationship between a categorical dependent variable and one or more independent variables, with different possible measurement scales.

M

Mantel-Haenszel method Provides a pooled odds ratio (or risk ratio or rate ratio) across strata.

McNemar test A test used to evaluate whether change occurs in paired two-level nominal data.

Measures of central tendency A typical value for a distribution of data, such as the arithmetic mean (average of a set of numbers), median (middle value), and mode (most frequent value). Other measures of central tendency are the midrange (sum of the lowest and highest values divided by 2) and the geometric mean (*n*th root of the product).

Measures of variation Measures of the extent to which a distribution is spread over the data range, such as the range (largest value minus the smallest value), interquartile range (third quartile minus the first quartile), variance (average of the squared differences from the mean), and standard deviation (square root of the variance).

Measurement error Difference between the true value and the actual value.

Median A number in which half the data values are greater than it and half the data values are less than it.

Meta-analysis A statistical examination of data from a group of independent studies covering the same subject, with the intent of providing an overall summary measure.

Minimum-variance unbiased estimator Termed a best estimator because, in addition to being unbiased, it has the smallest variance among all unbiased estimators.

Mode The number that most frequently occurs in a set of numbers.

Multinomial logistic regression A logistic regression model that involves a nominal dependent variable with more than two levels.

Mutually exclusive events A term that means two or more events cannot occur at the same time.

N

Natural logarithm Logarithm of base *e*.

Nominal data Data that fall into classes where there is no logical order or structure; unordered categories or classes; the simplest form of a scale of measure.

Nonparametric statistics Methods that are used when parametric assumptions are not valid, when the underlying distribution is not known, and the sample size is small.

Nonresponse bias Bias that results if subjects who do not respond to a survey differ from those who do respond in some meaningful way.

Nonresponse error The desired respondents do not participate; minimized by choosing a design that avoids invasive and uncomfortable tests, allays individual concerns, and provides incentives.

Normal distribution A probability distribution that is symmetric about the mean, with data around the mean more frequent in occurrence than data away from the mean, thus appearing bell shaped.

Null hypothesis A postulated belief about the population; it is what is currently believed—the status quo. It is a formal basis for a statistical test.

Odds ratio A measure of association between two dichotomous variables in a case-control study. It is derived by dividing the odds of exposure among cases by the odds of exposure among non-cases.

One-tailed (sided) test In hypothesis testing, we evaluate whether a parameter is either significantly greater than or less than a given value—not both.

One-way ANOVA Analysis of variance which involves one independent categorical variable.

Open-ended questions A question that requires more than a "yes" or "no" response but solicits elaboration.

Ordinal data Data measured on a scale that fits into categories where the order is informative but the relative positional distances are not quantitatively meaningful.

P

Paired design Baseline and follow-up measures taken on the same subjects or different raters evaluate the same thing. Paired studies involving numerical data are evaluated using the *t* test. Paired studies involving categorical data are evaluated using the McNemar test or Cohen's kappa *k*.

Parameter A measure from a population that is often unknown; usually unable to calculate its value.

Parametric statistics Statistical methods that assume that data derives from a population that can be modeled by a probability distribution with a specific set of parameters.

Pearson correlation coefficient A measure of the strength of the linear association between two continuous scaled variables, ranging from −1 (perfect negative association) to +1 (perfect positive association).

Person-time rate Number of cases occurring during a specified time period divided by the total person-time (days, months, or years) of those at risk of becoming a case.

Pie chart A chart that shows components of a whole.

Pilot testing A smaller preliminary study to assess effect size and variability for sample size calculations, feasibility, time, cost, adverse consequences, and instrument validity.

Point estimate The actual numerical value of an estimator.

Point prevalence proportion Prevalent cases divided by the population from which the cases originated at a point in time.

Poisson probability distribution A discrete probability distribution, which indicates the probability of a given number of events occurring in a specified interval of time, space, area, distance, or volume.

Poisson regression A form of regression in which we model count or rate data. The dependent variable is assumed to have a Poisson distribution.

Population A collection of individuals who share one or more personal or observational characteristics from which data may be collected and evaluated.

Power The probability that a statistical test will reject the null hypothesis when the null hypothesis is false.

Prevalence Proportion of cases, both new and old, of a specified health-related state or event at a given point in time.

Principal components analysis A statistical technique that assesses the interrelationships among several variables and explains these variables in terms of a smaller number of variables (principal components).

Probability A numerical description from 0 to 1 of how likely an event will occur.

Probability density function For a continuous variable, a function in which the interval over a region yields the probability that a random variable will occur in that region. For a discrete variable, a function in which the sum over the discrete set produces a probability of occurrence.

Probability distribution for a continuous random variable A probability density curve (also called a frequency curve) in which the areas under the curve represent probabilities.

Probability distribution for a discrete random variable A collection of probabilities along with their associated values that the distribution can take.

Prognosis A prediction of the likely course and outcome of a disease; generally based on selected prognostic indicators (signs, symptoms, and circumstances).

Proportion A part or amount in relation to a whole.

Proposal A document that consists of a protocol, as well as a budget, qualifications of the investigators, and other supporting information that is written for the primary purpose of acquiring external funding from a granting agency.

Protocol A detailed written plan of study.

***p*-value** The probability of obtaining a result at least as large as the one observed, given the null hypothesis is true.

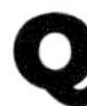

Qualitative data Information about the quality, nature, or essence of something, with information gathered and ordered into larger themes as the researcher works from the specific to the general; categorical data.

Quantitative data Information about quantities or numbers, measured on a numerical scale.

Quota sampling Sampling where the population is divided into exclusive subgroups that represent certain characteristics, the proportion of these subgroups in the population is identified, and samples are taken from these subgroups according to the proportions; a nonprobabilistic version of stratified sampling.

R

Random error A statistical error in the data attributable to chance, with the cause not immediately obvious. It occurs because of imperfect measurement.

Random experiment A process that is repeatable under stable conditions, with a set of possible outcomes that cannot be predicted with certainty.

Random variable A variable whose numerical value is determined by a chance mechanism, or a numerical result from a random experiment; generally denoted by X, Y, and Z.

Random sample A sampling method where each sample has the same probability as other samples to be chosen to be representative of the whole population.

Range The difference between the minimum and maximum values in a data set.

Rate base A value 10^n (where $n = 1, 2, 3, 4, 5, 6$) multiplied by a rate in order to express the rate as a number prior to a decimal point (e.g., 10 per 100 rather than 0.10).

Rate difference Consider three rates: R is the rate of the outcome in the whole group; R_o is the rate of the outcome in the non-exposed group; and R_e is the rate of the outcome in the exposed group. $R - R_o$ is the excess of the outcome in the population attributed to the exposure. $R - R_e$ is the excess of the outcome among the exposed group attributed to the exposure.

Rate ratio The ratio of two person-time rates obtained from a cohort study.

Rate A proportion with the added dimension of time.

Ratio The relationship between two quantities, normally expressed as the quotient of one divided by the other.

Ratio data Interval data with a true zero point. A ratio scale variable never falls below zero.

Rejection region (or critical region) In hypothesis testing, it is the range of values that leads the investigator to reject the null hypothesis.

Relative frequency The frequency of a given category divided by the total number of observations; the frequency in a given category compared with the total of all categories.

Reliability A measure that indicates whether a respondent's score on a variable would be the same if the survey was repeated.

Repeated measures ANOVA Equivalent to a one-way ANOVA, except the groups are not independent. It is an extension to the paired t test, but more than two groups are involved.

Residual An estimate of the random population error; $e_i = y_i - \hat{y}_i$

Response rate The number of completed surveys divided by the number of people who make up the total sample group. Usually expressed as a percent.

Risk difference The difference in risk for subjects exposed minus the risk of subjects not exposed.

Risk ratio The ratio of two attack rates from a cohort study. A measure of the risk of an outcome for those exposed compared with the risk of an outcome for those not exposed.

S

Sample space An exhaustive list of all possible outcomes of an experiment.

Sample A subset of items selected from a population.

Sampling distribution The frequency distribution of a statistic based on many random samples of size n from a single population.

Sampling error A statistical error that arises when the sample is selected in a way so that some of the sample is not representative of the entire population from which it was drawn; related to the design and size of the survey.

Sampling frame A complete list of people or items in a population from which a sample will be drawn.

Scales of measurement Various ways that variables are defined and categorized, such as nominal scale, ordinal scale, interval scale, and ratio scale.

Snowball sampling When existing study subjects recruit other subjects from among their network of associates.

Standard normal distribution See Z distribution.

Statistic A measure from a sample that is used in statistics.

Statistical hypothesis A statement about one or more parameters of a population that requires verification.

Statistical techniques Analytic approaches that utilize statistical methods to investigate a range of questions.

Statistical test The process in which we decide whether to reject the null hypothesis.

Statistics The science of data; involves collecting, classifying summarizing, organizing, analyzing, and interpreting data.

Stratified random sample Involves dividing the population into homogeneous subgroups (strata) and then taking a simple random sample from each stratum.

Student's *t* If X is normally distributed and a sample of size n is randomly chosen from the underlying population, then $t = \frac{\overline{x} - \mu}{s / \sqrt{n}}$ with $n - 1$ degrees of freedom.

Student-Newman-Keul (SNK) procedure A test for post hoc comparisons following a significant F test in ANOVA. Other post hoc tests include Duncan, LSD, Tukey, and Scheffee.

Subjective probability A type of probability based on a person's judgment about the likely occurrence of an event.

Survey A careful assessment or general view of behaviors, knowledge, beliefs, etc.

Survey sample A subset of the accessible population that comprises the participants in a study.

Systematic error Predictable, reoccurring inaccuracies in the same direction attributed to the instrument or process for measurement.

Systematic review A detailed plan and search strategy determined *a priori*, with the goal of identifying, appraising, and synthesizing relevant studies that address a particular research question.

T

***t* distribution** A theoretical probability distribution, which is symmetric, bell shaped, and has a mean of 0. It is similar to the standard normal distribution, except it has more area in the tails and the middle is not as high.

***t* statistic** The sample mean minus the hypothesized mean, divided by the sample standard error.

***t* test** A type of inferential statistic used to assess hypotheses about mean values, paired means, means from two independent populations, the Pearson correlation coefficient, Spearman correlation coefficient, and slope estimates from linear regression models.

Target population The large set of people to whom the results of a study are generalized.

Test statistic A quantity calculated from the sample that is used when making a decision about the hypotheses of interest.

Trial Any process that can be infinitely repeated with a specific set of possible outcomes.

Two-tailed (sided) test In hypothesis testing, we evaluate whether a parameter is either significantly greater than or less than a specified value.

Two-way ANOVA Assessment of how the means of a numerical dependent variable changes across the levels of two categorical independent variables.

Type I error Rejecting the null hypothesis when it is true.

Type II error Failing to reject the null hypothesis when it is false.

Unbiased estimator An estimator for which the expected value of a sample estimator equals the population parameter: $E(\text{Sample estimator}) = \text{Population parameter}$.

Validity The degree that a measurement, conclusion, or idea corresponds accurately to the truth.

Variable A characteristic that varies from one subject to the next and can be measured or categorized. It can take on a specific set of values.

Variance The sum of the squared deviations of each data point from the overall average of the dataset, divided by N for the population variance or $n-1$ for the sample variance.

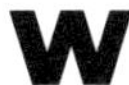

Wilcoxon rank sum test An alternative to the two-sample *t* test when the underlying populations are not normally distributed or their variances are not equal.

Wilcoxon signed rank test A nonparametric test that compares two samples from populations that are not independent. The test focuses on the difference in values for each pair of observations and does not require that the differences be normally distributed. The test takes into account both the magnitude of differences and their signs.

Wilks' lambda The multivariate version of the *F* test for a one-way ANOVA that examines the difference between two or more groups on multiple variables at once.

"Yes" or "No" questions A quick way to segment respondents.

***Z* distribution** A bell-shaped distribution where the mean is equal to 0 and the standard deviation is equal to 1. It is also called the standard normal distribution.

***Z* statistic** The sample mean subtracted by the hypothesized mean, divided by the population standard deviation (or standard error); a value in terms of standard deviations from the mean.

***Z* test** A statistical test based on the *Z* statistic that assumes the parameter of interest has a normal distribution under the null hypothesis.

Index

Note: Page numbers with "*f*" and "*t*" indicate figures and tables, respectively.

Q

R

S